THE PHYSICIANS' CRUSADE AGAINST ABORTION

Frederick N. Dyer

Science History Publications, USA
Sagamore Beach, Massachusetts
2005

First published in the United States of America
By Science History Publications/USA
a division of Watson Publishing International
P.O. Box 1240, Sagamore Beach, MA 02562

www.shpusa.com

Copyright 1999, 2005 Frederick N. Dyer

Library of Congress Catalog-in-Publication Data

The physicians' crusade against adbortion/ Frederick N. Dyer.
   p. cm.
Includes bibliographic references and index.
ISBN 0-88135-378-7 (alk. paper)
   1. Abortion—United States—History—Sources. 2. Abortion—United
States—History—Public opinion. 3. Physicians—United States—Attitudes. 4.
Public opinion—United States. I. Dyer, Frederick N.

HQ767.5.U5P49 2005
363.460973—dc22   200505088

Manufactured in the U.S.A.

In memory of

Dr. Joseph R. Stanton

*whose modern crusade against abortion saved thousands of
New England children from "legal" destruction in the womb.*

CONTENTS

ACKNOWLEDGEMENTS

The author wishes to acknowledge with thanks the contributions of

RICHARD J. WOLFE, former Curator of Rare Books and Manuscripts of the Countway Library of Medicine, whose editorial suggestions for an earlier book transmitted directly to portions of the current book and indirectly to the rest of it. Also current personnel at that Library, including Lucretia McClure and Jack Eckert, who provided information on John Preston Leonard and other early New England physicians.

ARLENE SHANER, Reference Librarian, Historical Collections, The New York Academy of Medicine, who consulted the Minutes of the Academy's meetings for 1867 and provided information on Augustus Kinsley Gardner. She also transcribed the fragile 1871 Report of the East River Medical Association of New York Committee on Criminal Abortions.

STEPHEN E. NOVAK, Head, Archives & Special Collections of the A.C. Long Health Sciences Library at Columbia University who provided information on John Preston Leonard's medical education.

CAROLYN KIRDAHY, Curator of Collections for the Museum of Science who laboriously searched the Boston Society of Natural History correspondence for possible letters from John Preston Leonard.

JOCELYNE RUBINETTI of the Methodist Library at Drew University, who provided copies of the March 1867 *Northwestern Christian Advocate* editorial and a transcript of a paragraph that could only be read directly from the microfilm.

FRED BURCHSTED, Reference Librarian, Research Services, Harvard Widener Library, who provided statistics from the original 1849 New York City Inspector's Report. These confirmed that Horatio Robinson Storer copied these data from Reese's 1850 editorial, "Criminal Abortionism in New York."

PROFESSOR THOMAS W. SPALDING, CFX, author of *Martin John Spalding: American Churchman*, who answered many questions regarding Archbishop Spalding's 1869 antiabortion efforts. Also Fr. Paul K. Thomas, Archivist, Archdiocese of Baltimore, who provided documents and information related to the Archbishop's 1869 antiabortion efforts.

CHRISTOPHER D. ELLITHORP, who provided information about Edwin Moses Hale and other homeopaths.

PATRICIA A. CARTER, M.D., retired South Carolina obstetrician who provided documentation and details of Samuel A. Cosgrove's successful effort to reduce the high rates of unnecessary "therapeutic" abortion in U. S. hospitals.

LIST OF ILLUSTRATIONS

(Illustration section follows page 146)

FIGURE 1   The Pioneer Antiabortion Crusaders: Hippocrates, John Brodhead Beck, Hugh Lenox Hodge, Gunning S. Bedford

FIGURE 2   EARLY CRUSADERS. Horatio Robinson Storer, David Humphreys Storer, David Meredith Reese, Augustus Kinsley Gardner

FIGURE 3   Horatio Storer's Books on Abortion Written for Popular Audiences

FIGURE 4   Cover of Storer's *Journal of the Gynaecological Society of Boston*

FIGURE 5   Edwin Moses Hale and the Pills He Provided the *Chicago Times'* Girl Reporter

FIGURE 6   Cartoon from the 1888 *Chicago Times'* Exposé

FOREWORD

In the middle of the nineteenth century, physicians became alarmed about an epidemic of induced abortion. One of these was the young Boston physician, Horatio Robinson Storer, who started the "physicians' crusade against abortion."[1] A major feature of this crusade was the lobbying of state and territorial legislatures to pass stringent antiabortion laws. The physicians were highly successful in this and the new laws remained in effect in most states with only minor changes until overturned in 1973 by *Roe v. Wade*.[2]

During the deliberations for *Roe v. Wade*, it was claimed that these laws were passed to protect women from a dangerous operation. Since physician-induced abortion was no longer dangerous, it was argued that there was no reason to maintain these laws. It was also claimed that concern for the unborn child was not an important factor leading to these laws.[3] A majority of justices accepted these false claims and the state laws were overturned.

In 1989, the Supreme Court decided the case of *Webster v. Reproductive Health Services*. It upheld Missouri's minor abortion restrictions that required viability tests after 20-weeks gestation and barred the use of public facilities for abortion services. A number of friend-of-the-court briefs were provided by groups who opposed Missouri's restrictions. One, signed by 281 professional historians, acknowledged "physicians were the principal nineteenth-century proponents of laws to restrict abortion," but denied that concern for the unborn was one of their reasons, claiming the life of the fetus "became a central issue in American culture only in the late twentieth century."[4] The brief claimed these physicians were concerned about protecting the health of women, regulating the medical profession, keeping women in traditional roles, and preventing the descendants of immigrants from becoming dominant in the population. The historians argued that these reasons now were obsolete or not credible and the Court should reaffirm the constitutional right to abortion they had announced in *Roe v. Wade*. However, James Mohr in his *Abortion in America* showed that almost all of these physicians opposed abortion because they saw it as the killing of a living human being.[5] Later in his book, Mohr confused the issue by discussing physicians' "professional" reasons for opposing abortion *before* their "personal" reason of defending the unborn.[6] He did this despite his admission that the "sincere belief" of physicians "that abortion was morally wrong" "helps to explain the intensity of their commitment to the cause."[7] Mohr signed the brief that contradicted the facts he had presented. He was chastised for this and withheld his name when the brief was resubmitted in the 1992 case, *Planned Parenthood of Southeastern Pennsylvania v. Casey*.[8]

Most recent books and articles discussing the history of abortion laws have emphasized the false statements made in the 1989/1992 historians' brief. The physicians' "professional" goals to eliminate the competition from irregulars and quacks and to control the practice of legitimate members have been particularly stressed.[9]

This book documents the true story of the passionate defense of the unborn by these physicians beginning with Hippocrates and continuing into the twentieth century. A 1999 biography of Horatio Robinson Storer tells an important part of this story, although Storer's crusade against abortion was only one of several major accomplishments of this pioneering surgeon and co-founder of American Gynecology.[10] Storer's antiabortion efforts are also described in the current book with a more complete discussion of the events, men, and ideas that influenced Storer. There also is a completely new discussion of Storer's probable influence while just a medical student on Dr. John Preston Leonard who condemned physician abortionists in an 1851 article in the *Boston Medical and Surgical Journal*. However, the bulk of this new book deals with the scores of antiabortion physicians whose efforts followed Storer's 1859 American Medical Association Report on Criminal Abortion. The concerns about abortion of Storer and these other physicians frequently will be presented in their own words. Had James Mohr provided such quotes in his *Abortion in America*, these physicians' motives might not have been subject to distortion.

The new laws against abortion prevented many women from even considering abortion. Another goal of the crusade was to inform women that a living human being existed from conception and physicians persuaded thousands, and, more likely, millions of women to continue pregnancies that they initially asked their physicians to end. The following chapter describes how these additional survivors of pregnancy are among the ancestors of almost every reader of this book with Protestant ancestors. Catholic women did not obtain abortions to any extent until well into the twentieth century.

However, despite the new laws and physicians' successful persuasive efforts, unnecessary abortion continued at a high rate and, as will be shown, it did not decline at the end of the nineteenth century as James Mohr claimed. One factor promoting abortion was the huge advertising revenues that abortionists and "abortion-drug" sellers paid to newspaper publishers. Another was the unwillingness of most Protestant ministers to address the issue. Not the least factor was the small group of physicians who performed abortions from the beginning of the epidemic. Some induced abortions to prevent the woman from suffering at the hands of incompetent abortionists or from her own hand. Others were motivated by the huge profits that could be made by providing an illegal operation that was detested by almost all of their colleagues.

After 1910, many physicians continued the crusade against abortion, but it was no longer strongly supported by the profession. A few physicians even worked to repeal the laws making abortion a crime. However, even physicians like Frederick J. Taussig, who in the late 1930s called for socioeconomic considerations in abortion decisions, still convinced many of the women who sought abortions to continue their pregnancies. This period from 1910 to 1973 might be referred to as "Physicians' Ambivalence about Abortion." It may be treated at a later time.

CHAPTER 1
FERVENT PHYSICIAN PLEAS FOR THE UNBORN

And now words fail. Of the mother, by consent or by her own hand, imbrued with her infant's blood; of the equally guilty father, who counsels or allows the crime; of the wretches who by their wholesale murders far out-Herod Burke and Hare; of the public sentiment which palliates, pardons, and would even praise this so common violation of all law, human and divine, of all instinct, of all reason, all pity, all mercy, all love,—we leave those to speak who can.[1]

These sentences first appeared in print in 1859 and were written by Horatio Robinson Storer two years after he started what has been termed the "physicians' crusade against abortion." Storer initially wrote "Of the mother, ..." in the first of a series of articles on "criminal abortion" written for his fellow physicians. These articles were included as an enclosure to an 1860 "Memorial" of the American Medical Association, written by Storer, sent to legislatures requesting that they pass stringent laws against unnecessary abortion.[2] Storer repeated this sentence in two widely-read books on abortion, the first "for every woman," and the second "for every man."[3] Storer also included the phrase in a book on criminal abortion written for both physicians and lawyers.[4] As will be seen, other physicians and even a judge would quote this phrase in their condemnations of unnecessary abortion.

Readers may be surprised to learn that induced abortion was common among married Protestant women when Storer began the "physicians' crusade."[5] The next chapters describe the sharp increase in abortions by these women and the reasons for it. When physicians became aware of this increase in "forced" abortion, nearly all viewed it as an epidemic that needed to be curtailed. They expressed their concerns in speeches, medical articles, letters to medical editors, editorials, and books, and, like Horatio Storer, they did not mince words.

A handful of American physicians preceded Storer in publishing condemnations of unnecessary abortions, the women who obtained them, and the men and women who induced them. Among the earliest was Hugh Lenox Hodge, Professor of Obstetrics at the University of Pennsylvania; who spoke about criminal abortion to his medical students on November 6, 1839. Hodge's Introductory Lecture included:

Would gentlemen that we could exonerate the moderns from guilt in this subject! It is, however, a mournful fact, which ought to be promulgated, that this crime, this mode of committing murder, is prevalent among the most intelligent, refined, moral, and Christian communities. We blush, while we record the fact, that in this country, in this city, where literature, science, morality, and Christianity are supposed to have so much influence; where all the domestic and social virtues are reported as being in full and delightful exercise; even here, individuals, male and female exist, who are continually imbruing their hands and consciences in the blood of unborn infants; yea, even medical men are to be found, who for some trifling pecuniary recompense, will poison the fountains of life, or forcibly induce labor to the certain destruction of the foetus, and not unfrequently of its parent.[6]

In 1854, Hodge again presented and published his 1839 Lecture.[7] Horatio Storer would praise Hodge for his lecture in his 1859 articles and Hodge would be one of seven influential physicians that Horatio selected to join him on the American Medical Association Committee on Criminal Abortion. This Committee was created in 1857 at the Association meeting in Nashville. The Committee presented their Report on Criminal Abortion two years later in Louisville.

Another probable factor in Horatio's crusade was John Preston Leonard, a young physician from nearby Rhode Island, who almost certainly was at least an acquaintance of Horatio. Leonard published an article, "Quackery and Abortion," in the widely read *Boston Medical and Surgical Journal* in January 1851.[8] Leonard accused regular physicians of performing unnecessary abortions and stated: "I believe that some who are promoted to *office in our medical societies* are of this order of quacks."[9] Horatio was a first-year medical student in January 1851. He almost certainly was helping his father review literature for two major reports, one on obstetrics and one on medical jurisprudence, and he would have read Leonard's article that also included:

Besides these bills of mortality, the records of criminal courts will furnish sufficient proof that this crime is every day becoming more prevalent. It is humiliating to admit that there are a class of physicians who, Herod-like, have waged a war of destruction upon the innocent. Though their motives are not the same as those which instigated that cruel king, they are no less murderers for that. If there is any difference, they are worse than Herod. He was influenced by popular clamor and bigotry; these quacks do all for money, and such could be hired to burn out the eyes of infant princes.[10]

Leonard's article was a blueprint for Horatio's future crusade in that it advocated bringing the American Medical Association into the fight and called for passage of stringent laws against abortion. Despite this, Horatio did not mention "Quackery and Abortion" when he discussed the factors that started him on his crusade. Horatio's certain awareness of Leonard's article, his possible contribution to it, and his failure to acknowledge Leonard will be discussed in Chapter 3.

When Horatio did give credit "for the thought of the present undertaking," it was to the Introductory Lecture that his father, David Humphreys Storer, Professor of Obstetrics and Medical Jurisprudence at the Harvard Medical School, presented in November 1855.[11] The title of David's lecture was "Duties, Trials and Rewards of the Student of Midwifery," and these were the major subjects addressed.[12] However, a final section condemned criminal abortion, described its bad effects on women's health, and implored physicians to use reason and moral suasion to reduce the crime. David's Lecture included:

> I do not presume to stand here as a moralist. I would attempt only to point out a few of the duties obligatory upon the physician, as such. I should, however, be faithless to the noble profession which occupies my every thought; I should be unworthy the confidence or esteem of my brethren did I refrain, while referring to this subject, to enter my solemn protest against the existing vice; to express, emphatically, the universal sentiment of horror and indignation entertained among the upright men of the profession in this community. Of *horror*, that the female can so completely unsex herself, that her sensibilities can be so entirely blunted, that any conceivable circumstances can compel her to welcome such degradation! Of *indignation*, that men can be found so regardless of their own characters, so perfectly indifferent respecting those of their cotemporaries, as to lend their services in such unholy transactions.
>
> To save the life of the mother we may be called upon to destroy the foetus in utero, but here alone can it be justifiable. The generally prevailing opinion that although it may be wrong to procure an abortion after the child has presented unmistakable signs of life, it is excusable previous to that period, is unintelligible to the conscientious physician. The moment an embryo enters the uterus a microscopic speck, it is the germ of a human being, and it is as morally wrong to endeavor to destroy that germ as to be guilty of the crime of infanticide.[13]

David's attack on criminal abortion was not well received by "others" on the faculty of the Harvard Medical School, although it may have been only Henry J. Bigelow, the Professor of Surgery, who objected.[14] David omitted the abortion portion when the Introductory Lecture was published and the Editors of the *Boston Medical and Surgical Journal* protested this failure to include the abortion condemnation. Their December 1855 editorial included:

> Deferring to the judgment of others, whose opinions we all delight to honor, Professor Storer has omitted the very paragraphs, which, in our judgment, should have been allowed to go forth as freely as they were spoken. To whom shall the community look for a verdict upon practices which disgrace our land and prevail to an extent that would hardly be credited, if not to physicians—and, chiefest among them, to medical teachers? For ourselves, we have no fear that *the truth*, as told by the writer of this Address, in reference to the *crime of procuring abortion* and the scarcely less heinous offence of

preventing impregnation, would do aught but good in this, or in any, city. It would appear that sheer ignorance, in many honest people, is the spring of much of the horrible *intra-uterine murder* which exists among us; why not, then, enlighten this ignorance? It would be far more effectually done by some bold and manly appeal like that to which we allude, than by the private and scattered influence of honorable practitioners alone.[15]

The pressure on David to suppress the abortion portion of his Lecture also did not sit well with his son. Horatio later wrote that this was one of the few times his father was to "show the white feather."[16] Horatio obviously was much less concerned about the objections of the medical faculty to raising the issue of criminal abortion, since a little more than a year after his father's Lecture, he commenced his crusade against abortion, or more correctly, commenced his crusade for the unborn children who were being destroyed in unnecessary abortion.

The first evidence of this campaign appeared in February 1857, and it may not be a coincidence that this was only one month after a Georgia physician, Jesse Boring, published an antiabortion article that included:

If I am not wholly mistaken, it will be seen that, of all the varieties of murder, that of the embryonic human being is the most atrocious and indefensible. It is a wanton, unprovoked and cruel deprivation of a human being, of the existence which God alone gave, and can of right, take away, and that being is not only inoffensive but utterly helpless.[17]

Horatio certainly had already made up his mind to take up his campaign, but Boring's article may have been a factor in the timing and nature of his crusade. Boring relied heavily on religious reasons for opposing abortion—"every abortion ... is in the sight of God, murder *out right*,"[18]—and Horatio may have seen this as an ineffective strategy for bringing physicians into the campaign, since many physicians were known to be skeptical about "the sight of God." Boring may also have been viewed as a competitor who could dilute the recognition that Storer no doubt expected he would receive as one result of a successful campaign against criminal abortion. Storer had repeatedly been acclaimed for his achievements as student, orator, author, editor of a major medical book, and natural scientist (he discovered new species of fish on a trip to Labrador), and Horatio no doubt expected his campaign against criminal abortion would bring acclaim as well.[19]

Horatio's contribution to the successful physicians' crusade against abortion was immense. Not only did he start the crusade and single-handedly carry out the major American Medical Association efforts of 1859 and 1860, his articles and books were quoted throughout the century and beyond in articles published in medical journals and in books written by physicians for their colleagues and for the public. However, reluctance to publicly discuss a crime that persisted at all levels of society blunted the fame that Storer surely deserved for the yeoman efforts that saved so many lives. Even a biographer who praised Storer did not specifically mention his efforts against abortion, referring instead to Storer's large contributions "where medicine touches morals."[20]

Was Storer motivated to protect the unborn or to achieve fame as the successful defender of the unborn? The answer no doubt is both, since Horatio would later describe recognition as a proper tribute for enthusiasm, hard work, and hard fights.[21] However, it is important to again stress what was *not* a high priority for Storer and for nearly all of the physicians crusading against abortion. We noted the historians' false claim that these physicians who successfully lobbied for laws against abortion were primarily motivated to protect the health of women, eliminate competition from "quacks," keep regular physicians in line and women in traditional roles, and prevent the descendants of Catholic immigrants from becoming dominant in the population. James Mohr signed the 1989 friend-of-the-court brief that made these claims despite the fact that he had repeatedly shown that these physicians opposed unnecessary abortion primarily because they saw it as morally wrong. Examples from Mohr's book include:

> The nation's regular doctors, probably more than any other identifiable group in American society during the nineteenth century, including the clergy, defended the value of human life per se as an absolute. Scholars interested in the medical mentality of the nineteenth century will have to explain the reasons for this ideological position. ... But whatever the reasons, regular physicians felt very strongly indeed on the issue of protecting human life. And once they had decided that human life was present to some extent in a newly fertilized ovum, however limited that extent might be, they became the fierce opponents of any attack upon it.[22]

> Most physicians considered abortion a crime because of the inherent difficulties of determining any point at which a steadily developing embryo became somehow more alive than it had been the moment before. Furthermore, they objected strongly to snuffing out life in the making. Only if a fully realized life—that of the mother—would surely be lost without their intervention could they morally justify the termination of another already developing life.[23]

> Physicians who personally believed abortion to be morally wrong— and their many fervent writings on this subject must be taken as evidence of their sincerity—must have been frustrated by the persistent lack of public support for their position.[24]

However, Mohr discussed this "fervent" moral opposition to abortion by physicians *after* discussing "professional" reasons for physician opposition.[25] He may have done this to exaggerate the reasons for opposing abortion that were obsolete when he wrote in the 1970s and to diminish the importance of the primary moral reasons that were not obsolete.

Well, in a nutshell, that is the story. Physicians, led by Horatio Robinson Storer, opposed the dramatic increase of abortion that occurred in the middle of the nineteenth century and did it primarily because they believed unborn children must not be sacrificed unless the life of the mother was truly at stake. Hundreds of physicians took up the crusade and their efforts continued into the twentieth century. Although the campaign may not have greatly reduced the rate of abortion from its level in 1857, it kept that rate from swelling to much greater levels. What remains to be shown are the factors that led to these physicians' passionate efforts, the strategies and tactics they used in the campaign, and the obstacles that prevented their crusade from being totally successful.

One item related to their crusade deserves early stress because it has particular relevance to almost every reader. This is the children who survived pregnancy because of the new laws the physicians helped enact and because of physicians' successful persuasion of many women to refrain from abortions. These additional "survivors" of pregnancy may have made up five percent or more of the children born during the century when physicians were actively opposing unnecessary abortion. However, to be conservative and to simplify the math, assume that three percent of the children of the single generation while Storer was actively involved in antiabortion work owed their existence to the physicians' crusade.[26] By chance, the .97 proportion of this generation who were *not* "Storer's survivors" would marry each other at the rate of .97 x .97 = .9409. This means that 94.09 percent of the next generation would not have had one or both of "Storer's survivors" for a parent. However, it also means that 5.91 percent of that generation *would* have had one or both of "Storer's survivors" for a parent.

Similarly, the .9409 proportion without "survivor" parents would marry each other at the rate of .9409 x .9409, which, when rounded, equals .8853. This means that 88.53 percent of the next generation would not have had one or more of "Storer's survivors" for a grandparent, but 11.47 percent *would.* Similar calculations show that in the next generation, 21.6 percent of children would have had one or more of Storer's survivors as a great-grandparent, and 38.6 percent of the next generation (approximately our current generation) would have one or more of "Storer's survivors" as a great-great-grandparent.

However, the abortion reductions produced by the "physicians' crusade" were not limited to a single generation and three percent probably is a low estimate for the number of additional children born because of the campaign. If one assumes five percent for two generations beginning in 1860, the 38.6 percent figure for our current generation becomes a whopping 72 percent! This exponential increase in succeeding generations of people with "Storer's survivors" as ancestors may surprise you. *If you have primarily Protestant ancestors, you can be fairly certain that your own existence was one result of the successes of the physicians' crusade for the unborn.*

As will be shown, Catholic women did not participate in the epidemic of induced abortion in any numbers until well into the twentieth century. Horatio Storer and other physicians credited the Catholic confessional for this. If your ancestors were largely Catholic, you can be thankful to the priests of your great-great-grandmother, great-grandmother, and grandmother for your existence.

CHAPTER 2
EARLY MEDICAL OPPOSITION

Physician opposition to unnecessary abortion did not begin with Hodge, Leonard, the Storers, or the other physicians who contributed to the founding of the physicians' crusade. Medical opposition goes back at least to Hippocrates, a Greek physician who lived in the fifth and fourth centuries B.C. and who is known as the "Father of Medicine." Hippocrates wrote, or is given credit for writing, the Hippocratic Oath, which specifically prohibits the physician from inducing abortion. One translation by Francis Adams includes the sentence: "I will give no deadly medicine to any one if asked, nor suggest any such counsel; and in like manner I will not give to a woman a pessary to produce abortion." Another translation by Ludwig Edelstein reads: "I will neither give a deadly drug to anybody if asked for it, nor will I make a suggestion to this effect. Similarly I will not give a woman an abortive remedy." For many centuries, the Hippocratic Oath was sworn to by medical students before they began medical practice and this frequently was the case in the nineteenth.

Horatio Storer and scores of other physicians who wrote articles condemning unnecessary abortion referred to the Hippocratic Oath in support of their position. The importance of Hippocrates to their crusade may be best shown by the fact that in 1954, Alan F. Guttmacher would falsely discredit Hippocrates as part of his attempt to make many more abortions legal.[1] Guttmacher claimed that another Greek physician who *recommended* an abortion technique was the Hippocrates of the Hippocratic Oath. However, Guttmacher earlier had acknowledged that the two physicians differed.[2]

Storer and other physicians also frequently referred to another early condemnation of induced abortion by Thomas Percival, an English physician who set down a body of *Medical Ethics* in 1803.[3] Percival's *Ethics* included: "To extinguish the first spark of life is a crime of the same nature, both against our Maker and society, as to destroy an infant, a child, or a man; these regular and successive stages of existence being the ordinances of God, subject alone to His divine will, and appointed by sovereign wisdom and goodness as the exclusive means of preserving the race, and multiplying the enjoyments of mankind."[4]

A New York physician, John Brodhead Beck, quoted Percival's "To extinguish the first spark ..." in his 1817 dissertation, "Infanticide," that was republished as a chapter in his and his brother's textbook, *Elements of Medical Jurisprudence*.[5] The *Elements* was first published in 1823 and was used as a text at the Harvard Medical School when Horatio Storer was a student.[6] Horatio mentioned Beck's "admirable" chapter when he provided a history of medical opponents of abortion in the first of nine articles about criminal abortion in the *North-American Medico-Chirurgical Review.*[7]

Beck condemned unnecessary abortion and also discussed the inappropriateness of the laws of England and other countries that treated abortion as a less serious crime at early stages of the pregnancy.[8] Beck showed the fallacy of claims that the fetus was not alive early in pregnancy that were the basis for these different penalties. He wrote:

> The foetus, previous to the time of quickening, must be either dead or living. Now, that it is not the former, is most evident from neither putrefaction nor decomposition taking place, which would be the inevitable consequences of an extinction of the vital principle. To say that the connexion with the mother prevents this, is wholly untenable: facts are opposed to it. Foetuses do actually die in the uterus before quickening, and then all the signs of death are present. The embryo, therefore, before that crisis, must be in a state different from that of death, and this can be no other than life.[9]

Beck also mentioned that abortion was resorted to by the unmarried "to avoid the disgrace which would attach to them from having a living child; and sometimes it is even employed by married women, to obviate a repetition of peculiarly severe labour-pains."[10] His "sometimes" in reference to the married, is evidence that the "epidemic" of abortion among married Protestant women had not begun when he wrote his dissertation in 1817.

Percival's and Beck's opposition to abortion at any stage of pregnancy was referred to by the British physician, Michael Ryan, in the 1836 edition of his *A Manual of Medical Jurisprudence and State Medicine*. Ryan strongly approved their views and contrasted them to the views of four British physicians, "Dr. Gordon Smith, Dr. Good, Dr. Paris, and Dr. Copeland," who indicated that punishment *should* be less for women obtaining abortions prior to "quickening."[11] Horatio Storer quoted Ryan's criticism of these four physicians in the fourth of his 1859 articles, "Its Proofs."[12] However, Horatio almost certainly became aware of Ryan's views nine years earlier, since David Humphreys Storer included a quote from Ryan's *Manual* in "Medical Jurisprudence," the paper David presented to the Massachusetts Medical Society on May 28, 1851.[13] Horatio almost certainly helped prepare this paper and would have read Ryan's condemnation of criminal abortion. Horatio also would have been highly aware of his father's antiabortion views that existed "long ere" David's 1855 Introductory Lecture.[14] We can be certain that Horatio was strongly opposed to unnecessary abortion by 1851 and probably earlier.

In his seventh 1859 article, "Its Obstacles to Conviction," Horatio made note of two early physicians who worked to strengthen their state laws on abortion. Horatio discussed how Levin Smith Joynes had petitioned the Virginia legislature to eliminate the quickening distinction in their abortion statute.[15] Joynes was successful and abortion at any time during the pregnancy became punished by fine and imprisonment in 1849.[16] William Henry Brisbane was working in 1857 to change the Wisconsin laws on abortion and he included a copy of the new statute in a March 1859 letter to Storer.[17] Storer praised Joynes and

Brisbane for their efforts, but followed this with the observation that "total silence" was far more likely to have been heard by legislators and officers of justice
from the medical profession.[18] As will be seen, this "total silence" would change
to a physician uproar in the decades after 1859.

When Storer made reference to earlier antiabortion efforts of physicians he
did not mention one of the earliest efforts of U.S. physicians to influence abortion laws. John Brodhead Beck's brother, Theodric Romeyn Beck, was one of
the "principal behind-the-scene revisors" when New York added a special section on abortion to its new law code in 1828.[19] This made it a crime to "willfully
administer to any pregnant woman, any medicine, drug, substance or thing
whatever, or shall use or employ any instrument or other means whatever, with
intent thereby to procure the miscarriage of any such woman, unless the same
shall have been necessary to preserve the life of such woman, or shall have been
advised by two physicians to be necessary for that purpose."[20] Theodric practiced medicine in Albany where he would have had ready access to New York
legislators. One key legislator also was a long-time friend and their correspondence discussed Theodric's medical input to legislation.[21] Mohr suggested that
John Brodhead Beck also made medical input to the abortion legislation via
Theodric.[22]

Storer probably was not aware of this successful lobbying effort that occurred in another state two years before he was born. Storer also did not make
reference in 1859 to the efforts of another early physician opponent of abortion,
Gunning S. Bedford, Professor of Midwifery and the Diseases of Women and
Children at the University of New York. However, Horatio was aware of Bedford, since, in the same 1859 series of articles where Storer praised other physician opponents of abortion, he cited abortion frequency data from a July 1850
editorial, "Criminal Abortionism in New York," that heaped praise on Dr. Bedford.[23] Horatio may have omitted reference to Bedford because he was concerned
that associating the Roman Catholic Bedford with the antiabortion campaign
would lead some physicians to view it as a Roman Catholic effort instead of one
requiring the attention of all medical and moral men. Another possibility is that an
early dispute between Bedford and the physicians who started the American
Medical Association caused Horatio to ignore Bedford. Bedford had claimed
(vainly) that participants in the 1846 organizational meeting of the Association
were not sufficiently representative of the United States.[24]

Bedford's efforts certainly deserved mention. In 1844, Bedford published
an article, "Vaginal Hystereotomy," that described his womb-opening operation
and also condemned the notorious New York City abortionist, Anna Caroline
Lohman, who called herself, "Madame Restell."[25] Restell began performing
abortions in the late 1830s and extensively advertised her drugs and services.
One of her clients was in critical condition during extended labor. Earlier in her
pregnancy, the woman had inserted a whalebone through her vagina in an unsuccessful attempt at self-abortion and the injuries she produced caused scar
tissue to completely close the opening of the womb. Bedford discovered this
after the woman was in labor for 29 hours. He opened the womb surgically, the
child was born, and the infant and mother both survived to good health.

Bedford insisted on learning what had closed the womb and the woman confessed to the unsuccessful abortion attempt. She indicated that Madame Restell had offered to produce the abortion with a whalebone, but she could not afford Restell's fee and administered the whalebone herself. In his discussion of the case, Bedford described Restell as "a monster who speculates with human life with as much coolness as if she were engaged in a game of chance." He learned from the patient that Restell had caused five earlier miscarriages with drugs, but drugs failed in the latest pregnancy. The patient also claimed to know "a great number of females who were in the habit of applying to Madame Restell for the purpose of miscarrying and that she scarcely ever failed in affording the desired relief." Bedford continued:

> It, indeed, seems too monstrous for belief that such gross violations of the laws both of God and man should be suffered in the very heart of a community professing to be Christian, and to be governed by law and good order. Yet these facts are known to all who read. This creature's advertisements are to be seen in our daily papers; there she invites the base and the guilty, the innocent and the unwary, to apply to her.[26]

Two months after Bedford's March 1844 paper, a *Boston Medical and Surgical Journal* editorial mentioned Bedford and claimed that Boston also had a large criminal abortion problem. It included:

> Madam Restell, the vampire of New York, the most infamous of her sex, if any reliance is to be placed in the expression of the press and the specific recital of Dr. Bedford, has deprived as many human beings of the right of birth, as any individual in the criminal calendar of the world. She has likewise an office in Boston, where her medicines are in constant request. But Madam Restell is not the only depredator on human happiness and life in the city of Boston. There are men—in external organization, but not in character—who are celebrated among the vile attendants at the court of infamy, for their success in exterminating foetal life. Their criminal assistance is even sometimes sought after by married women who cannot render a shadow of excuse to the tribunal of public scorn for their heartless depravity.[27]

David Humphreys Storer surely was aware of this editorial and Horatio may have been as well, since he already was contemplating pursuit of his father's career.[28] The editor's "even sometimes sought after by married women" suggests that married women did not yet predominate among those seeking abortions in Boston in 1844.

A pair of Boston abortion trials at the same period showed a major defect in Massachusetts' abortion laws. In 1843, a woman abortionist, Luceba Parker, was brought to trial in Massachusetts for having successfully produced an abortion in a married woman. Parker was convicted but the Massachusetts Supreme

Court did not uphold the conviction because it had not been proven that the woman, though pregnant, was "quick with child."[29] Shortly after the Parker case, another abortionist, Dr. Alexander S. Butler, was indicted for murder after an abortion that caused the death of an unmarried woman. The woman's lover also was indicted for arranging the abortion. However, neither was convicted because it was an "unquickened" abortion and this was not a crime.[30]

The Massachusetts Legislature quickly made abortion attempts at any time in the pregnancy punishable and the *Boston Medical and Surgical Journal* published the "important act."[31] These two Massachusetts trials and the associated change in abortion law were prominently displayed in the newspapers, one of which, the *Boston Atlas*, was published by Horatio's uncle, Thomas Mayo Brewer. They almost certainly were the subject of discussions between Horatio and his father and perhaps between Horatio and his uncle who also had a medical degree. As a result, Horatio in his early teens would have become aware that married women as well as unmarried women were obtaining abortions, that both women and men abortionists were a problem, that differences in the criminality of early and late abortions were "absurd," and probably also that medical men could persuade legislators to correct deficiencies in abortion statutes. He certainly was aware of all these facts by 1857 when he started the physicians' crusade against abortion.

CHAPTER 3

"QUACKERY AND ABORTION" AND OTHER FACTORS LEADING TO STORER'S CRUSADE

We mentioned Horatio's early intention to follow his father in becoming a physician. He also began early to follow his father in pursuit of natural history. David Humphreys Storer produced taxonomies and descriptions of fish that were widely acclaimed and his contributions to ichthyology may be better known today than his work as Professor and Dean at the Harvard Medical School.[1] When the 20-year-old Horatio published a paper on the fish he discovered in Labrador, he dedicated one of the new species to his father "in slight token of remembrance and gratitude for the very many pleasant hours we have spent together in the study of nature."[2] Horatio's natural history interests also were whetted and shaped by daily contact as a Harvard student with other outstanding natural scientists such as Louis Rodolphe Agassiz. Not the least stimulus for natural history pursuits occurred when Horatio was six. John James Audubon visited the Storer home and Horatio listened to Audubon's tales of the birds and other wildlife of Labrador.[3] These inspired Horatio to set up the voyage to Labrador where he discovered the new fish.

At Harvard as an undergraduate, Horatio was curator, vice-president, and president of the Harvard Natural History Society and he routinely brought scientists to speak at Society meetings.[4] On June 14, 1850, the speaker was Charles Frédéric Girard who helped Horatio classify the new fish species. Horatio's classmate and friend, Hermann Jackson Warner, wrote in his diary: "lecture from Girard—thinks that the study of the embryo is to work great revolutions in practical medicine."[5] One might hazard the guess that Girard was pointing out that the human embryo was being destroyed when physicians used means, such as dilation of the cervix, to restore "stopped menses." There was no reliable way of determining if a woman were actually pregnant in the first few months of a pregnancy and many of women's visits to physicians to restore menstruation were made to end pregnancies, although the woman would not admit her suspicion or awareness of pregnancy. Given this interpretation of Girard's "lecture," it might have been another stimulus for Horatio's eventual decision to work to end destruction of human life in the womb.

However, a recently located copy of Girard's talk indicates that this probably was not what Girard was saying.[6] He discussed the physical similarity between blood cells and embryos and jumped to the conclusion that this may have a bearing "upon the practical medicine," giving as his only example "the possibility of curing the consumption." Girard's vain attempt to show the relevance of his theorizing for practical medicine suggests that the attempt was made to satisfy Horatio who probably asked his "friend Girard"[7] to discuss the implications of "the study of the embryo" for "practical medicine."

Two weeks before Girard's talk, Hermann Jackson Warner found Horatio dissecting a "most disgusting foetus." Warner added in his diary that Storer "meditates dissection of foetus' for his father for the next two or three years."[8] It is likely that this "most disgusting foetus" was a victim of criminal abortion, perhaps "delivered" by his father or another physician following the initiating actions of an abortionist or of the woman. This dissection could have been another stimulus for Horatio's antiabortion views and may have prompted him to ask Girard to discuss how human embryos were frequently being destroyed in "practical medicine."[9] If Girard actually addressed this issue, it was not mentioned in the written version of Girard's speech.

A few weeks after Girard's talk, the *New York Medical Gazette* published the editorial that praised the antiabortion efforts of Gunning S. Bedford. The *Gazette* editor, David Meredith Reese, quoted extensively from the 1849 Report of the New York City Inspector, Dr. Alfred W. White. A table reproduced from this Report showed a five-fold increase over 45 years in the rate of stillborn children and fatal premature births, or, as Dr. White referred to them, "human beings that never breathed."[10] Statistics were provided for five-year periods and the sharpest increase occurred from 1840 to 1845. Dr. White did not name criminal abortion as the source of these increases in the following quoted by Reese, but he came close:

"This is a state of mortality from these accidents truly alarming which, while no remedy in this connection can be advised, demand our most serious consideration. What of crime and recklessness there is in this sum dare not be expressed, for we cannot refer such a hecatomb of human offspring to natural causes. *An honest and fearless expression of the causes or circumstances attending these events, on the part of the medical attendant, would bring into this department an amount of valuable knowledge that might be useful in checking this horrible and increasing waste of life.*"[11]

Reese continued:

We have italicized this last sentence, and cordially assent to the implied rebuke it contains against our profession, very many of whom, while they deplore the evil and appreciate truly the horrible crimes of the guilty parties, yet still lack the moral courage to expose the authors of these secret infanticides and murders, for such they are in a multitude of examples, and might, if followed up, be fastened on the criminals.[12]

Reese then contrasted Dr. Bedford with the "many" physicians who lacked "the moral courage." He praised Bedford for the "fearless manner in which he has publicly exposed the principal offender who has outraged her sex and insulted humanity by her shameless avowal of this terrible iniquity." This obviously was

"Madame Restell." Reese also noted that Bedford's expose was "extensively copied by the public press," and that it led to arraignment and conviction of "one of the guilty parties."[13] This was Restell who was convicted in 1847 for performing an abortion on a young woman. Following a series of unsuccessful appeals, Restell began her sentence of a year in the city penitentiary in June 1848. Although not mentioned in Reese's editorial, Dr. Bedford was one of the witnesses for the prosecution in Restell's trial.[14]

It is likely that Horatio read Reese's *Gazette* editorial shortly after it appeared, given its relevance to his father's two upcoming presentations and Horatio's long history of assisting his father's academic, scientific, and professional efforts, including the "most disgusting fetus" dissection that Warner mentioned.[15] He eventually read it, since a table showing the increase of stillborn and premature births was reproduced in an 1858 paper and in his second 1859 article on criminal abortion.[16] Although Horatio cited the original 1849 Report of the City Inspector, his source for the data was Reese's editorial. This is shown by a minor difference between Horatio's table and Reese's table. Horatio recalculated a ratio of stillborns to the population that appeared incorrect in Reese's table. Reese's (or the *Gazette* typesetter's) actual error was to quote 76,770 instead of 75,770 from the 1849 Report as the population of New York in 1805.

David Humphreys Storer was chosen to present the next Annual Address to the Massachusetts Medical Society in May 1851. It is not clear when David selected the topic of medical jurisprudence, but certainly by November 11, 1850 when Horatio discussed medical jurisprudence with Warner.[17] This and a subsequent conversation with Warner about David's medical jurisprudence paper discussed below, show Horatio's involvement with his father's effort. Criminal abortion was a key issue in medical jurisprudence and David and Horatio would have been particularly interested in Reese's July 1850 "Criminal Abortionism in New York" and Leonard's January 1851 "Quackery and Abortion."

No direct evidence has been located that Leonard was a friend or even an acquaintance of Horatio, but there are strong reasons for believing this was the case. One was their mutual strong interest in the western regions. Leonard made a trip to California in 1849 and published two letters dealing with the medical profession and medical conditions in the region.[18] These letters were described in Leonard's obituary in the *Boston Medical and Surgical Journal* as "not only new, but of a reliable character, and were extensively read and prized."[19] Horatio wrote a prize-winning dissertation, "The History and Resources of the Valley of the Mississippi," in the spring of 1850 that made references to California, including "the star of our westward extending empire can set but in the ocean."[20] Horatio repeatedly referred to his infatuation with the West in his later writing and he traveled to Texas in 1858 and to California in 1871.[21] He no doubt "extensively read and prized" Leonard's letters and may have visited nearby Greenville, Rhode Island for firsthand accounts of California after Leonard returned. Leonard sent a long article on diarrhea to the *Boston Medical and Surgical Journal* from Greenville in May 1850.[22] However, he probably was back before May since his wife gave birth to a daughter on November 25, 1850 and there is no evidence that she accompanied Leonard on his California trip.[23]

Leonard made a general reference in "Quackery and Abortion" to Reese's *Gazette* editorial as one piece of evidence for abortion's high prevalence.[24] However, although Gunning Bedford and his bravery was a major feature of that editorial, Leonard did not mention Bedford. Horatio's similar use of the Reese abortion frequency data and failure to mention Bedford in his 1859 articles may not be a coincidence. Horatio may have influenced the writing of "Quackery and Abortion."

Horatio began medical school in September 1850 and had access to the *New York Medical Gazette* in the Harvard Medical School's library. He may have made Leonard aware of Reese's editorial and its data. Horatio may have contacted Leonard after the editorial was published in early July, but before September 2 when Horatio started a medical school journal that did not mention Leonard.[25] However, Horatio's journal entries were brief and this may not have indicated that there had been no contact with Leonard after September 2. Warner, wrote in his diary on January 25, 1851 that Horatio "[t]alks of his invitations to Newport, Baltimore."[26] Storer's journal included no mention of Rhode Island or Maryland invitations or trips before or after January 25. This shows how little of Horatio's plans and activities found their way into Horatio's medical school journal.

Leonard died on July 1, 1851[27] from typhus fever contracted while examining emigrants aboard a boat that docked at Boston.[28] He was two months shy of his 32nd birthday. Leonard had moved from Greenville, Rhode Island to Middletown, Connecticut only one month before his death.[29] Leonard's last Boston visit augurs for many earlier Boston visits and opportunities for Leonard and Storer to meet when he lived much closer to Boston. Horatio's medical school journal ended three weeks before Leonard's death and thus any possible activities of Horatio related to Leonard's last Boston visit, his illness, his death, his funeral, or his obituary went unrecorded.

Leonard's obituary indicated he was "well known to the medical profession in the United States" and "a prominent correspondent to this Journal for many years."[30] He obviously was at least "well known" to the editor of the *Journal* and probably to other medical men in nearby Boston. The obituary praised Leonard for his "numerous and valuable contributions to science."[31] Earlier medical articles by Leonard dealt with cases of fever, cyanosis, and the essential elements and qualities of epidemics.[32] Horatio and his father were dedicated to medical science and Leonard's "numerous and valuable" articles would have made him an attractive figure. They almost certainly were among those in "the medical profession in the United States" to whom Leonard was "well known."

These various factors suggest a relationship, possibly a strong friendship between Horatio and Leonard. It is conceivable that Horatio encouraged Leonard to write "Quackery and Abortion" and that Horatio may have contributed to it. It also is conceivable that Horatio or his father may have contributed to Leonard's obituary for the *Boston Medical and Surgical Journal*, whose editor, Jerome Van Crowninshield Smith, was an amateur ichthyologist like David and Horatio.[33] The strong praise of the California articles suggests Horatio's input. The obituary failed to mention Leonard's last article, "Quackery and Abortion," and this may be because the charges Leonard made against regular physicians in that article upset Boston physicians, including "some who are promoted to *office in our medical societies*." Leonard also specified the tools used by abortionists and for self-abortion and this probably was badly received, given some later comments by Dr. Walter Channing (See Chapter 7).

Despite all of these indications that Horatio was aware of Leonard and Leonard's article and perhaps involved in the article's preparation, Leonard was not mentioned in any of Horatio's future writing about physicians who spoke out against abortion. What is more, Horatio would write in 1865 that his father was the man "who, in New England, first appreciated the frequency of criminal abortions, pointed out their true character, and denounced them."[34] Perhaps Horatio was so anxious that his father receive the credit for starting him on the physicians' crusade that he ignored Leonard. What is more, David actually may have stimulated Horatio's plan to crusade against abortion with this occurring *before* "Quackery and Abortion" was written. When Horatio gave credit to David he may have referred to the November 1855 Introductory Lecture because this was David's first public demonstration of his antiabortion stance. To have acknowledged Leonard's earlier article with its antiabortion crusade recommendations, would have identified a different New Englander who "first appreciated the frequency of criminal abortions." Leonard was from New England and in fact referred to himself as "[b]eing a true Yankee myself" in "Quackery and Abortion."[35] Leonard was long dead by 1859, when Horatio first acknowledged antiabortion contributors, and by 1865, when Horatio credited his father as first in New England. Horatio may have rationalized that there was no problem in ignoring Leonard's contribution.

"Quackery and Abortion" appears to have been Leonard's only published article dealing with quackery or criminal abortion. This may indicate that Leonard was influenced to write about criminal abortion by Horatio or someone else of strong antiabortion bent. But for his early death, Leonard might have continued with antiabortion efforts and he might have been the founder of the "physicians' crusade." On the other hand, Leonard discussed in his article his willingness to "join such a crusade" against abortionists, not his willingness to lead it.[36] Perhaps he was aware of Horatio's (or someone else's) plan to lead physicians in a crusade against abortion. Admittedly, it is stretching things to assume that Horatio, a first-year medical student in 1850, was already planning his crusade against abortion.

Leonard began his article with a testimony to the rising status of the medical profession, an unlikely claim that medical progress was "nowhere more marked than in the United States," and a primer on the American Medical Association and its contributions that are easy to interpret as the comments of a first-year medical student whose father was a member of the fledgling American Medical Association.[37] A pair of quotes from *Hamlet* in "Quackery and Abortion" also could reflect Horatio's influence. Horatio indicated in his journal he was at a "Shakespeare Club" meeting on December 10, 1850 and "read Shakespeare" on December 24.[38] However, Leonard may have been as versed on *Hamlet* as Horatio. A great-granddaughter of Leonard owned two books that came from Leonard, "his set of Shakespeare and his Cheselden's *Anatomy of the*

Human Body."[39]

We earlier mentioned Leonard's implication of regular physicians in the practice of criminal abortion, including "some who are promoted to *office in our medical societies.*" We also noted that he claimed this "class of physicians" had like Herod "waged a war of destruction upon the innocent," and "[i]f there is any difference, they are worse than Herod." Leonard also called for new state laws making unnecessary abortion a much more serious crime.[40] Horatio's campaign against abortion would have the same goal of increasing legal penalties for criminal abortion, and, if Horatio did not plant this call for strict laws in Leonard's article, Leonard may have planted the idea in Horatio.

Leonard also called on the American Medical Association to take actions to inhibit the crime. He noted that they had taken some steps against irregular physicians and "quacks," but he decried the fact that the Association "has not yet struck any decided blow on that most diabolical kind of quackery, that high-handed villany [sic], which characterizes the *abortionist.*"[41] This call for the Association to strike a "decided blow" against abortionists also may have influenced Horatio or been influenced by Horatio. As will be shown, Horatio would petition officials of the Association to form a Committee on Criminal Abortion within weeks of the commencement of his 1857 campaign. Leonard and Storer appear to be the only physicians who called on the American Medical Association to address criminal abortion by 1857.

Leonard made other points in his article that are important for an understanding of the "epidemic" of criminal abortion that prompted the "physicians' crusade." One was a stern warning about the "dangerous situation" faced by the new physician without a medical practice. Leonard indicated this new doctor is a likely candidate for requests for illegal abortion, "especially if thought to be in need of money." Leonard cautioned such new physicians to treat these offers with disdain. "[I]f they fall here, just as they are to be introduced into legitimate practice," Leonard wrote, "they fall forever; their sins will surely find them out."[42]

Leonard also pointed out the rapidity with which news of the availability of an abortionist was communicated and the futility of the new physician's attempt to conceal a criminal abortion.

> It is said that a woman cannot keep a secret. Whether this is so or not, the man who procures abortions is generally well known. He needs no hand-bills, placards, or other advertisement; he is soon notorious. Inglorious fame! Who would have such a disgraceful notoriety? Who would thus disgrace his profession; who would sell his claim to honor and principle; who would shed innocent blood for a few pieces of silver? After a man has thus degraded himself, after he has sunk so low, can he expect to retrieve his character? Who ever knew such a man to reform? If he is susceptible to feelings of remorse, like Judas he will go out and hang himself to hide his own shame.[43]

Leonard also foreshadowed numerous medical articles over the next decades by describing his patients who were impaired or died because of abortionists. He wrote:

> I shall not stop to give the history of these lamentable cases which have come under my observation, and terminated fatally as the consequence of procured abortion—those fatal cases of puerperal peritonitis, caused by the bloody hands of *doctors* and ***M.D.'s***; but if the confessions of the dying are to be relied upon, I know men who have carried on this shameful and iniquitous business, and have not only been the murderers of infants, but the instruments also of consigning their guilty mothers to premature graves, "unhouselled, unanointed, unannealed."[44]

The "puerperal peritonitis" from "bloody hands" charge suggests that the writer was familiar with Oliver Wendell Holmes' 1843 paper, "The Contagiousness of Puerperal Fever." Holmes was one of Horatio's professors at the Harvard Medical School. Leonard obtained medical degrees from the Berkshire Medical Institute in western Massachusetts (1846) and from the College of Physicians and Surgeons of New York (1848), but not from Harvard.[45] However, Leonard lived close to Boston and may have known Holmes or at least been knowledgeable about Holmes' controversial paper that indicted physicians for spreading childbed fever long before germs were understood.

Leonard's charges became more specific against a "regular abortionist" who had inserted a marble-sized lead ball into the "*os uteri*" to induce abortion. "For the information of the villain who was guilty of this double massacre (should his eye fall upon this page)," Leonard continued, "I will state that the operation succeeded—succeeded in destroying a foetus of five months, and in impairing the health of the girl so that she continued to suffer from uterine disorder, and finally died in about three years afterwards."[46]

Leonard asked "every respectable physician" to expose the abortionists, but not "our patients, those who place their lives and reputations in our hands." (Storer would similarly proscribe the revealing of patients' abortion secrets in 1865.)[47] Leonard pleaded for medical societies and medical associations to expel the "assassinators" from their ranks and for individual physicians to inform the authorities "whenever opportunity may offer." As mentioned, he indicated his willingness "to join such a crusade, however unpleasant the war may be."[48]

Leonard concluded:

> The evil is one of such magnitude that I have felt it my duty to make this communication. If by it any one shall be persuaded from falling into criminal quackery, certainly good will come out of it. Or if those who make laws and regulations for medical men shall be induced to render the crime punishable, and this action be taken any sooner because the medical public have thus had their attention directed to the subject, I shall have no cause to regret that I have incurred the displeasure of those practitioners who have been styled *abortionists*,

or that I have made the admission, through the medium of your Journal, that there is *criminal quackery in the medical ranks.*[49]

Although Horatio surely was aware of Leonard's claim that regular physicians were procuring unnecessary abortions, Horatio would virtually deny that regular physicians were involved in the practice in the reports and articles that he wrote from 1857 to 1860. However, in almost every other respect, Horatio's strategies and tactics were foreshadowed by those Leonard outlined in his 1851 article. If Leonard were implicating some of the powerful Boston physicians as abortionists with his claims and offending them thereby, Horatio may have refused to similarly implicate and offend them in 1857. Horatio was seeking the approval of these physicians for his Suffolk District Medical Society Report on Criminal Abortion (or hoping they would not attend meetings and cast a negative vote). The Suffolk District Medical Society was the society of all regular physicians in Boston and any who were more-or-less abortionists would have been members.

Horatio's unwillingness to implicate regular physicians in the crime of abortion may also help explain his unwillingness to mention Leonard and "Quackery and Abortion." Horatio may have worried that even mention of Leonard or Leonard's article in Suffolk meetings and the Suffolk Report would be tantamount to repeating the article's strong indictment of regular physicians. This may explain his silence about Leonard in 1857. It doesn't account for it in his later writing.

Criminal abortion itself was omitted in David Humphreys Storer's paper, "Medical Jurisprudence," that was presented at the Annual Meeting of the Massachusetts Medical Society on May 28, 1851. The 31-page address mentioned the connection of medical jurisprudence to "midwifery" in an introductory paragraph.[50] This certainly would have been an opening for a discussion of criminal abortion, but no further discussion of midwifery appeared. David certainly was aware that criminal abortion was relevant to his paper. He even noted in his 1851 "Report of the American Medical Association Committee on Obstetrics" that a paper on criminal abortion would be left to the Association's Committee on Medical Jurisprudence, since to include it would be to "encroach upon their province."[51] It is puzzling that he did not discuss criminal abortion in the "province" of his own paper on medical jurisprudence. If Boston physicians were disturbed by "Quackery and Abortion" and its indictment of regular physicians, David may have avoided the topic of criminal abortion because he did not want to renew their distress. He also might have believed such references would embarrass "some who are promoted to *office in our medical societies*" whom David knew would be in his Massachusetts Medical Society audience.[52]

On October 20, 1851, medical jurisprudence came up again in conversation between Horatio and Hermann Jackson Warner. Warner reported that Horatio lent him a copy of his father's Massachusetts Medical Society address and that Horatio discussed his father's plan to write a book on the subject of medical jurisprudence, "but his eyes are bad & his time is much professionally occupied."[53] This comment is more evidence that it was Horatio's eyes that reviewed literature for David's two major 1851 Reports.

While Horatio was in medical school there were other references to criminal abortion in Boston that would have increased his awareness of the problem. In May 1851, the *Boston Medical and Surgical Journal* published a note about the trial of an irregular physician from Boston who was charged with manslaughter in the death of a woman on whom he attempted an abortion.[54] In the same issue there was mention of a woman who died from drinking "two ounces of oil of tansy for the purpose of procuring abortion."[55] Walter Channing, Professor of Obstetrics and Medical Jurisprudence at the Harvard Medical School, read a paper on the death of a woman who was "taking medicines for abortion, especially those sold by a woman named Restell."[56] The woman's efforts led to a sudden enlargement of the uterus that was untreatable and quickly proved fatal. The case was unlike anything that Channing had ever seen and he no doubt discussed it with his medical students.

After Horatio obtained his M.D., an editorial from the *New York Medical Gazette* was republished in the March 1854 *Boston Medical and Surgical Journal*. This dealt with a new arrest of Madame Restell along with the "wealthy seducer and paramour" who had financed three Restell abortions for a young woman. "All the parties are in custody," wrote editor Reese, "and, but for a lamentable defect in human laws, they should be hanged together on the same gallows, as a warning against this fiendish and awfully frequent crime, which is perpetrated in this city to an extent enough to 'make the cheek of darkness pale.'" Reese also noted that Restell would actually receive little punishment under current laws and accurately speculated that "her bloody gains" might prevent conviction altogether.[57]

The *Boston Medical and Surgical Journal* provided another strong reminder to Boston physicians of the prevalence of criminal abortion in an October 1854 editorial.[58] It included:

> We are pained and mortified to know that members of the medical profession, in good standing in the general estimation of the world, are occasionally detected in this nefarious practice. It is sometimes made a source of profitable business, falsely classed professional. It is villainous, criminal, destructive to the moral character, and hazardous to the future prospects of those who embark in it. It is better to starve with a fair fame, than to hazard one's happiness, in this world and the next, by participating in so murderous a deed. No sophistry can do away with the fact, that whether the lamp of life is extinguished in the womb or at any period after birth, with an avowed and willful intention of taking the life of the foetus or infant, it is murder, and the perpetrator of it cannot expect to escape the vengeance of offended heaven.[59]

These editorials would have been read by David Humphreys Storer and may have been stimuli for his inclusion of a veiled reference to criminal abortion in an address to graduating medical students in March 1855 and for his open discussion of the subject in November 1855. Horatio's reading of these two edi-torials would have been delayed. He and his bride traveled to Europe in Decem-ber 1853 and, after spending time in Italy, France, and England, arrived in Edin-burgh late in the spring of 1854. They remained there until returning to Boston in June 1855. Horatio was studying with and assisting Scotland's most famous physician, Dr. (later Sir) James Young Simpson. Letters home indicated that Horatio was providing Simpson's lecture materials and diagrams to his father to assist David in developing medical lectures for his new Professorship at the Harvard Medical School that began in the fall of 1854 (Walter Channing had retired).[60]

The editorials may have been a factor leading Hugh Lenox Hodge to repeat his 1839 lecture in November 1854. His lecture was republished and included only minor changes. We earlier presented paragraphs describing Hodge's horror that women would destroy their own progeny and that some physicians assisted them. Hodge described illegitimacy as the major reason that physicians faced requests for abortion from men and women "respectable and polite in their gen-eral appearance and manners," "under the vain hope of preserving their reputa-tion by this unnatural and guilty sacrifice." However it was not just the unmar-ried:

> Married women, also, from the fear of labor, from indisposition to have the care, the expense, or the trouble of children, or some other motive, equally trifling and degrading, have solicited that the embryo should be destroyed by their medical attendant. And when such individuals are informed of the nature of the transaction, there is an expression of real or pretended surprise that any one should deem the act improper—much more guilty; yea, in spite even of the solemn warning of the physician, they will resort to the debased and murderous charlatan, who, for a piece of silver, will annihilate the life of a foetus, and endanger even that of the ignorant or guilty mother.[61]

Hodge indicated that it was the duty of the physician to persuade these women seeking abortion to have their babies:

> Often, very often, must all the eloquence and all the authority of the practitioner be employed; often he must, as it were, grasp the con-science of his weak and erring patient; and let her know, in language not to be misunderstood, that she is responsible to her Creator for the life of the being within her system.[62]

An implication of this was that the physician sometimes, perhaps frequently, succeeded.

Hodge closed with the following additional discussion of the unique role of physicians in reducing criminal abortion.

They alone can rectify public opinion; they alone can present the subject in such a manner that legislators can exercise their powers aright in the preparation of suitable laws; that moralists and theologians can be furnished with facts to enforce the truth on this subject, upon the moral sense of the community, so that not only may the crime of infanticide be abolished, but that criminal abortion be properly reprehended, and that women, in every rank and condition of life may be sensible of the value of the embryo and foetus, and of the high responsibility which rests on the parents of every unborn infant.[63]

David Humphreys Storer would provide a similar claim and discussion of the physician's important role a year later in his own Introductory Lecture. However, David did not mention the need to influence legislators to prepare "suitable laws" and, in fact, claimed: "The laws of the land, with all their penalties annexed, can do but little to abolish the crime."[64] David did not mention Hodge's Lecture in his own, but David almost certainly was aware of it. Even if he had not seen the pamphlets published in 1839 or 1854, he would have read the review of Hodge's 1854 lecture in the April 1855 *American Journal of the Medical Sciences*, the country's premier medical journal.[65] The reviewer was David Francis Condie, a Philadelphia physician who had published the definitive *Treatise on the Diseases of Children* in 1844. Condie first praised Hodge's inculcation in his listeners of the "deep responsibilities and incumbent moral obligations" of men entering the medical profession. Condie then called attention to Hodge's "leading theme," criminal abortion, and praised Hodge for his "plainness of language and warmth of indignation." "If his language and feelings, in this respect, shall be responded to by the profession generally, throughout the breadth and length of our land," Condie continued, "we shall, at least, absolve ourselves from all participation in the guilt incurred by those who, having gained admittance into our ranks, are willing, for a price, to prostitute themselves as panderers to vice by the criminal induction of abortion; while, at the same time, we may be the means of diminishing the frequency of the crime, if we shall be unable entirely to suppress it."[66]

After providing a full page of quotes from Hodge's lecture, Condie claimed "the induction of abortion, to subserve a selfish or wicked purpose" was "a crime tantamount to that of murder." He decried the newspaper "advertisements, couched in scarcely equivocal language, proffering to those who would avail themselves of them, the services of the professed abortionist." He concluded:

It is, indeed, surprising with what impudence—with what an entire contempt of every moral principle and obligation, men who profess themselves to be practitioners of "the healing art," and who, perchance, are the unworthy possessors of a collegiate diploma, proclaim themselves to be ready, for a trifling compensation, to induce abortion. We were recently shown a letter containing an order for such medical books to be sent to the writer, as would prove useful to him in facilitating his practice as an abortionist; or, as he more hypo-critically expressed it, would instruct him in the best and safest means for relieving females from the exposure and disgrace that an unfortunate pregnancy would necessarily entail upon them.

If it be a fact that the laws of Pennsylvania are insufficient to remedy the evil—if they consider it rather in the light of a misde-meanor than as a crime, it is high time that our Legislature should be called upon to make such enactments as will insure the conviction and adequate punishment of all who are concerned in the perpetration of this most demoralizing form of murder.[67]

A much different view of Hodge's 1854 lecture was provided by the New Jersey physician, Isaac Skillman Mulford.[68] Mulford indicated:

This production is marked by the great comprehension and breadth of its views, as well as by much energy and vigor of style. In it he lays down the proposition, that the ovum is possessed of vitality even from the period of conception, and consequently, that any attempt to destroy it is equally criminal, in every respect, at this as at any subse-quent period.[69]

Mulford commented that he had once shared and publicly expressed the same view, but "subsequent consideration has led him to doubt as to the entire correctness of such a view of the subject." He claimed "nature sometimes fails in her purposes; her attempts to attain a certain result proving to be abortive, a true conception does not take place; a living, growing being is not produced in the womb, but instead thereof there exists a mere rude, unformed, unorganized mass of matter."[70] Mulford's position was that abortion was prohibited only af-ter the contents of the womb are definitely known to be a living being and "[t]he most common manifestation of this is that which takes place at the time usually called the 'quickening.'" He concluded: "These considerations have led the writer to doubt whether it would be wise to sweep away at once all the ancient landmarks that have so long stood in this portion of the field of medical sci-ence."[71] Mulford's letter may have been the only published apology for early abor-tions in a medical journal until the late 1880s and that apology may have been written by a lawyer (See Chapter 23). Mulford's letter may have been one stimu-lus leading David Humphreys Storer to add the subject of criminal abortion to his Introductory Lecture, since David specifically addressed and condemned the "generally prevailing opinion" that abortion "is excusable previous" to present-ing "unmistakable signs of life."[72]

Eight months before his Introductory Lecture, David made a reference to the taboo subject of criminal abortion in an address to graduating Harvard medi-cal students, although the word "abortion" was not mentioned.[73] David comple-mented the new Harvard graduates on completing their medical degrees and provided advice for tolerating the long period that it would take to develop a thriving practice. This included:

> Alone, depressed, wretched, he receives a request for professional advice, accompanied with a remuneration, which to him is immense, which will relieve his necessities for months. This service he can render; and, with it, his employer alone need be conversant. This may be your position, as it has been that of others. Hesitate not a moment; allow not the struggle to commence, even, between your destitution and your conscience. As yet, you have committed no crime. You are penniless, you feel perhaps friendless; but you are still yourselves. Return the gold to the tempter, untouched; and thus teach him that your integrity is priceless. However frequently such demands may subsequently be made, the remembrance of the joyous satisfaction with which you indignantly repelled the first advance will prompt you, without a moment's delay, to pursue a similar course.[74]

John Preston Leonard had provided a similar caution to the struggling new physician and did it much more openly. Scores of physicians over the next decades presented similar warnings to the impoverished new physician.

Horatio returned to Boston on June 7, 1855 just in time to assume duties as an attending physician at the newly reopened Lying-in Hospital in Boston.[75] Later that summer, a reminder of Boston's abortion problem appeared when Dr. Francis Minot, published an article on the treatment of a married woman who had undergone a surgical abortion by "an empirical practitioner."[76] Also in this period preceding David's November Introductory Lecture, three deaths of Boston women that were initially attributed to natural causes were subsequently shown to have resulted from injuries received in procuring abortion.[77]

The annual Introductory Lecture marked the commencement of the Harvard Medical School term and was a major event for the physicians and medical students in Boston. The title of David's Lecture was "Duties, Trials and Rewards of the Student of Midwifery," and the beginning and major portion of the lecture did deal with obstetrics. He described how it was the most demanding work that a physician could undertake and he warned students unwilling to make the huge sacrifices involved, that it was their duty to find another profession.[78] Following this discussion David added:

> I should feel that I had been guilty of an unpardonable neglect were I to omit to glance at a subject the importance of which, each succeeding year, has been more forcibly impressed upon my mind. I had hoped that, *long ere this*, some one of the strong men of the profession,— strong in the affections of the community, strong in the confidence of his brethren,—would have spoken, trumpet-tongued, against an existing, and universally acknowledged evil. I have waited in vain. The lecturer is silent, the press is silent, and the enormity, unrebuked, stalks at midday throughout the length and breadth of the land. It is time that

this silence should be broken. It is time that men should speak. It is no presumption in the humblest individual to point out a much-needed reformation, however others may doubt the expediency of his course, if he thinks by thus doing he shall awaken in any mind the slightest attention to the subject; particularly if he sincerely believes that anything which can be found to be wrong can be rectified, that anything which ought to be done *can be* done sooner or later, whether it affects an individual, a community, or a race.[79]

The claim that "lecturer," "press," and "strong men of the profession" were silent, is perplexing. Hugh Lenox Hodge was "one of the strong men of the profession" and David certainly was aware of Hodge's lecture and its review by another strong man of the profession, David Francis Condie. The *Boston Medical and Surgical Journal* certainly had not been silent, having reproduced Reese's scathing editorial in March 1854 and published its own in October 1854. This claim of silence, almost suggests that someone was composing the abortion portion of the Introductory Lecture who had been out of the country in 1854 and the first half of 1855 and was unaware of these editorials, Hodge's republished Lecture, and Condie's review. Another possibility is that it was being composed by someone well aware of all these, but someone who did not want to call attention to pioneers in the antiabortion crusade because he wished to have major credit for starting the crusade go to the Storer family. More on this possibility later.

Another feature of David's Introductory Lecture was his description of the sharp increase in diseases that women were experiencing because of the increase in criminal abortion and the duty of physicians to persuade women to refrain from the criminal act, if not for moral reasons, then to preserve their health.[80] Physician persuasion was key to curtailing abortion for David:

The laws of the land, with all their penalties annexed, can do but little to abolish the crime. Compulsory measures may meet individual cases, and cause a temporary respite in a limited circle, but in order to produce an effect co-extensive with the transgression, that course should be pursued, the lenity of which proves its sincerity. Reason should be dealt with; moral suasion should be used, and no one can exert a greater influence than the physician; for no one is compelled like him to witness the misery, to see the distress which is acknowledged by the sufferer to have been thus produced, to hear the disclosures as they reluctantly fall from the lips of the dying penitent. We can do much—we can do all. If our profession will feel and act as one man; if they cannot all regard the subject in the same light as I have, as respects its morality, but will look at it merely as a cause of physical suffering to the mother; if they will upon all proper occasions freely express their convictions of its injurious effects, of its present danger, of its detrimental consequences,—a triumphant result must follow.[81]

Although tissue damage associated with invasion of the uterus was one basis for disease associated with induced abortion, David argued that the failure of the organs of pregnancy to complete their normal course of events also was a factor. He also believed that prevention of conception by any means left the reproductive organs in an interrupted state and similarly subject to disease. Thus, in addition to an antiabortion portion of David's Introductory Lecture, there was a brief anti-contraception portion.[82] As will be seen, both portions would be frequently praised and echoed in the writing of Horatio.

As mentioned in Chapter One, the antiabortion segment was omitted when the Introductory Lecture was published and this led the editors of the *Boston Medical and Surgical Journal* to criticize the "others" who persuaded David to leave his discussion of abortion out of the pamphlet. Horatio would credit his father's Introductory Lecture and these editors "by whom the effort then made was so warmly and eloquently seconded" "for the thought of the present undertaking," i.e., for the thought of campaigning against unnecessary abortion.[83]

The suppressed portion was finally published as "Two Frequent Causes of Uterine Disease" in 1872 in the sixth volume of the first medical journal devoted exclusively to gynecology.[84] This was the *Journal of the Gynaecological Society of Boston* that was started and edited by Horatio (See Chapter 15). Horatio not only was responsible for the long-delayed publication of the abortion portion, he probably made input to it when it was being composed in 1855. We earlier noted Horatio's involvement in his father's professional activities while still a medical student and his sending instructional material from Scotland to assist David in his new Professorship. Horatio continued to assist his father's teaching after Horatio returned to Boston in June 1855.[85]

It is even possible that the antiabortion section was Horatio's idea. David had been unwilling to mention abortion by name in his March 1855 address to graduating students when Horatio was in Edinburgh. After Horatio had been back in Boston for five months, David was willing to openly discuss criminal abortion. If Horatio were primarily responsible for the abortion portion of his father's lecture, this could explain "David's" new candidness about the subject and could account for why David allowed the section to be omitted when the lecture was published. This also could account for why his father did not persist in antiabortion efforts after the Introductory Lecture.

Conflicting with all of this "evidence" that Horatio made input, even large input, to his father's Lecture was its expressed opinion that "laws ... can do but little to abolish the crime." This was a totally different perspective on abortion legislation from that of Horatio a year later when he began the crusade, and, if Horatio influenced Leonard's "Quackery and Abortion," a totally different perspective from five years earlier. As will be seen, Horatio would emphasize reform of Massachusetts' abortion laws in his 1857 Suffolk District Medical Society Report on Criminal Abortion and reform of the laws of the rest of the country in 1859 in the American Medical Association Report on Criminal Abortion.

Whether original with David and the inspiration for Horatio's "physicians' crusade," as Horatio repeatedly claimed, or whether more-or-less authored by Horatio, the antiabortion segment of this Introductory Lecture is a landmark event in the successful "physicians' campaign against abortion." Leonard's "Quackery and Abortion" is another such landmark, even if it were only an influence on Horatio, but particularly if Horatio had some responsibility for it.

CHAPTER 4

STORER'S CRUSADE BEGINS

Horatio did not begin the physicians' crusade against abortion for more than a year after his father's Introductory Lecture. However, abortion no doubt was on his mind in January 1856 when he offered ways to control vomiting during pregnancy at a meeting of a Boston medical society.[1] Abortion was often induced to eliminate pregnancy-associated vomiting when the vomiting was so severe that starvation threatened. Abortion also may have been on Horatio's mind in May 1856 when he traveled to Detroit to attend the Ninth Annual Meeting of the American Medical Association.[2] No discussion of abortion appeared in the published *Transactions*, but Horatio surely met John Berrien Lindsley of Tennessee who was key to Horatio being nominated as Chairman of the Committee on Criminal Abortion the next year when the Association met in Nashville. It is possible that the initial plans for the future Committee were laid in Detroit in May 1856.

Shortly after returning to Boston, Horatio probably read the article, "A few Observations on the Attributes of the Impregnated Germ," published in June 1856.[3] Horatio would praise this article and its author, R.H. Tatum, in his 1859 article, "Its Obstacles to Conviction."[4] Tatum emphasized that even as independent life existed from conception, an immortal soul also existed from conception:

> In the death of a developed human being, body returns to its mother dust, but the indestructible—the mind—wings its flight to Him who gave it. So with the little *embryo*, when it has laid aside its "mortal coil," it puts on immortality around the throne of its mighty Creator. And there it shall remain to confront the fiend, that may have sent it on its uncalled errand.[5]

Tatum claimed that it was physicians' "imperative duty to direct the attention of legislators to the importance of enacting a statute" to protect this "sentient being." "The death of an embryo either by direct physical force or the administration of some noxious substance," he wrote, "should be declared murder in the first degree."[6] Tatum also claimed it was the duty of physicians to "inculcate" this view that the fetus was alive and immortal from conception "in the popular mind." "By a knowledge of this fact," Tatum continued, "many might be deterred from producing abortion, and many be induced to reject the syren [sic] overtures of the seducer."[7]

Horatio also praised the article, "Some of the Legal Relations of the Foetus in Utero," by Levin Smith Joynes, a Professor at the Medical College of Virginia.[8] Joynes wrote his article because of Tatum's call for making abortion a capital crime. Joynes argued that this would never lead to a conviction and he called for a lesser penalty that would lead to verdicts of guilty. While Joynes was at it, he pointed out his 1849 success in eliminating the quickening distinction in Virginia law.

As mentioned in Chapter 1, another probable stimulus for Horatio's "undertaking" was the article, "Foeticide," by Jesse Boring that was published only one month before Horatio began his crusade. Boring was a Methodist minister and medical doctor who was described in his paper as "Professor Obstetrics, &c., Atlanta Medical College."[9] Boring followed Hodge and Tatum in referring to the embryo's immortal soul. Horatio probably viewed such claims that God would punish the abortionist and the woman seeking abortion as detrimental to a crusade aimed at suppressing the crime, since there were many irreligious women and abortionists who would not have accepted these as valid. He may have also worried that some religious opponents of abortion would leave the solution of the problem of criminal abortion and the punishment of abortionists to God, instead of actively working to achieve these ends.

The first hard evidence of Storer's crusade appeared in February 1857. John Keith, a Boston lawyer, provided a letter in response to Horatio's request for information on the Massachusetts laws "respecting procuring abortion, &c." Keith indicated that should the woman die as a consequence of an attempt at abortion, the offence was punishable by not more than twenty years nor less than five years of imprisonment. If she survived, the imprisonment was not more than seven years and not less than one year. Keith also indicated: "the law makes no distinction between the pregnancy before & after quickening."[10]

This information was part of Horatio's homework for a long presentation he made on the subject of criminal abortion at the February 28 meeting of the Suffolk District Medical Society. The Secretary was Luther J. Parks, Jr., and there was bad blood between Parks and Horatio related to disagreements about medical treatment of women patients.[11] Parks' dubious rendition of Horatio's remarks, omitting even the month of the meeting, was not published in the *Boston Medical and Surgical Journal* until May 7.[12] This was two days before a special meeting of the Suffolk District Medical Society called to review the Society's Report on Criminal Abortion that was proposed on February 28. Had it not been for the special meeting, these Minutes probably would never have been published. They included:

> [Horatio Storer] desired to bring before the Society a subject which imperatively demanded its early and decisive action. Somewhat over a year ago, the present professor of obstetrics in the University (Dr. Storer, Sen.) had called attention, in a public inaugural address, to the alarming increase of *criminal abortion* in this community, and to the fact that the initiatory steps towards suppressing the crime should come from physicians. When the address alluded to was subsequently published, so much of it as bore upon this question, as also upon a kindred one, the prevention of pregnancy, was suppressed—in deference to the request of other gentlemen of the College Faculty, but entirely against the author's will. That gentleman had since been repeatedly called upon for a reiteration of his views; many months had, however, now

elapsed, and as there seemed little or no probability of such being done at present, if at all, his son, after duly ascertaining this fact, had no hesitation in at once bringing the subject before the Society; it being acknowledged by all, in the least degree conversant with this matter, that immediate action was necessary. ...

Dr. S. referred to our statutes on this subject, and to the ignorance prevalent in the community respecting the actual and separate existence of foetal life in the early months of pregnancy. He dwelt on the moral and absolute guilt of the parties offending, and on the necessity of prompt and efficient action by the profession, and called upon the Society, as representing the physicians of Boston, to take such steps as would alike further ensure the innocence in this matter of all its members, and show to the community the sincere abhorrence with which they viewed the crime.[13]

Horatio's father was at the meeting and

expressed his satisfaction that the subject was at last to be brought before the community. He held without abatement the views he had formerly expressed regarding it; the crime, if it existed to the extent all would allow it did exist, should be repressed, and it was the duty of physicians to expose and to denounce it. ... He disclaimed any collusion with his son in thus bringing up the matter, but was delighted it had been done, and had no doubt of the ultimate result.[14]

One must be cautious in judging whether the phrase, "if it existed to the extent all would allow it did exist," was really David's comment or whether it was Parks' lack of certainty about abortion's high prevalence. David had expressed no such doubts about the prevalence of the crime in his Introductory Lecture. However, if David really were not as certain about the frequency of abortion as Horatio, this also supports the possibility that Horatio had had much influence on the abortion remarks of that Lecture.

The Minutes also indicated that Horatio proposed a Resolution: "That a Committee be appointed to consider whether any further legislation is necessary in this Commonwealth, on the subject of *criminal abortion*, and to report to the Society such other means as may seem necessary for the suppression of this abominable, unnatural, and yet common crime." Horatio consented to adding: "And that said report, when accepted by this Society, shall by it be recommended to the Massachusetts Medical Society as a basis for its further action."[15] The amended Resolution passed unanimously, and the Chair appointed Horatio, Henry Ingersoll Bowditch, and Calvin Ellis as the Committee with Horatio designated Chairman.[16]

Parks' Minutes of the February meeting did not capture an exchange between Horatio and the foremost physician of Boston, Jacob Bigelow, which Horatio described in an autobiographical letter in 1901. Horatio indicated it was at the Suffolk District Medical Society that he "first entered the anti-abortion lists." "I

was at once challenged and given the lie by Dr. Jacob Bigelow," Horatio continued, "who I have always supposed brought me into the world."[17]

With the blessing of the Suffolk District Medical Society, Horatio began a
huge letter writing campaign that produced responses from physicians in twenty
states and territories providing information on their laws related to criminal abortion.[18] One deserves particular emphasis because it gives evidence of Horatio's
plan to make his campaign a national one. The 1857 Annual Meeting of the
American Medical Association was scheduled for Nashville in May. In addition to
a request for Tennessee statutes on abortion, Storer apparently requested creation
of a Committee on Criminal Abortion at that Meeting. This request no doubt was
what the following letter indicated would "be attended to duly at the meeting."

> Nashville March 20
>
> H. Storer
> Roxbury
>   Dear Dr
>   Yours to Dr Lindsley is recd. He is absent north—may be in Bos-
> ton next month early.
>   Your letter is filed & will be attended to duly at the meeting
> though we shall expect you at the Association.
>   There is no statute on the subject of Crim. Ab. in this state, & no
> decisions in our Courts, as there has never been a case of the crime.
>   Good for Tennessee!
>   Very truly yours,
>   James W. Hoyte[19]

The other physician responses to Horatio's requests typically included
condemnations of induced abortion and strong support for Horatio's efforts
along with the requested law data. Charles A. Pope from St. Louis noted that
punishment of abortionists in his state "seems to be wholly disproportionate to
the sin and enormity of this offence." He continued: "I am glad that you are
directing your attention to this important subject and doubt not it will receive
full justice at your hands. When fully considered and your conclusions known, I
should be glad to obtain them, as I can easily have them embraced in our own
statutes."[20]

William H. Brisbane, an ex-slave-owner turned minister and physician,
provided a response that included:

> It is my *present intention* to endeavor to get a law passed by our
> legislature to meet the case, much too common, of administering
> drugs & injections either to prevent conception or destroy the
> embryo. It is an undoubted fact that, especially in high life, & in the
> middle rank of society, many wives (& often with the connivance of
> their husbands) take measures of this kind. It is not probable that any
> law could be enforced in such cases; but the fact of the existence of a

law making it criminal, would probably have a moral influence to prevent it to some extent. And perhaps in some cases it might be enforced against those who furnish knowingly & designedly the means of procuring the destruction of the embryo or foetus.[21]

The letter from C.W. LeBoutillier, of Minnesota, included:

The practice of producing abortion is frequently resorted to in our vicinity, and it is not unfrequent for married women of high social position to apply for medicines which will produce abortion and it is with regret that I say that Regular physicians have in many instances, assisted in this damnable practice. The law as it stands is to us worthless & unless it is amended the evil will not soon cease.[22]

Although there were three members of the Suffolk District Medical Society Committee on Criminal Abortion, Horatio apparently took full responsibility for writing its Report. He had completed a draft by April 20, 1857 when fellow committee member, Henry Ingersoll Bowditch, provided a letter with his reactions to it. Bowditch agreed that "making the woman an accomplice is perfectly just." Bowditch argued that Horatio should drop references to prevention of pregnancy and also omit the draft abortion statute that Horatio had appended to the report.[23] Horatio heeded Bowditch's suggestion to omit contraception, but he retained the draft abortion statute.[24]

Horatio read his Report to the Suffolk District Medical Society on April 25.[25] The Report was printed and distributed to Society members early in May with a cover letter announcing "a Special Meeting for action on the report" on May 9, 1857.[26] The Report began by describing the high frequency of criminal abortion in Massachusetts and indicating that "it is probably steadily increasing."[27] Horatio noted that there were no official statistics to support this, but it was recognized by authorities that many reports of stillbirths were really instances of criminal abortion. He also noted "that in no less than *fifteen* instances during the past half-year has the Chairman been called to treat the confessed results, near or remote, of criminal abortion; and, of these patients, all without exception were married and respectable women."[28]

Horatio noted that criminal abortion escaped "punishment by law" and had "found public and unblushing defenders, who have so blunted the moral and religious sense of the people, that many respectable women do not hesitate to avow their belief that abortion is no crime." He called on physicians to make the public aware of the nature of the fetus and the crime associated with its destruction. Physicians were "the guardians of the public health" and were the people most apt to learn of the crime. They should "declare its true nature, its prevalence, and its deplorable consequences; to denounce it in unmeasured terms, and, where possible, to point out and to enforce efficient means for its suppression." "In private, among his families; in public from his professor's desk, from the pages of his journal, or from the witness' stand," the Report continued, "the physician is called upon by every dictate of humanity and religion to condemn it."[29]

Horatio claimed "the profession can control the crime through the laws" and he devoted the remainder of the Report to how this could be done. He called for stringent laws against abortion that were "faithfully enforced." They should prevent as well as punish the crime and thus needed to "be simple, easily understood, and not be evaded." He quoted the current Massachusetts statutes and identified why he believed they had led to few indictments and even fewer convictions.[30] One reason was the necessity to show that "malice or want of lawful justification" existed. Another was the need to prove that the woman was pregnant. Still another was the limitation on aborting agents to a "poison, drug, or medicine, or noxious thing." He called for a statute that clearly pointed out that the only excuses for induced abortion were "to save the life of the mother, or of the foetus within her womb." It also should specify that this could only be determined "by experienced physicians" and that at least one other physician must agree that abortion was necessary.

The Report continued with a discussion of the meager punishment for the crime and the major reason for this, the failure of the law to consider the true victim. He wrote:

> The law is predicated on an entirely erroneous idea. The real intent is seldom against the life of the mother; in almost every instance, she is herself, not merely an accessory, but one of the principals—in what? Not an attempt at the murder of herself,—for that would be simply absurd,—but the murder of her child.
>
> The law is here fundamentally wrong. It utterly ignores the existence of the living child, though the child is really alive from the very moment of its conception, and from that very moment is and should be considered a distinct being; this the law does not, however, recognize.[31]

Horatio noted that civil law, unlike "moral" law, recognized the child's existence before birth. He also pointed out that the "perils and dangers" of the uterine existence were no reason for reducing the "criminality" of fetal destruction as some had argued. He noted that the perils "which threaten the new-born child" were as great or greater and these "would hardly be allowed to invalidate a charge of infanticide."[32]

Horatio then argued that the purposeful destruction of a living fetus was "clearly MURDER," but "there are those who will not allow that it should be punished as such." He called for its reclassification from a simple misdemeanor to at least a felony. He also proposed, following an article of the French penal code, that medical persons be punished more for inducing abortion than those not associated with the medical profession. Horatio also called for a greater crime if the woman seeking abortion were married.[33]

Another plea of Horatio was that anyone who even advocated abortion be charged with a crime. "Much of the public indifference and error on the subject of criminal abortion," he wrote, "is owing to the influence of certain misguided or brutal men, who by their publications or lectures, have given rise to a belief that the induction of abortion is alike the prerogative and duty of the married."[34] Horatio then provided the following paragraph that described physician actions that contributed to the rise of criminal abortion. As will be seen, Charles Edward Buckingham would request that everything from "the frequent repetition ..." to the end of the paragraph be dropped.

> The resort to craniotomy, where, in some cases at least, the child's life might by other means be saved; the frequent repetition of that opera-tion, or of the premature induction of labor before the seventh month, in the same patient, in accordance with the rule, almost universally ac-knowledged, but still often WRONG, that the child's life is as nothing in comparison with that of its mother; the neglect of attempts at resus-citating still-born children, especially where, as the phrase goes, "it is a mercy" if the child were born dead; the fear sometimes shown by medical men to denounce the crime in fitting terms to patients who have confided to them their sin; the occasional carelessness in treat-ment and mistakes in diagnosis, where proper attention and examina-tion would have shown the unmistakable signs of pregnancy; the rely-ing upon a single and unaided opinion, in cases where not one life only, but two, may be involved,—are all instances of apparent disregard of foetal life, that serve with the community as incentives to abortion.[35]

Horatio called for coroners to be selected from physicians and for physicians to become more familiar "with the true principles and with the details of Obstetric Jurisprudence."[36] Horatio predicted this would lead to increased certainty of pun-ishment and that this in turn would sharply reduce the incidence of the crime.

Horatio followed with the draft abortion statute that incorporated the changes and additions he had recommended. "But enforce this law," Horatio continued, "and the profession would never allow its then high place in the community to be unworthily degraded; nor, as now, would those be permitted, unchallenged, to remain in fellowship, who were generally believed guilty or suspected of this crime."[37] Although Horatio Storer had been told of numerous physicians who were inducing unnecessary abortions by Hodge, Leonard, editors of the *Boston Medical and Surgical Journal*, his physician correspondents, and others, Storer made only this one brief reference to actual or suspected physician abortionists. As suggested earlier, he may have downplayed the problem of physician abortionists to keep probable opponents of the Report, abortionists or their supporters, from attending the Society meeting on May 9, 1857 where the Report was considered.

At that meeting, Jacob Bigelow, claimed that criminal abortion "had been well considered by the legislature when the present laws were passed, and perhaps they could not be improved."[38] He objected to the Committee's dropping of the requirement to prove pregnancy. He also pointed out that a physician could go to prison for treating amenorrhoea if abortion should follow, even though it were impossible to determine that pregnancy existed. Bigelow's final objection was to the Committee's plan to increase the severity of punishment. This he felt would increase the difficulty of obtaining convictions for the crime, noting that "juries sometimes will not bring in a man guilty of murder because the punishment is so severe." "As to the punishment of the woman," the Minutes continued, "Dr Bigelow thought her perhaps the least culpable of all; less so than the physician, for she has frequently the fear of shame and disgrace to urge her on; much less so than her seducer who escapes easily while she suffers severely." Bigelow thus showed his belief that induced abortion was largely confined to the unmarried.

Horatio countered that the Committee "had considered all these objections and differed in opinion." He noted that "several distinguished lawyers" indicated that convictions were not possible with the present law. "As to the punishment of the woman," the Minutes continued, "Dr Storer thought that the seducer did not generally share in the crime of procuring abortion." The Minutes also reported:

> As to "proving the existence of pregnancy," a large proportion of these cases occur during the first few months of utero-gestation, when this can not be positively done. The existence of "malice" is also a difficult thing to prove. Dr Storer thought it much easier and much more apt to promote the ends of justice, that the government should be obliged merely to prove the deed, and the prisoner be made to show its necessity.[39]

A Dr. Moore indicated his approval of "the sentiments and opinions contained in the report." He argued that the woman obtaining the abortion should be punished and described a woman who had requested him to perform an abortion. He refused and she "performed the operation on herself by means of a whalebone."

It then was Buckingham's turn. He first emphasized "that regular practitioners do not countenance the production of abortion save in extreme cases, and do not practise it; that the statements to the contrary are made by irregular practitioners to justify themselves." He indicated his agreement with Dr. Bigelow's objections and cited his additional concern about the greater punishment for married than single women. He acknowledged that married women had more abortions than single women, but noted that once a woman made the decision to abort there was no stopping her, "if she can't get drugs she will operate on herself as in Dr Moore's case." The Minutes then described Buckingham's objections to the paragraph in the Report that countered the frequently accepted belief that "the child's life is as nothing in comparison with that of its mother." Buckingham saw this as "going back too far, to the Roman Catholic laws; making an excuse for the operation of Cesarean Section, a capital and very dangerous operation." Horatio was reported to have responded:

> The Committee thought it their duty to report the paragraph objected to, and was surprised that Dr. Buckingham should object to it. In cases of deformed pelvis abortion is frequently produced in order to save the life of the mother; it has sometimes been done as often as five times in the same patient. He thought that the lusts of man or woman should not be pandered to in this way. The man should be castrated or the child have a chance. The mother is responsible if she puts her own life in danger

and the crime is against the child. In regard to Dr. Buckingham's statement that if a woman can't get drugs she will operate on herself, Dr. Storer said that was her own risk; *the Committee act for the child*; the mother is a willing agent and must answer for herself.[40]

The members then decided that still another meeting of the Society was needed to deal with the report. It was moved and carried "that the report be recommitted with instructions to the Committee to make alterations if they thought necessary, and report at the next *regular* meeting" that was scheduled for May 30, 1857.[41]

CHAPTER 5

WAR BETWEEN THE MEDICAL JOURNALS

Charles Edward Buckingham wrote a guest editorial which appeared in the *Boston Medical and Surgical Journal* on May 28 and which he signed "B."[1] It was highly critical of the Committee Report and we can be sure that it was available for Boston physicians to read two or more days before the meeting of the Society on May 30.[2] It began as an announcement of the upcoming meeting.

> At the regular meeting of the Suffolk District Medical Society, this month, the Report upon Criminal Abortions will come up for final action. That Report has been printed and distributed among the members, who, before that time, will doubtless have read it, and formed their opinions. The affair was too hastily got up, and ought not to pass in its present form. The writer of it seems to have thrown out of consideration the life of the mother, making that of the unborn child appear of far more consequence, even should the mother have a dozen dependent on her for their daily bread. It cannot be possible that either the profession or the public will be brought to this belief. *Argue as forcibly as they may, to their own satisfaction, the Committee will fail to convince the public that abortion in the early months is a crime, and a large proportion of the medical profession will tacitly support the popular view of the subject.*[3]

Buckingham indicated that physicians should concentrate their efforts on changing public attitudes about criminal abortion. He also pointed out problems associated with calling abortion "murder."

> But allowing the committing of abortion to be murder, and the writer is not prepared to deny that, although he is less disposed to assert it than he was, before this subject was broached by the Committee, with what consistency can it be proposed to inflict any punishment less than capital for it? Or how can they make it less a murder, if performed upon an unmarried woman, than upon a married one?

"Let the Suffolk District Society utter their protest as strongly as they please," he concluded, "but the making of laws is as much out of their province as the mending of watches."[4]

As will be seen, Horatio and his father were outraged by this guest editorial, not only at "B.", but at the *Boston Medical and Surgical Journal* editors for publishing something which the Storers *accurately* saw as calculated to prevent acceptance of the Society's Report on Criminal Abortion, and, *inaccurately* saw as libeling physicians. Horatio immediately sought the help of the *New-Hampshire Journal of Medicine* and the *American Medical Gazette*, both of whose editors were in New York.

Although the official Minutes of the Society's May 30 meeting have been lost, several sources indicate that Buckingham's guest editorial came under intense criticism. The most comprehensive account of the meeting was by "Medicus" and published in *The Medical World*, a short-lived journal edited by Dr. Jerome Van Crowninshield Smith. Medicus described Horatio's reading of the revised Report and continued:

> But, as this was, in effect, *a new report*, and, as it was difficult to trace the parts which were left out, and those which were retained from the former Report, Dr. Buckingham moved that this new Report, with the Resolutions, be laid upon the table, and printed, to be acted upon at a future meeting.
>
> Dr. Storer, Sen., was very much surprised that any member of the Society should hesitate for a moment to adopt this Report. He assailed, with considerable severity, the following sentence, in the *Journal* of May 28th, 1857: "Argue as forcibly as they may, to their own satisfaction, the Committee will fail to convince the public that abortion in the early months is a crime, and a large proportion of the medical profession will tacitly support the popular view of the subject." He (Dr. Storer, Sen.,) was surprised that any member of the profession should write thus, and especially, that the man who would make such a statement should not put his whole name to the article, ...
>
> Dr. Buckingham, (with no small share of the dauntless courage of his father, in the days of the "New England *Galaxy*,") arose and said he was the author of the article in the *Journal,* and he did not shrink from assuming the responsibility of all that was there said. He believed it was all true, and was ready to defend it; and that it contained no such sentiments as Dr. S. had tried to make it contain, &c.
>
> Dr. Storer read it again, and renewed his former statements. ...
>
> After an expression of various opinions, (sometimes half a dozen speakers at once,) the report was accepted. ...
> Medicus.[5]

Medicus' report of the meeting did not identify the specific objections of David Humphreys Storer to Buckingham's "Argue as forcibly ..." statement. David (and no doubt Horatio) had interpreted the statement as claiming that "a large proportion" of physicians *shared* the public view that abortion was not a crime. David claimed this was "a libel on the profession," since it was well known that virtually all regular physicians believed unnecessary abortion was criminal. David and Horatio were concerned that this published "deliberate falsehood" about how physicians regarded induced abortion "would tend to prejudice the profession, wrongfully and dangerously, in public opinion."[6] This we learn from the

New-Hampshire Journal of Medicine for July which reported the Suffolk Society's abortion doings and strongly criticized the *Boston Medical and Surgical Journal* for publishing "B."'s piece.

"B."'s intended meaning of the words "tacitly support the popular view" was given in a June 11 *Boston Medical and Surgical Journal* editorial. The Editors repeated the "Argue as forcibly ..." sentence, then wrote:

> We are willing to allow that this is capable of a construction which would imply a "libel" on the profession; but it is also capable of another, and which, to all who know either the writer of the article or the editors of this Journal, will, we believe, be the one most naturally suggested. We should be not a little, and most disagreeably surprised, did we think there was even *one*, in the profession or out of it, who could for a moment imagine we admit that any honorable physician panders, ever so slightly, or even "tacitly," to the procurement of criminal abortion. But that, either from sheer ignorance or a lack of high moral sense, ... the public do not consider "abortion in the early months" a crime, is only too evident—and what we understood by the expression which has excited so much feeling, is that the profession, or a "large proportion" of it, has not hitherto considered, and does not now consider, it worth while to waste time upon people who will not be convinced, and who are nearly always wholly uninformed, upon the *morale* of the act, at least. By admitting the article in question, we in no degree compromised ourselves, or expressed an opinion contrary to the above; neither does the article betray such sentiments on the part of the writer.[7]

If "B." had said "tacitly *endure* the public view of the subject," or even "tacitly *accept* ...," there would have been no misunderstanding at the time (or now). However, "tacitly *support* the popular view" that early abortion was not a crime, makes it easy a century and a half later to believe that "B." was actually saying that most physicians did not believe that early abortion was a crime. "B." made a poor selection of words, as he himself was to indicate in a subsequent letter asking his critics to look at his complete article.[8] James Mohr was to write in 1978 that "B." "was finally driven to claim that his statements had been misinterpreted ..."[9] "[F]inally driven to claim" suggests, even implies, that "B." was forced to claim something *counter* to his actual belief. However, despite the appearance to the contrary, "B." almost certainly was not claiming that the medical profession supported early abortions or viewed them as not being criminal.

The July *New-Hampshire Journal of Medicine* editorial almost certainly was based on "correspondence" from Horatio to its editor, Edward Hazen Parker. The editorial began:

> Criminal Abortion.—We have watched with much interest the progress of the movement lately commenced by the profession in Boston against Criminal Abortion. This movement has now secured the sanction of the State Medical Society of Massachusetts, and as it will doubtless be *par-*

ticipated in by physicians of other States we are inclined to think its history from the outset, obtained from current numbers of the Boston Medical and Surgical Journal, and from the correspondence of a friend may prove not unacceptable to our readers.[10]

The "sanction of the State Medical Society of Massachusetts" was obtained at its meeting in New Bedford on June 3. However, it was a weak sanction, if it could be considered such at all. According to the Minutes of the New Bedford meeting, Horatio described the actions of the Suffolk District Medical Society related to the increased frequency of abortion and proposed a Resolution for the Massachusetts Medical Society which would lead to a Committee "to bring before the next Legislature the alarming increase of criminal abortion in this Commonwealth, and to request in the name of this Society a careful revision of the Statutes upon that crime."[11]

The Minutes of the New Bedford meeting also indicated that there was much discussion where "several of the Fellows advocated the proposition, and others opposed any action which would involve the Society in seeking additional legislation." "Drs. Foster Hooper, of Fall River, J. Bigelow, J. Ware, J.C. Dalton, E. Hunt, C. Gordon, and H.R. Storer" were appointed as a Committee "with instructions to report to the Councillors, that they may bring the matter before the Society at its next annual meeting."[12] The *New-Hampshire Journal of Medicine* version of the New Bedford proceedings predicted that the make-up of the Massachusetts Medical Society Committee was such that they would "not rest till they have secured all they desire. They aim at an open and general condemnation of the crime by the profession, and at thus removing the imputation now so generally considered as resting on its fair name."[13] As we will see, the Committee made their report when the Councillors met in February 1858 when Horatio was away from Massachusetts, and Horatio repeatedly would claim that the Report should have been made to the entire Society six months later.

The following final paragraphs of the *New-Hampshire Journal* editorial show that the antiabortion crusade was viewed as a "war," and indicate why Editor Parker at the outset predicted the movement against criminal abortion would be "participated in by physicians of other States."

We feel that we may well be pardoned for first speaking at length as we have, of the connection of our Massachusetts brethren with this subject, as the war seems first to have fairly begun with them; and will only say in addition, that we have personal knowledge that the evil is no less prevalent in our own community. ...

Dr. H. R. Storer has taken a stand in this matter alike creditable to his head and his heart, and we feel that he will receive the hearty thanks of every *true* physician.

That his efforts are appreciated by the profession at large, is evident, from the fact that he was appointed by the American Medical Association at its late meeting at Nashville, as Chairman of a Special Committee "on Criminal Abortion, with a view to its general suppression," to report next year at Washington, and may be regarded as an earnest, that the work now begun, *will be carried forward.*[14]

John Preston Leonard had referred to the crusade against abortion as a "war" in January 1851.[15] Perhaps he had heard Horatio describe it as such, even as Parker probably heard it so labeled by Horatio in 1857.

Although Horatio was already aware that he had been selected Chairman of the American Medical Association Special Committee on Criminal Abortion, he received a July 4 letter from John Berrien Lindsley of Nashville notifying him of this. It included:

> The Nominating Committee objected to raising so large a special committee as you wished, but very cordially appointed you Chairman. As such you have the privilege of selecting such Co-adjutors as you may wish. The subject *is* very important as well as interesting, and the Washington meeting will be a good time to bring it up. We all anticipate a very large turn out next year, which will make up for the small attendance at our[,] for the present[,] inaccessible city.[16]

The power of nomination of "Co-adjutors" was a boon in that it allowed Horatio himself to select those men he believed could best advance the antiabortion effort.

The furor associated with the Suffolk District Committee Report continued. The *Boston Medical and Surgical Journal* responded on July 23 to the editorial in the July *New-Hampshire Journal of Medicine.*[17] They criticized Editor Parker for either discussing something he did not have first-hand knowledge of or of surrendering his editorial function to an actual participant in the Massachusetts Society's criminal abortion discussions. They stuck by their definition of "tacitly support" as "tacitly endure" and rather successfully showed that their editorial positions on the question of criminal abortion had not changed from strong opposition. They also called for physicians to help dispel the ignorance that caused people to "allow, or seek for the perpetration of the crime."

The *New-Hampshire Journal of Medicine* responded in August with "Criminal Abortion; The Boston Medical and Surgical Journal and its Attempts at Bullying."[18] The editorial pointed out that it had acknowledged the information in their July editorial had come "in part from conversation and correspondence with a personal acquaintance and friend, resident in" Massachusetts. The editorial reiterated the claim that "B."'s controversial sentence would be interpreted by nine out of ten impartial readers as indicating that the profession would agree with the public's view of abortion's criminality, not quietly put up with a view they disagreed with. The editorial added: "Such was our impression before we had written or had heard a word upon the subject, and we are glad that 'B.' has been denounced by one of the New York Journals, as in this matter 'heretical alike to truth and good morals.' Are the Boston editors prepared to quarrel with all who have so thought?"[19]

The *Boston Medical and Surgical Journal* did not continue the exchange, but published another letter of Buckingham that repeated his claim that he had been misinterpreted. Buckingham also cast aspersions on the *New-Hampshire Journal's* "personal acquaintance and friend," claiming he "stands in such a relation to the profession that his evidence would not, by itself, be considered of much worth among the profession in Boston."[20] Although unnamed, it was obvious that Buckingham was referring to Horatio.[21]

The New York journal that "denounced" Buckingham was the *American Medical Gazette*. Their denouncement began:

> The following two articles are inserted connectedly, that our readers may see how this important topic is regarded by the medical mind in Boston. The first, being a report of the Committee, is, in our opinion, well considered, and a truthful exposition of a topic which ought to be regarded of the highest interest to the profession and the public. Its ethics are sound and in conformity with the morale of the profession, which has always been on the side of true religion. But the second we regard as heretical alike to truth and good morals, this being a critique on the report of the Committee, and foreshadowing a hostile demonstration to the latter when it shall come before the Society.[22]

This was followed by the Suffolk District Report on Criminal Abortion and "B."'s original guest editorial from the *Boston Medical and Surgical Journal*. Horatio provided at least the Committee Report to the Editor, David Meredith Reese, and he no doubt also described the problem the guest editorial posed for acceptance of the Report, namely, "foreshadowing a hostile demonstration to the latter." "Foreshadowing" and the words that followed, "*when* it shall come before the Society,"[23] are evidence that Horatio provided material to Reese, and no doubt also to Editor Parker of the *New-Hampshire Journal*, *after* "B."'s guest editorial appeared, but *before* the Suffolk District Medical Society meeting only a few days later on May 30. Horatio must have realized that the *Gazette* and *New-Hampshire Journal* could not do anything in time to influence the Suffolk District Medical Society vote on his Report. Perhaps he was counting on these journals' help in a later reconsideration of the Report if it were rejected on May 30.

Reese's support of Horatio's efforts followed this editor's earlier strong concerns about criminal abortion in his 1850 and 1854 editorials. Reese also presented a "Report on Infant Mortality in Large Cities" at the same 1857 American Medical Association meeting that created the Committee on Criminal Abortion.[24] Reese's city of New York had an immense problem of infant mortality, much of which was associated with poverty and unsanitary conditions. However, another reason for "infant" mortality was criminal abortion. Reese's Report included:

> Without entering into any unnecessary detail upon this delicate and ungracious topic, it may suffice to allude only to the ghastly crime of abortionism, which has become a murderous trade in many of our large cities, tolerated, connived at, and even protected by corrupt civil authorities, and often patronized by newspapers whose proprietors insert conspicuously the advertisements of these male and female vam-

pires, for a share in the enormous profits of this inhuman traffic in blood and life. These murderers, for such they are, are well known to the police authorities; their names, residences, and even their guilty customers and victims are no secret to the authorities; they have their boxes at the post-office, loaded down with their correspondence and fees; take their seats at the opera; promenade our fashionable thoroughfares, and drive their splendid equipages upon our avenues in proud magnificence, while the "blood of the slaughtered innocents" is crying against them for vengeance.[25]

In his May 1859 article, "Its Victims," Storer would write that Reese "deserves unqualified commendation" for his Report's "direct and earnest dealing with the subject."[26]

Other medical journals were to get involved in Boston's abortion controversy. In August 1857 the *Atlanta Medical and Surgical Journal* reproduced the July *New-Hampshire Journal of Medicine* article, preceding it with the following:

CRIMINAL ABORTION OR FOETICIDE
> We are glad to see that the attention of the profession is becoming fixed upon this subject, and we hope that it will not be allowed to rest until it is placed in its proper position in the scale of crime.
>
> The laws upon this subject throughout, we believe, the entire world, show an utter ignorance or disregard of one of the most positive facts in Physiology, the effect of which has been to corrupt and degrade our species, and to destroy an almost incalculable amount of human health.
>
> The product of conception should be looked upon as a living being, and its wanton destruction should be held as *murder*, whether it be with a view of concealing the evidence of a departure from virtue, or resorted to by the married for the purpose of getting rid of the cost or trouble of families.[27]

The Michigan-based *Peninsular Journal of Medicine* also entered the discussion. An August 1857 editorial claimed: "We are confident that no considerable number of the members of the regular profession in any manner countenance, or even tacitly support, the popular sentiment on this subject, as stated by one of the journals."[28] The Editor, Edmund Potts Christian, followed this restatement of Buckingham's controversial phrase by claiming that physicians were still remiss, since they were not using their unique power to *change* the popular sentiment they did not support. Christian continued:

> [H]erein lies the true duty of the physician. It may not be his business, he may think, to preach its wickedness; that he leaves to spiritual advisers; nor to make the laws, or to bring prosecutions, or to threaten punishment; that he leaves for the makers of the law, its administrators, and the friends or relatives. But it is his duty to show the physical evils that

must result, that cannot be entirely averted. This is a duty he can dele-
gate to no one. We do not say he is travelling [sic] out of the line of his
duty in dwelling on these other points, but if he neglects this, he comes
sadly short of his duty.[29]

However, two months later Christian questioned whether he had been correct
in his August comment "that no considerable number of the members of the regular profession in any manner countenance, or even tacitly support, the popular
sentiment on this subject."[30] Christian provided and commented on a newspaper
report of a Chicago trial of an abortionist. Dr. Nathan Smith Davis was reported to
have testified that production of abortion by mechanical means was "in the highest
degree dangerous, and also as highly injurious to the system in its subsequent effects." "Out of twenty cases of abortion that came under his knowledge," the
newspaper article continued, "he could not recollect a single case where permanent and serious injury was not the result." The newspaper also reported that Professor Daniel Brainard, founder of Rush Medical College, testified "to the effect
that the production of abortion by mechanical means which rupture the membranes was not at all dangerous or injurious to life, if proper care were taken of the
person subsequently." The newspaper included the comment: "The medical testimony given in the court was in the highest degree conflicting, illustrating the old
adage that 'doctors differ.'"[31]

Christian agreed with Davis and took Brainard to task with two-and-one-half
pages of quotes of authorities, all claiming that mechanical production of abortion
was nearly always accompanied by serious health problems or death. Christian
suggested that Brainard's claim reflected a deficient moral view:

And when he thus dogmatically gives an opinion so opposed to the
teaching of the best, and, indeed, of all authors on the subject, as we
think we can show, we are inclined to ask ourselves if we uttered a mistaken opinion, that very few members of the regular profession in any
manner countenanced, even tacitly supported, the popular sentiment as
regards the danger; and if we find such opinions among the teachers,
how much more shall we not among the pupils; and, indeed, we fear
there are no small number who construe their ideas of the immorality of
the business according to their views of the danger.[32]

Brainard had studied under Alfred Velpeau during his early trips to France
and Velpeau was "the surgeon whom he most admired."[33] Velpeau claimed "the
fetus has no independent life and no claims upon our consideration on any such
account—that it is, in short, nothing more than a vegetable."[34] Daniel Garrison
Brinton heard Velpeau say this during Brinton's early study of medicine in Paris.
Brinton disagreed, but Brainard undoubtedly heard similar descriptions of the
fetus and may have found them more or less agreeable.

Both Brainard and Davis were professors at the Rush Medical College.[35] The
students no doubt were receiving very different views from the two men on the
morality and dangers to health of induced abortion. Probably some opted for the

Brainard view that led to fewer restrictions on their medical and surgical practice and to greater fees. Davis would leave Rush Medical College two years later for the new Chicago Medical School and Brainard's views on abortion may not have had opposition.[36] One result may have been the high rate of criminal abortion in Chicago that was to vex many of the city's physicians for decades (see Chapters 22 and 26).

CHAPTER 6

NEWSPAPER ABORTION ADVERTISEMENTS, BIGELOW'S TREACHERY

We noted physician complaints about the newspaper advertisements of abortionists, including Gunning Bedford's 1844 tirade against Madame Restell and David Meredith Reese's 1850 and 1854 editorials. David Francis Condie mentioned such advertisements in his 1855 review of Hodge's Lecture and Reese again referred to them in his 1857 "Report on Infant Mortality in Large Cities." There also were veiled advertisements for drugs that were claimed to end pregnancy. The advertised drugs typically were ineffective or only effective with women who were predisposed to miscarriage. On the other hand, some of the potions produced poisoning so severe that the body took the defensive measure of miscarriage, even in women who were not predisposed. Medical journals published articles and editorials describing deaths from such potions and discussing the controversial question of whether or not there actually were any drugs that would end pregnancy. One of the earliest appeared in the *Boston Medical and Surgical Journal* for November 22, 1831.[1] The editor claimed that women without a predisposition to miscarriage could not have abortions induced by any medicine and that even ergot had no effect prior to labor. The editorial concluded with the views of half a dozen other authorities, all denying the existence of abortifacients.

The *Journal* again dealt with these drugs in 1844. Jerome Van Crowninshield Smith was the editor and he decried the opinion of "some magnates in the profession" that "abortion could not be effected by medicine."[2] He noted that this was contrary to the belief of most physicians and claimed there were "half a dozen unprincipled scoundrels, at least, in Boston, whose fees for accomplishing just what is declared to be impossible, are surprisingly large." Smith was worried that communication of this false medical opinion would lead to increasingly open conduct by these "unprincipled scoundrels."[3] The *Journal's* attention to these drugs and to a death that resulted from their administration,[4] almost certainly was a factor in the passage of the 1845 Massachusetts law penalizing the administration of such drugs.

Madam Restell and others sold medicines that were claimed to produce abortion. When these failed, Restell and some of these men and women provided instrumental abortions. In 1847, Restell's husband, under the name, "Dr. A.M. Mauriceau, Professor of Diseases of Women," published *The Married Woman's Private Medical Companion*.[5] He no doubt selected the pseudonym, Mauriceau, because two centuries earlier a French physician, Francois Mauriceau, was the outstanding obstetrician of his time. The *Companion* made the claim that induced abortion often was appropriate and the book was largely an advertisement for "Portuguese Female Pills." These were described as: "The most successful specific, and one almost invariably certain in removing a stoppage, irregularity, or suppression of the menses (monthly turn)." "Mauriceau" added that they "appeared to be infallible, and would, undoubtedly, even produce miscarriage if exhibited during pregnancy." He also claimed the pills sometimes were used to end a pregnancy when the pelvis was malformed and "the woman incompetent to give birth at maturity." The 1847 edition indicated that whole boxes of the pills were five dollars and half boxes were three dollars.[6]

"Mauriceau's" *Companion* also advertised "M. Desomeaux's Preventive to Conception" and would forward packages of the "celebrated preventive" that "neutralizes the fecundating properties in semen" "to all parts of the United States."[7] Last, but hardly least, the book told that Professor Mauriceau had safely and painlessly induced abortion and the title page prominently displayed: "Office, 129 Liberty St., New York."

Edition after edition of the book appeared with one as late as 1864 and it probably was not the last. A Brooklyn physician in 1866 reported that a book "explaining and advising the process of abortion by one method or another" had sold over 400,000 copies (See Chapter 11). This probably was "Mauriceau's" *Companion*.

In 1857, there was a sharp increase in the frequency of medical editorials and medical articles protesting advertisements for abortion services and drugs claiming to produce abortion. The *Boston Medical and Surgical Journal* printed a letter of an Ohio physician under the heading "Abortion Advertisements."[8] The Editors preceded the letter by stating their belief that such drugs did not work since if they did, "we should not so often meet with cases of injury and death from the use of instruments employed with this wicked design." The letter included:

> "These advertisements have become so villainously common that one can hardly find a weekly newspaper whose columns are free from the nuisance; which, while they recommend abortions in an indirect manner, do not fail to impress upon the minds of the public that miscarriage can be produced, certainly and safely, with drugs! The following will serve as a specimen of the whole class. It is taken from a paper published and extensively circulated in Northern Ohio:—
>
> "'Ladies in want of a pleasant and safe remedy for irregularities, obstructions, &c., should use Dr. Miller's Female Monthly Powders. It has been said that these powders will produce miscarriage. Without admitting the truth of this assertion, I must confess that it is the inevitable consequence of their use during the early months of pregnancy. Therefore ladies who desire an increase of family should not use them. If after this caution any lady in a certain situation should use them, she must hold herself responsible for the abortion which will surely follow. Price $5.'...

"Whether any of the advertised articles are capable of producing miscarriage, I cannot say; but I am quite sure that many more cases of that nature have come under my observation in the past six months (which is about the time since these notices came in vogue in this vicinity), than in the preceding six years. This may be merely a coincidence, or the result of an epidemic tendency; but whatever the cause, those who circulate such advertisements are none the less culpable. If legislatures will not protect the public from such swindling, the medical profession should take the matter in hand. They can at least do something toward setting the mind of the public right."[9]

Significant in the above was the belief of the physician that these advertisements actually taught women that induced abortion was an appropriate way to solve the problem of an unwanted child. The correlation between the onset of these advertisements and the increase in frequency of abortion cases supports the notion of a causal relationship. As will be seen, numerous physicians would echo this claim that these advertisements legitimized abortion in the minds of the public.

Two editorials condemning criminal abortion and newspaper advertisements for means to induce abortion were published in the September and October 1858 numbers of the *Buffalo Medical Journal and Monthly Review*. They were written by its 22-year-old editor, Austin Flint, Jr. The first began:

Criminal Abortions.—The periodical medical press, which usually meets the eye of the medical man only, is the sole organ of defence which is used against this terrible crime which is now so rife in what is considered an enlightened and virtuous community, and seems lately to have thrown off even the decency of concealment. Why are we thus left alone to exclaim against this burning outrage? Why is it that the daily press, which assumes to be the guardian of the public welfare, and the religious press, which assumes to be the custodian of the public morals, are silent on this revolting theme? We need not ask the reason why, when we take up any of the daily papers which come into the heart of every family, and are read at the fireside of every home. They are filled with the iniquitous advertisements of quacks, who, not contented, like our "consumption cures," and scrofula exorcisers, with a traffic in the health of a credulous public, must attack its moral, as well as physical integrity. On us, then, devolves the sole duty of fighting against this fearful evil; and so rapidly is it spreading, that we must awake and do something. Let the matter be brought before our City, County, State, and National Associations! Let our legislatures be memorialized, if we have no laws which can touch these money-thirsty and blood-thirsty scoundrels; and let laws be made so that they may be exterminated, root and branch![10]

Flint provided a long example of one advertisement for "$1.00 per box" pills from a daily paper that the *Maine Medical and Surgical Reporter* had repro- duced a few months earlier.[11] Flint claimed such "flaming advertisements are undermining the strongest element of a Christian and enlightened society— female delicacy and purity."[12] He indicated that women were convinced by the ads that abortion was easy, safe, and not immoral. He continued:

> Females have now come to regard the production of abortion as one of the most innocent and natural things in the world; and our indigna- tion cannot be unmingled with pity, when we are coolly asked to as- sist in getting rid of an embryo, with as much *"sang froid"* as we are asked to vaccinate. Our horror and indignation is not in the least un- derstood, and the fair petitioner goes away entirely unconvinced of the nature of the crime which she wishes to commit.[13]

Flint claimed abortion was not only murder, but, given "the entire help- lessness of the victim," it was worse than murders committed in the height of passion, murders to avenge a crime, or even murders to steal. He called on phy- sicians *"en masse"* to demand from their legislatures "a law to prevent this hor- rible destruction of human life and public morals." He also called on his fellow *medical editors* to make a strong united effort to remedy the problem of criminal abortion.[14]

Flint's statement of many of the recommendations Horatio Storer would make a few months later in the American Medical Association Report on Crimi- nal Abortion, including memorials to legislatures to provide better abortion laws, suggests that Storer motivated Flint to editorialize on the subject. Horatio, who knew Flint "intimately,"[15] spent several months in Texas early in 1858 and returned to Boston by July 22.[16] He may have visited Buffalo during his return or sometime afterwards.

In his second editorial, Flint continued this discussion, but noted the futil- ity of convincing "the public that there was any great amount of crime in de- stroying the vitality of a newly impregnated ovum." He indicated things were different when abortion was still desired by the woman later in pregnancy after she "begins to feel that she has a living being within her." The public could eas- ily be taught that this late abortion was a crime, and Flint condemned such a woman who experienced movements of her unborn child but still felt "horror" instead of "fond anticipation" at the prospect of its birth.[17]

Flint indicated that James Platt White of the Buffalo Medical College had asked the Buffalo Medical Association to determine whether existing abortion statutes were properly enforced and to identify new legislation that might be needed "for abolishment of this great and growing evil."[18] Storer also knew White "intimately,"[19] and it is possible that Horatio stimulated White's effort. The Buffalo Medical Association resolved to undertake "any measure which may be deemed necessary and expedient to lessen these horrible offences against the morality of the community" and Flint called for other medical socie- ties and associations to join in these efforts.[20] According to James Mohr: "Regulars of the state of Maine immediately endorsed the Buffalo resolves against 'this great and growing evil.'"[21]

Flint noted that one newspaper, the *Brooklyn Daily Times*, had provided an editorial that concurred with and repeated Flint's September observations about the frequency and criminality of induced abortion. The *Times* editor, Walt Whitman, did this at the request of Flint's "esteemed correspondent, Dr. N.L. North." Flint copied Whitman's editorial that not only condemned the "advertisements of professed abortionists," but also claimed that any publisher who printed them was a participant in their crime.[22]

Flint concluded by repeating his hope that physicians would eliminate the "vile announcements" of the abortionists. He wrote:

> We do not advise a Quixotic attempt to have abortionists hung, drawn and quartered, but merely wish to begin the matter by keeping their vile announcements out of respectable daily papers; and if this cannot be done we are powerless indeed; if it can be done, and we have the most enduring faith in its possibility, are we men, are we Christians, are we good physicians, if we fail to make the effort?[23]

In 1912, the Editor of the *Buffalo Medical and Surgical Journal*, Arthur L. Benedict, noted that Flint's September 1858 editorial "called upon the profession and the lay press to cooperate in a campaign" against criminal abortion and "emphatically denounced" religious papers for carrying abortifacient advertisements. According to Benedict, this and subsequent editorials "illustrated the progressive spirit of the western New York physicians, as voiced in their *Journal*."[24] Austin Flint, Jr. was still alive and probably became aware of this praise. He died at age 79 in New York City in 1915 "while putting on his coat in preparation for a speaking engagement."[25]

Edmund Potts Christian included criticism of newspaper advertisements in his "Report to the State Medical Society on Criminal Abortions."[26] Christian blamed "ignorance and abnormal sentiment" on the subject of abortion for the deficient laws that provided inadequate and differing penalties for the crime and for the reluctance to convict women who obtained abortions. He noted that this "ignorance and abnormal sentiment" "pervades all ranks," including the press:

> Newspaper proprietors exhibit it in a lamentable degree, or else are thrice guilty in accepting pieces of silver as the price of innocent blood. We refer to the glaring advertisements to be daily perused in prominent corners of even the most respectable journals, of safe and ready means of effecting this purpose. For example, such as the following: "This medicine, to married ladies, is invaluable, as they (it) will, in all cases, bring on the monthly flow with regularity." Thus is the crime encouraged and fostered.
>
> The dealing in lotteries of any kind is contrary to our laws, and even their advertisement is prohibited, and why is it that such advertisements as these—far more pregnant with evil, with wickedness,

with perdition, are tolerated and so openly displayed—destructive to
morality and debauching to innocence?[27]

Following the tumultuous reception of Horatio's Suffolk District Medical
Society Report and his call for the Massachusetts Medical Society to address the
legislature about deficiencies in abortion statutes, Horatio continued medical society presentations and medical publishing through 1857.[28] However, at the end of
the year he was concerned about chest symptoms and feared he had contracted
tuberculosis. As a result, he headed for Texas in January 1858 and remained there
(or somewhere away from Boston) for at least six months. Letters to the Smithsonian Institution before the trip indicated that he planned to conduct natural history investigations.[29] Only a single confirmation has been located that these Texas
natural history investigations occurred. Horatio's uncle, Dr. Thomas Mayo
Brewer, noted in his discussion of Cassin's Sparrow in Volume 2 of *North American Birds*: "An egg of this species, taken in Texas by Dr. H. R. Storer, the identifi-
cation of which, however, was incomplete, is more oblong than the eggs of *P.
oestivalis*, and smaller, measuring .72 by .58 of an inch."[30]

A month after Horatio left Boston, Horatio's nemesis, Jacob Bigelow,
thwarted Horatio's hopes to have the Massachusetts Medical Society petition the
Massachusetts Legislature for stricter abortion laws. Jacob and Horatio were two
of the seven members of the Massachusetts Medical Society Committee on Criminal Abortion that was theoretically chaired by Dr. Foster Hooper. The Minutes of
the Councillors' February meeting indicated:

> The Committee ... reported that they do not recommend any application
> to the Legislature on the subject, believing that the Laws of the Com-
> monwealth are already sufficiently stringent, provided that they are
> executed, and offered the following Resolutions, which on motion of
> Dr. Fiske, of Fiskedale, were taken up separately and unanimously
> *adopted.*
>
> *Resolved,* That the Fellows of the Massachusetts Medical Society
> regard with disapprobation and abhorrence all attempts to procure abor-
> tion, except in cases where it may be necessary for the preservation of
> the mother's life.
>
> *Resolved,* That when any Fellow of this Society shall become
> cognizant of any attempt unlawfully to procure abortion, either by per-
> sons in the profession or out of it, it shall be the duty of such Fellow
> immediately to lodge information with some proper legal officer, to the
> end that such information may lead to the exposure and conviction of
> the offender.
>
> *Resolved,* That no person convicted of an attempt to procure
> criminal abortion can, consistently with its By-Laws, any longer remain
> a Fellow of this Society.[31]

Bigelow, almost certainly drafted the Report, given the similarity of the unusual letter "g" in Bigelow's signature and "g"s in the rest of the document.[32] Also

Jacob's signature was *not* over a penciled name, unlike the other signatures on the document. Horatio strongly disagreed with the Committee's conclusion that existing abortion laws were adequate and would repeatedly protest their action in his absence and without his knowledge. A year later, Horatio would remark in the American Medical Association Report on Criminal Abortion, "Mere resolutions [condemning the crime] and nothing more, are therefore useless, evasive, cruel."[33] However, the three Resolutions of the Massachusetts Medical Society certainly showed that there was no acceptance or tolerance of unnecessary induced abortion by these physicians, despite their unwillingness to petition the Legislature.

Storer returned sometime before July 22, 1858.[34] He apparently was no longer concerned about his health. In October, he submitted an article on uterine tents that was published a few months later.[35] Uterine tents were small pieces of sponge or other material that expanded when they became moist and which were used to dilate the cervix to allow diagnosis and treatment of uterine disease. Horatio provided a strong caution against their use if there were any chance of pregnancy.

> It might seem superfluous to add a caution, lest by tents abortion be accidentally and unintentionally induced. Two cases in the practice of friends, however, have satisfied me that the risks are much greater than they might seem. Upon this point I shall speak more fully in another connection,* and here merely state, as the safer rule, that ... tents should not be used, or the uterus otherwise disturbed, where the woman is at all liable to pregnancy by marriage or other chance, till the short time sufficient to establish the diagnosis has been allowed to elapse.[36]

Despite this sounding a little like the advertisements warning pregnant women not to take the pill being sold, this was not intended to show practitioners a new way to produce abortion. However, it probably actually did have this effect. The footnote indicated Horatio had made up his mind to write extensively on criminal abortion for the *North-American Medico-Chirurgical Review.*

CHAPTER 7

STORER'S ARTICLES AND THE AMA REPORT

Of the 1858 activities of Horatio Storer of which we are aware, the presentation of his first paper to the prestigious American Academy of Arts and Sciences on December 14, 1858 must be considered the highlight.[1] Horatio had only recently been elected to the Academy and his nominators included Louis Rodolphe Agassiz.[2] His paper was entitled "On the Decrease of the Rate of Increase of Population Now Obtaining in Europe and America" and this reduced rate of increase of the American population was a puzzle in 1858. "I was led to the true answer to the question," he wrote in 1897, "not as a medical jurist, philanthropist, or social reformer, but solely as a gynecologist."[3] He noted that he was "struck by the prevalence of certain forms of pelvic disease after abortion, and by the frequency with which patients in easy circumstances acknowledged to me in such cases that there had been an enforced shortening of pregnancy." He asked his colleagues to make similar inquiries of their patients and "soon a body of evidence that justified me in suggesting that criminal abortion, and this alone, afforded the missing link." Horatio then described the "perfect whirlwind of surprise and indignation in Boston" created by his presentation.

> I was told that to expose them publicly would but increase the evil; was upbraided and condemned for exhibiting, even in the privacy of a scientific society, this blot on the good name of New England, and was begged to postpone publication outside of the medical profession until I had obtained from it a more general corroboration of the position that I had assumed. In deference to the judgment of so many of my seniors and friends, I delayed the publication of the Academy paper, and it did not appear till nearly ten years after, in Silliman's New Haven Journal, *The American Journal of Science and Arts*, for March, 1867.[4]

Horatio first documented the large drop in births in America from earlier years. He also noted the higher birthrate of recent largely Catholic immigrants compared to the "native" Protestant population. He noted that the reduction of the increase in the population could not be explained by contraception. "We are to consider these pregnancies, not as prevented," he continued, "but as terminated without the birth of a living child."[5]

Horatio provided a wide range of statistics supporting his claim that many pregnancies were being ended on purpose. One class showed the sharp rise in stillbirths relative to living births. However, a more telling statistic was the large rise in the ratio of premature stillbirths to stillbirths at term. In Massachusetts there were two premature stillbirths per stillbirth at term for the period 1850-1855. This compared to one premature stillbirth per five stillbirths at term for 1848-1855 in New York City and this compared to only one in ten in 1838-1847 for that city. The implication was that the rate of criminal abortion in Massachusetts was much higher than in New York City.[6]

Horatio concluded:

> The immense proportion of living births to the pregnancies in the foreign as compared with the native and protestant population of Massachusetts, already referred to, is to be explained by the watchful protection exercised by the Catholic church over foetal life. However we may regard the dogma on which this rests, the sanctity of infant baptism, there can be no question that it has saved to the world millions of human lives. But of the various corroborative testimony to which I have alluded, and of other matters I shall elsewhere speak.
>
> Were mankind, in following the advice that has been quoted from past and present authorities in political economy, content merely to practice greater abstinence and greater prudence in sexual matters, less blame could justly be laid. But when we find infanticide and criminal abortion thus justified, rendered common and almost legitimated, we may well oppose to the doctrine of these cruel teachers the words of the indeed admirable Percival, "To extinguish the first spark of life is a crime of the same nature, both against our Maker and society, as to destroy an infant, a child, or a man."[7]

Horatio's "I shall elsewhere speak" referred to his agreement with Dr. Samuel D. Gross, the editor of the *North-American Medico-Chirurgical Review*, to publish a series of articles on "obstetric jurisprudence." Gross, the foremost surgeon of his time, provided a preview in his December 1858 number that included:

> Commencing with criminal abortion in our January number, Dr. Horatio R. Storer will present our readers with a series of important papers on obstetric jurisprudence, to which no one in this country has paid so much attention as himself, and which in point of fact has never been, as such, touched upon. ... Dr. Storer has taken a very decided and praiseworthy position in the matter, and we hope these papers will serve to awaken the attention of and prepare the minds of the profession for the report on criminal abortion in this country, which Dr. Storer is to make to the American Medical Association.[8]

Horatio identified the different topics of his series of papers in the first article. They would "show the real nature and frequency of the crime: its causes; its victims; its perpetrators and its innocent abettors; its means and its proofs; its excuses, the deficiencies and errors of existing laws, and the various other obstacles to conviction; and, above all, so far as the present series of papers is concerned, the duty of the profession toward its general suppression."[9] For the most part, Horatio's nine articles corresponded to this list of topics.

The first article began:

By the Common Law and by many of our State Codes, foetal life, per se, is almost wholly ignored and its destruction unpunished; abortion in every case being considered an offence mainly against the mother, and as such, unless fatal to her, a mere misdemeanor, or wholly disregarded.

By the Moral Law, THE WILFUL KILLING OF A HUMAN BEING AT ANY STAGE OF ITS EXISTENCE IS MURDER.[10]

Horatio then provided three premises:

First.—That if abortion be ever a crime, it is, of necessity, even in isolated cases, one of no small interest to moralist, jurist, and physician; and that when general and common, this interest is extended to the whole community and fearfully enhanced.

Secondly.—That if the latter assumption be true, both in premise and conclusion, neglected as the crime has been by most ethical writers and political economists, hastily passed over by medical jurists, ... either it cannot in the nature of things be suppressed, as by these facts implied, or its suppression has not been properly attempted. Discarding the former of these alternatives as alike unworthy of belief and proved false by facts hereafter to be shown, it will appear,

Thirdly.—That the discussion now broached is neither supererogatory nor out of place; further, that it is absolutely and necessarily demanded.[11]

A footnote following "jurists" read:

So far as the writer is aware, there exists, in this or any other language, no paper upon the subject at all commensurate with its importance. The chapters devoted to it in medical text-books, though some of them admirable so far as they go, especially that of Beck, are defective and often erroneous; while but little information of any value can be found elsewhere. In the French periodicals have appeared articles on special points hereafter referred to; in Great Britain able arguments regarding the commencement of foetal life have been made by Radford, (1848;) and in this country, with remarks on the frequency of the crime, by Hodge, of Philadelphia, (1839 and 1854,) and by the present Professor of Obstetrics in Harvard University, (1855.) To the latter, his father, and to the journalists (Drs. Morland and Minot of Boston,) by whom the effort then made was so warmly and eloquently seconded, the writer acknowledges his indebtedness for the thought of the present undertaking.

No mention of Leonard's 1851 "Quackery and Abortion" that provided a virtual blueprint for "the present undertaking."

Horatio then discussed a number of real and apparent objections to discussion of abortion. First was the "natural dislike of any physician to enter upon a subject on some points of which it is probable that a portion of the profession is at variance with him." It should be noted, however, that Horatio did not give as a reason for opinions "at variance with him" *actual support of abortion* by these physicians, only their "disbelief in the alleged increase in abortion" or their preference for "reliance on Providence of itself to abate the evil." Other possible objections to discussion of criminal abortion included the physician's "reluctance" to tell his patients the "most unwelcome truth" about abortion, "thus not merely condemning, but to their own consciences at least, criminating them;" his risk of losing practice because thought more scrupulous than other physicians; his reluctance to come into "contact with the law, even though for ends of justice," and, finally, his "grave doubts lest the statements made, though simple and true, should yet appear so astounding as to shock belief, or so degrading as to tend to lessen all faith in natural affection and general morality."[12]

However, "more than counterbalancing them all" were these arguments *for* speaking out against abortion:

That medical men are the physical guardians of women and their off-spring; from their position and peculiar knowledge necessitated in all obstetric matters to regulate public sentiment and to govern the tribunals of justice.

That the discussion by them of this crime may very probably be the means, in great measure, of ultimately restraining or suppressing its perpetration.

That such will undoubtedly tend to save much health to the community and many human lives.

And, that, were there no other reason, it is clearly a duty.[13]

Horatio went on to show how the Common Law and many American statutes failed to recognize abortion as an offence against the fetus. Following this, he pointed out that the very frequency of induced abortion and the high "character and standing" of many of the mothers upon whom abortion was induced were evidence "that the public do not know, or knowing deny, the criminal character of the action performed." He continued:

It having now been shown, directly and by temporary assumption, that the law and public sentiment, both by its theory and its practice, alike deny to unjustifiable abortion the imputation of crime, it remains for us to discuss this question abstractly, and to prove not merely that they are wrong, but that the offence is one of the deepest guilt, a crime SECOND TO NONE.[14]

Horatio's key to proving "that the offence is one of the deepest guilt," was to show that the "foetus" was both separate from the mother and alive from conception. Common sense was the first means used. He wrote, "the mother and the child within her, in abstract existence, must be entirely identical from conception to birth, or entirely distinct." Common sense also required that the "foetus, previous to quickening, as after it, must exist in one of two states, either death or life." Since the state of death was never followed by a return to the state of life, "and we can conceive no other state of the foetus save one, that, namely life, must exist from the beginning."[15] This approach probably was copied from John Brodhead Beck.

Although "quickening" was thus demolished as the commencement of human life, it served a key role in many state laws as a marker of when abortion became a crime or a more serious crime and Horatio singled it out for special discussion. To show that movement of the fetus occurred much earlier than when this movement was felt, he cited the sounds that these movements produced and the visible movements of fetuses born premature to quickening. "Quickening," Horatio concluded, "is therefore as unlikely a period for the commencement of foetal life as those others set by Hippocrates and his successors, varying from the third day after conception, to that of the Stoics, namely birth, and as false as them all."[16]

The following were the concluding paragraphs of his first installment:

> If we have proved the existence of foetal life before quickening has taken place or can take place, and by all analogy, and a close and conclusive process of induction, its commencement at the very beginning, at conception itself, we are compelled to believe unjustifiable abortion always a crime.
>
> And now words fail. Of the mother, by consent or by her own hand, imbrued with her infant's blood; of the equally guilty father, who counsels or allows the crime; of the wretches who by their wholesale murders far out-Herod Burke and Hare; of the public sentiment which palliates, pardons, and would even praise this so common violation of all law, human and divine, of all instinct, of all reason, all pity, all mercy, all love,—we leave those to speak who can.[17]

As we earlier noted, the second paragraph would be used repeatedly in Horatio's writing and quoted by other opponents of abortion.

We mentioned that Horatio was upset that Jacob Bigelow had provided the Report of the Massachusetts Medical Society Committee on Criminal Abortion to the Councillors of that Society while Horatio was away and without Horatio's input or signature. Horatio wrote a letter in complaint a week before the February 1859 annual meeting of the Society's Councillors. He requested "that the whole matter may be either resubmitted to the same Committee, with instructions to again report at an adjourned meeting of your body before the next Annual meeting of the Society, or that the Councillors will themselves hear the remonstrant or permit him to submit a minority report."[18]

The Councillors' response was reported in the Minutes of their February 2, 1859 meeting:

The Corresponding Secretary read a communication from Dr. H.R. Storer requesting a reconsideration of the vote, by which the Council at the stated meeting in February 1858 accepted the Report of the Committee appointed at the Annual Meeting of the Society in 1857 to consider the Resolution offered by Dr. Storer and the whole subject of the increased frequency of the procuring criminal abortion, and permit him to submit a minority report.

Dr [M.S.] Perry moved that the prayer of the petitioner be granted. Considerable discussion ensued upon the introduction of this motion, when upon motion of Dr. J.C. Dalton of Lowell, the consideration of the subject was indefinitely postponed.[19]

Horatio would not let the Councillors forget their indefinite postponement.

In March 1859, a long article, "Effects of Criminal Abortion," by Walter Channing was published in the *Boston Medical and Surgical Journal*.[20] Channing, the former Professor of Obstetrics at the Harvard Medical School,[21] was not at his literary or scientific best. He rambled, first and last discussing nitrate of silver as a successful remedy for vomiting in pregnancy and, in between, describing several cases of induced abortion that required medical treatment. All but one were married woman. One woman attempted to abort herself, left a wire permanently embedded at some internal location, survived this without problem, and, as it turned out, was not pregnant after all. Channing was unwilling to describe other instruments that his patients had used, but mentioned the wire "as it was believed, it would not be likely to be imitated."[22] Leonard had specified the implements used by abortionists and by women themselves in his "Quackery and Abortion" and perhaps this had led to "imitation" and criticism of the *Boston Medical and Surgical Journal* for allowing such explicitness. If so, this may have provided Horatio with a reason, or excuse, to avoid mentioning Leonard or "Quackery and Abortion" when he gave credit to other pioneer antiabortion physicians.

Channing listed a dozen uterine diseases that had followed induced abortion and indicated that sterility had followed on one occasion. He provided no advice in the article on how "this infamous crime" could be reduced and claimed attempts to prosecute the crime were futile. "Men and women are arrested and tried," he wrote, "but you can get no convictions." Channing had been told that one abortionist "in a certain place" "actually carries these abortions about in his pocket, and showed one or more" to Channing's confidante.[23] This gruesome hearsay no doubt was included to show the indifference of abortionists to the laws against abortion.

The second article of Horatio's series in the *North-American Medico-Chirurgical Review*, "Its Frequency, and the Causes Thereof," also appeared in March.[24] As Horatio noted, many of his statistics were taken from his December 1858 "decrease of the rate of increase" paper and this was also true for much of the supporting text. He indicated that although requests to regular physicians for abortion were not that frequent, the same was not true for the "quacks," and their willingness to comply led to much work by regular physicians "to treat its acute and immediate effects." Horatio's own medical practice had disclosed the frequent incidence of uterine disease when there was a history of induced abortion and he "was able, in consultation, to point out similar cases in the practice of gentlemen who, at that time, had denied the legitimacy of his conclusions."[25]

Horatio indicated that maternal deaths from criminal abortion were not infrequent, although "in but few of the fatal cases really occurring, is foul play ever thought of."[26] Only a fraction of the attempts at abortion caused the woman's death and their not infrequent occurrence was cited as evidence of a very large number of such attempts. Horatio noted that criminal abortion not only was "of alarming frequency," "but that its frequency is rapidly increasing." He concluded the section: "Every effort that might possibly check this flood of guilt will, if delayed, have so much the more to accomplish."[27]

The first of the "causes" which Horatio addressed was the "low *morale* of the community as regards the guilt of the crime." In addition to the primary factor of ignorance about the actual existence of "foetal life" early in pregnancy, Horatio described other erroneous physiological beliefs that contributed. One was the notion that it was detrimental to a woman's health to bear a large number of children and the other was that "the fewer one's children, the more healthy they are likely to be and the more worth to society."[28]

Horatio then took Thomas Robert Malthus, John Stewart Mill, and other political economists to task for the key role that they inadvertently played in fostering criminal abortion. They were among the strongest proponents of the benefits to the state and the individual of a reduced population and these political economists probably had been mentioned when his patients admitted to a history of induced abortion.[29]

Horatio next discussed "fear of child-bed" as a cause of abortion. This captured not only Horatio's commitment against abortion, but also his strong commitment to use of anesthetics during labor.[30] "Fear of child-bed, in patients pregnant for the first time, or who had suffered or risked much in previous labors," Horatio wrote, "might formerly have been allowed some weight in excuse, but none at all in these days of anaesthesia."[31]

In the final paragraph of his March installment, Horatio returned to the "cause" of public ignorance of the status and life of the fetus. "[Where] ignorance is so evidently and so extensively its foundation," he wrote, "those who, possessing, yet withhold the knowledge which by any chance or in any way would tend to prevent it, themselves become, directly, and in a moral sense, responsibly accountable for the crime."[32]

A month later, David Meredith Reese provided an editorial, "Dr. Horatio R. Storer, of Boston," in his *American Medical Gazette* that included:

> Dr. Storer deserves the thanks of the profession, and the public gratitude for the thorough exposure he has made, and continues to make, of this giant iniquity, as it exists in our country, as well as in foreign lands; the statistics of criminal abortionism, the world over, having been cited by him in these valuable contributions to Medical Jurisprudence. We honor him for the manly and fearless independence he manifests, in denouncing as murderous, and worthy of the highest penalty known to our laws, every principal or accessory to criminal abortion. The demonstra-

tion he makes of the frequency of this crime, and this among every class of our population—by facts and figures, as shown in our bills of mortality—exhibits proof that the "slaughter of the innocents" in our own country exceeds, in cruelty and extent, any records of this crime in ancient or modern history. When will legislation and reform arrest this terrible iniquity?[33]

Horatio planned to read the Report of the American Medical Association Committee on Criminal Abortion at the Annual Meeting of the Association in Louisville. It is not clear when he actually drafted the Report, but it may have been ready by March 11, 1859 when Horatio sent letters to a number of prominent physicians around the country. One was to a District of Columbia physician, Alexander J. Semmes, whose response included:

Your letter of the 11th instant has been duly received, and I take my earliest occasion to make reply. I fully agree with you in your sense of the importance of bringing the subject of Criminal Abortion before the profession, and the proper authorities of society generally, in such imposing form as to lead to such measures as may effectually check the farther growth of so great an evil, and if possible put such an extinguisher upon it as to prevent its becoming a characteristic feature in American "civilization." ... [I]t will afford me great pleasure to do all in my power to assist you in your investigations.[34]

Another letter from a future Committee member repeated some of the words of Horatio's request:

> St. Louis, March 18th '59
>
> Horatio R. Storer, M.D.
> Boston.
> Dear Dr.
> Your kind letter asking me to join in rendering your report on Criminal Abortion to the Am. Med. Association was received on yesterday. I will do so most cheerfully, and hope that your efforts "at the revision and more consistent wording of our laws upon the subject, and to abate the prevailing ignorance of the true character of the crime" may meet with abundant success.
> I shall endeavor to meet you if possible in Louisville in May next.
> With sincere regards to your Father and Mother and the rest of your family I remain
>
> Yours very truly
> Charles A. Pope[35]

Only ten days after mailing his letter indicating his willingness "to assist," Alexander Semmes mailed another letter that shows that Horatio had provided Semmes a draft of the Report on Criminal Abortion. Semmes wrote:

> The Report seems to me to say all that is needful for the occasion, while it, at the same time, avoids any degree of that prolixity which might obstruct its favorable consideration.
>
> The Report is clear, pointed and condensed, that nothing from me can improve or amend it.
>
> It will give me the greatest pleasure to sign my name to the Report, which you can do for me.[36]

Hugh Lenox Hodge's letter agreeing to sign Horatio's Report also suggested a key tactic of the physicians' crusade. It included: "I return your Report and shall be gratified to have my name attached to it, trusting that your praiseworthy efforts will meet with their due rewards. Perhaps the probability of success might be increased, if the general association would strongly recommend that each state med. association would press the subject on the legislative bodies of their respective states."[37] Other letters allowing their signatures to be added to the report were received from Drs. A. Lopez of Mobile,[38] Henry Brisbane of Wisconsin,[39] Thomas Blatchford of New York,[40] and Edward H. Barton of South Carolina.[41] Thus the American Medical Association Committee on Criminal Abortion, formed at Nashville in May 1857, was rounded out less than a month before its Report was presented at Louisville on May 3, 1859.[42]

Horatio's respondents' strong approval of his draft report probably indicates minor changes at most were required for the version read in Louisville. It began: "The heinous guilt of criminal abortion, however viewed by the community, is everywhere acknowledged by medical men. Its frequency—among all classes of society, rich and poor, single and married—most physicians have been led to suspect; very many, from their own experience of its deplorable results, have known."[43] Additional evidence of abortion's frequency were "comparisons of the present with our past rates of increase in population, the size of our families, the statistics of our foetal deaths, by themselves considered, and relatively to the births and to the general mortality."

Horatio then moved to the reasons for the large number of abortions. These included the "wide-spread popular ignorance of the true character of the crime," the innocent abetment of abortion by physicians who "are frequently supposed careless of foetal life," and "the grave defects of our laws, both common and statute, as regards the independent and actual existence of the child before birth, as a living being." As "[a]bundant proof upon each of these points," Horatio called attention to his articles in the *North-American Medico-Chirurgical Review.*

The Report then moved to the duties of physicians toward reduction of criminal abortion. "The case is here of life or death—" he continued, "the life or death of thousands—and it depends, almost wholly, upon ourselves." He called on physicians to enlighten the public about fetal development, to avoid any appearance of negligence "of the sanctity of foetal life," and to establish an "obstetric code; which ... would tend to prevent such unnecessary and unjustifiable destruction of human life."

He then turned to the deficient laws on abortion and called on physicians "as citizens" to improve them. "If the evidence upon this point is especially of a medical character," he continued, "it is our duty to proffer our aid, and in so important a matter to urge it." When the faulty laws reflected "doctrinal errors of the profession in a former age," he called on physicians "by every bond we hold sacred, by our reverence for the fathers in medicine, by our love for our race, and by our responsibility as accountable beings, to see these errors removed and their grievous results abated." The Report concluded:

> In accordance, therefore, with the facts in the case, the Committee would advise that this body, representing, as it does, the physicians of the land, publicly express its abhorrence of the unnatural and now rapidly increasing crime of abortion; that it avow its true nature, as no simple offence against public morality and decency, no mere misdemeanor, no attempt upon the life of the mother, but the wanton and murderous destruction of her child; and that while it would in no wise transcend its legitimate province or invade the precincts of the law, the Association recommend, by memorial, to the governors and legislatures of the several States, and, as representing the federal district, to the President and Congress, a careful examination and revision of the statutory and of so much of the common law, as relates to this crime. For we hold it to be "a thing deserving all hate and detestation, that a man in his very originall, whiles he is framed, whiles he is enlived, should be put to death under the very hands, and in the shop, of Nature."[44]

Following the signatures of the eight members, three Resolutions were offered for consideration by the Association.[45] These were repeated in the Minutes of the American Medical Association meeting for the first day, May 3, that included:

> The Committee, appointed in May, 1857, on Criminal Abortion, submitted a report written by Dr. Storer, of Boston, which was read by Dr. Blatchford, of New York, and referred to the Committee on [sic] Publication. The following resolutions appended to this report were unanimously adopted:—
> "*Resolved*, That while physicians have long been united in condemning the act of producing abortion, at every period of gestation, except as necessary for preserving the life of either mother or child, it has become the duty of this Association, in view of the prevalence and increasing frequency of the crime, publicly to enter an earnest and solemn protest against such unwarrantable destruction of human life.
> "*Resolved*, That in pursuance of the grand and noble calling we profess, the saving of human lives, and of the sacred responsibilities thereby devolving upon us, the Association present this subject to the

attention of the several legislative assemblies of the Union, with the prayer that the laws by which the crime of procuring abortion is attempted to be controlled may be revised, and that such other action may be taken in the premises as they in their wisdom may deem necessary.

"*Resolved*, That the Association request the zealous co-operation of the various State Medical Societies in pressing this subject upon the legislatures of their respective States, and that the President and Secretaries of the Association are hereby authorized to carry out, by memorial, these resolutions."[46]

Horatio was too ill to travel to Louisville to present his Report and this must have been a huge disappointment to him. We are aware of Horatio's illness because of the following letter:

Louisville 3 May 59

Dear Dr

I have ordered the paper sent to you daily during our associate existence. You will see that your report was read and the resolutions unanimously adopted. Your report was highly spoken of, not a dissenting voice in any direction. I am sorry my dear Dr to hear from Dr Townsend the cause of your not being with us. I do hope my dear yoke fellow (though I am not the oldest ox) that your illness will be of short duration, and that a little relaxation will restore you to your wanted measure of health and professional ability.

Dr Reese of the N Y Gazette took a deep interest in the subject and so do many others.

Yours truly
Thos W Blatchford[47]

Blatchford's failure to mention the name of Horatio's illness may indicate something not readily discussed. A decade later, Horatio wrote an article on surgical treatment of hemorrhoids and referred to his own frequent bouts with the problem.[48] What is more, Blatchford's prescription of "relaxation" is not an unusual one for this condition. It is easy to imagine Horatio was "sitting on pins and needles" in Boston while his Report was being read at Louisville.

Another letter from Blatchford two days later included the following: "I cannot tell you the number of Gentlemen who have spoken to me about your Report since I read it nor can I begin to tell you the high encomiums, bestowed upon it without a single drawback. I thought you would like to know it. To know that our labors are appreciated by our brethren when those labors have been bestowed in the cause of humanity is a precious cordial for one's soul in this old and thankless world."[49]

David Francis Condie also praised Horatio's Report on Criminal Abortion. This was part of Condie's review of the published *Transactions of the American Medical Association* for 1859 and Storer's Report was one of the few things in the *Transactions* that Condie praised. He wrote:

> The report denounces, in the most explicit terms, the procurement of abortion, as no trifling offence against public morality and decency—no mere misdemeanor—no unjustifiable risking of the life of a pregnant female for the attainment of some paramount good—but a crime of the most heinous character on the part of all concerned in it; being no less than a wanton and murderous destruction of a living human being; a deliberate taking away of life, justifiable in no instance by any defensible motive, nor counterbalanced by any possible benefit that can result from it under any supposable contingency; but, in all cases, a crime of the first magnitude, deserving of unmitigated detestation.[50]

Condie continued by describing the sharp increase of criminal abortion and he noted that "even the mothers of families" resorted to abortion "to relieve them from the suffering and confinement incident to childbirth, and from the care, the responsibility, and the expense that would be entailed upon them by a family of children." He discussed the three causes that Storer had enumerated: ignorance of the true character of the crime, the widespread public belief that the profession itself is "careless of foetal life," and the defects of abortion statutes. Condie then quoted three paragraphs of the Report giving Storer's recommendations for the profession's duties to overcome these three causes. He concluded his review with the three resolutions unanimously adopted by the Association.[51]

Storer's series of papers in the *North-American Medico-Chirurgical Review* continued with three in the May issue, the first being, "Its Victims."[52] Horatio provided French data showing that the ages of aborted fetuses were concentrated between the third and sixth months. He indicated that the women obtaining abortions covered all child-bearing years and that only a minority were unmarried women concealing their pregnancies. What is more, they were not largely uneducated and poor women as was commonly believed. He continued:

> we are compelled to admit that Christianity itself, or at least Protestant-ism, has failed to check the increase of criminal abortion. It is not astonishing to find that the crime was known in ancient times, as shown by evidence previously given, nor that it exists at the present day among savage tribes, excused by ignorance and superstition; but that Christian communities should especially be found to tolerate and to practice it, does almost exceed belief.[53]

Horatio pointed out that Catholics outside of France rarely sought or obtained abortions. Horatio also discussed how Catholic guarding and supervision of foetal life, while reducing abortions, had also led to the death of women during childbirth, when craniotomy was delayed to insure that the foetus was dead. Horatio then showed how to prevent this unnecessary death of the mother through "intra-uterine baptism" which was a part of Catholic doctrine and reduced in the eyes of the Church the tragedy of death of the child. Horatio chided physicians who "from fear of ridicule or dislike to sanction what they do not believe in, would shrink from such a duty." "I am not ashamed to acknowledge," he continued, "that for myself, though no Catholic, I have performed this intra-uterine baptism, where delivery without mutilation was impossible. ... [I]t was ... simply my duty."[54]

Horatio indicated that women who immediately survived attempts at criminal abortion often succumbed within the next week or two from delayed hemorrhage or peritonitis. Horatio then provided a "long and fearful list" of problems, including pelvic cellulitis, various fistulae, adhesions of the os or vagina, inflammatory or malignant diseases of the uterus and ovary, "each, too frequently incurable" which were the direct consequence of "intentional and unjustifiable abortion." The article concluded:

> We have seen that in some instances the thought of the crime, coming upon the mind at a time when the physical system is weak and prostrated, is sufficient to occasion death. The same tremendous idea, so laden with the consciousness of guilt against God, humanity, and even mere natural instinct, is undoubtedly able, where not affecting life, to produce insanity. This it may do either by its first and sudden occurrence to the mind; or, subsequently, by those long and unavailing regrets, that remorse, if conscience exist, is sure to bring.[55]

In his fourth article, "Its Proofs,"[56] Horatio pointed out that an absence of local wounds and mutilations in the patient did not preclude an intentional abortion, and, referring to a case he had reported to the Society for Medical Observation in February, neither did their presence imply that violence had occurred.[57] He then described the following indicators of probable criminal intent:

> If violent purging or vomiting have been resorted to without any apparent reason, or to a greater extent than ordinarily prescribed or required; or if leeches have been applied to the thighs, to the number of an hundred or more ... there is certainly ground for suspicion.[58]

> If the cervix, the portion of the uterus most frequently wounded, is found punctured or lacerated, while the ovum is still retained, there is reason for suspicion; if the membranes are torn and extensively detached, while the cervix is but little dilated, such is increased; and it is made almost a certainty, if with the latter condition, nothing remain of the ovum in the uterine cavity but lacerated fragments. Here the abortion would probably not merely have been intentionally induced, but by the direct introduction and agency of instruments.[59]

On excuses for induced abortion, Horatio claimed:

the plea of Drs. Gordon Smith, Good, Paris, and Copeland, that as a foetus born before the seventh month has a slender chance of surviving, its murder should be viewed with leniency, [cannot] be allowed. Such arguments, that the perils and dangers to which the foetus is naturally subjected should lessen the criminality of attempts at its destruction, are without foundation, and when advanced by physicians are utterly unworthy the profession.[60]

Horatio cited Michael Ryan's 1836 edition of *A Manual of Medical Jurisprudence and State Medicine* following mention of these four British physicians. As noted earlier, Horatio's father had quoted from and cited Ryan's *Manual* in his May 1851 "Medical Jurisprudence." Horatio almost certainly helped prepare his father's paper and may have resolved at (or by) that earlier period to crusade against unnecessary abortion.

In his fifth article, "Its Perpetrators," Horatio noted that in France "where the abortion is not induced by the mother itself, the offenders are women."[61] "With us," Horatio indicated, "the same statement is, without doubt, equally true." After noting that the mother was out of the reach of most state laws against abortion, Horatio wrote:

If the mother does not herself induce the abortion, she seeks it, or aids it, or consents to it, and is, therefore, whether ever seeming justified or not, fully accountable as a principal. We have already seen the position these mothers hold in the community, high as well as low, rich as well as poor, intelligent and educated as well as ignorant, professedly religious as well as of easy belief, not single alone, but married.[62]

Harsh as Horatio was on women seeking abortion, he was harsher on their accomplices. Among these he included "friends and acquaintances; nurses; and midwives and female physicians." Among the men, "husbands; quacks and professed abortionists, druggists; and worst of all, though fortunately extremely rare, physicians of regular standing." Horatio was to take each "class" in turn starting with the female friends and acquaintances:

It has been said that misery loves companionship: this is nowhere more manifest than in the histories of criminal abortion. In more than one instance, from my own experience, has a lady of acknowledged respectability, who had herself suffered abortion, induced it upon several of her friends, thus perhaps endeavoring to persuade an uneasy conscience, that, by making an act common, it becomes right. Such ladies boast to each other of the impunity with which they have aborted, as they do of their expenditures, of their dress, of their success in society. There is a fashion in this, as in all other female customs, good and bad. The wretch whose account with the Almighty is heaviest with guilt, too often becomes a heroine.[63]

Horatio indicated that nurses were apt to be approached by women to perform or assist in an abortion and were "not always found proof against an offered fee. He claimed midwives and female physicians were even more likely than nurses to be sought out by women seeking abortion and some also would be more than tempted by an offered fee:

> By these remarks we would not be supposed endeavoring to excite prejudice against female physicians and midwives, as such, or advocating their suppression. We are now merely considering this crime of abortion, in relation to which they are peculiarly and unfortunately situated. At present everything favors their committing the crime; their relations to women at large, their immunities in practice, the profit of this trade, the difficulty, especially from the fact that they are women, of insuring their conviction.[64]

Horatio had less to say about male accomplices. Husbands he saw as aware of their wives' abortion, but rarely performing it and probably rarely compelling it, although he would claim otherwise a few years later in his *Is It I? A Book for Every Man* (See Chapter 14). "Professed abortionists" were men who prepared and distributed drugs, "against the use of which, 'at certain times,' the public are 'earnestly cautioned.'" Horatio then criticized the newspapers, including religious newspapers, who carried the advertisements for these nostrums and, as a result, were "so constantly and so dangerously an accessory to the crime." He presented the Massachusetts statute prohibiting such advertisements and noted it was not enforced. "The press, if it choose, may almost annihilate the crime;" Horatio continued, "it now openly encourages it."[65]

Horatio's final discussion was of regular physicians and abortion:

> It has been often alleged, and oftener supposed that *physicians in good standing* not unfrequently, and without lawful justification, induce criminal abortion. This statement, whatever exceptional cases may exist, is wickedly false. The pledge against abortion, to the observance of which Hippocrates compelled his followers by oath, has ever been considered binding, even more strongly of late centuries. The crime is recognized as such in almost every code of medical ethics; its known commission has always been followed by ignominious expulsion from medical fellowships and fraternity. If this direct penalty be at any time escaped, it is only through lack of decisive proof, bare suspicion even of the crime insuring an actual sundering of all existing professional friendships and ties; a loss that subsequent proof of innocence could hardly restore. Such is the unanimous feeling of the profession; to its credit be it said, that, with but a single exception,* and this to his eternal disgrace, its writers are all agreed, abstractly considering the subject, on the sanctity of foetal life.[66]

Horatio's footnote read: "*Jörg, of Leipsic, who speaks of the human foetus as 'only a higher species of intestinal worm, not endowed with a human soul, not entitled to human attributes.'" This was Johann Christian Gottfried Jörg (1779-1856) a prolific author of medical books and articles. It is somewhat surprising that Alfred Velpeau did not come in for similar criticism.

Horatio's next article in the series was "Its Innocent Abettors."[67] Horatio first discussed how some physicians resorted to premature labor for reasons other than to save the life of the mother or of her child. Craniotomy also was employed far too often, according to Horatio, and he discussed whether the fetus justified Caesarean section in cases where pelvic irregularities prevented birth of a living child. A Caesarean section was more frequently fatal to the mother than not, although some operators were highly successful in saving both mother and child. Horatio indicated that at least one authority claimed the operation should be forced on the woman who repeatedly became pregnant, even though fully aware of her inability to normally bear a live child. "The question now so plainly put," Horatio wrote, "is one for the profession soberly to discuss and to answer."[68]

Referring to Henry Ingersoll Bowditch only as "one of the most eminent practitioners of the Eastern States" and "my friend," Horatio quoted a paragraph from Bowditch's letter of April 20, 1857 asking whether a physician might not "use common means for amenorrhoea if the menses have been absent six weeks" when a mother's "health, and possibly life," might be endangered by another pregnancy. "Covering, as these questions do, much of the ground already gone over," Horatio began, "we may answer them at once, and decidedly in the negative."[69]

Other rules for physicians were to immediately perform Caesarean section to extract every foetus old enough to survive in cases of maternal death; to make every effort to prevent threatening miscarriages and to resuscitate still-born children; to avoid "operations of any kind on pregnant women, even tooth-drawing, that might be delayed;" and to avoid "the careless or unnecessary use of ergot" which Horatio believed could produce premature labor. To do otherwise in these situations would not show the highest valuation of the unborn and newly born and people might conclude that abortion was no crime.[70]

"We proceed to the other relations of criminal abortion," Storer continued, "more especially to those immediately pertaining to the claims and course of justice." This led to Horatio's next installment, entitled "Its Obstacles to Conviction."[71] Horatio described how Massachusetts' statutes against abortion were among the most "wisely and completely drawn." However, not one of the 32 trials for abortion since they were enacted had led to a conviction. Horatio also mentioned the failure of the Massachusetts Medical Society Committee Report to recommend changes in these laws to the legislature and reiterated his January 1859 "earnest protest against the plainly erroneous opinion avowed in that report." He contradicted their stated belief that the crime could never be controlled by law, claiming that legislation failures were caused by the ignorance of legislators, judges, attorneys, and jurors about the criminality of criminal abortion. What is more, the "only source possible for enlightenment" was the medical men from whom they "have hitherto found but few bold and honest statements, and these unindorsed by the mass of the profession."[72] As discussed earlier, Horatio singled out Drs. Tatum and Joynes of Virginia, and Dr. Brisbane of Wisconsin as among the few physicians who did boldly and honestly speak out on the subject. He praised these physicians for their input to recent changes in their states' abortion laws. However, he noted that "total silence" from the medical profession was far more likely to have been heard by legislators and officers of justice. Horatio indicated that this "first and great cause," the silence of physicians, "is by no means an essential one."[73]

Horatio discussed the various laws against abortion, presenting the statutes "at length" for the states and territories that had them. He noted their problems starting with "the absurd distinction between the foetus of an early and a later age" that he indicated was the largest of the obstacles to conviction. He also noted that in almost all these statutes "the offence is considered a trifling one, except as affecting the person or life of the mother." Horatio indicated that some statutes encouraged the crime, since a crime existed only if the mother were injured. "We have seen," Horatio noted, "that the surest and most efficient means of producing abortion are those where no injury whatever is inflicted upon the mother."[74] Horatio noted that only three states would punish the women, regardless of her involvement in the decision or act. Two states referred to the abortionist as "he," perhaps preventing any prosecution of female abortionists. Horatio then described the common law's schizophrenic treatment of the fetus, noting "that while it recognizes the distinct existence of the foetus for civil purposes, it here considers its being as totally engrossed in that of the mother."[75]

Horatio concluded with the following quote from Charles Albert Lee who annotated the American Edition of *Guy's Principles of Forensic Medicine*:

> "It is to be hoped," has forcibly been written, "that the period is not far remote, when laws so cruel in their effects, so inconsistent with the progress of knowledge and civilization, and so revolting to the feelings and claims of humanity, will be swept from our statutes."[76]

Lee wrote this as an addendum to Guy's discussion and criticism of the "absurd distinction" that still existed in some American laws between quick and non-quick pregnancies. Horatio probably read the American Edition of Guy's *Principles* during 1850 or 1851 when his father was preparing "Medical Jurisprudence." If so, Lee's call for legislative change may have been another stimulus for Horatio's "thought of the present undertaking."

"Its Obstacles to Conviction" was quickly acclaimed in the *British Medical Journal*. "Dr. Storer;" the editors wrote, "shows plainly that the legislation in America on the subject of criminal abortion is in a most imperfect state."[77]

Horatio's final two articles appeared in November. The first, "Can It be at all Controlled by Law?," began by giving an "unqualified answer in the affirmative."[78] He noted that this was not the case "anywhere," but this was because "laws against abortion do not as yet exist, which are in all respects just, sufficient, and not to be evaded." Horatio then stressed that a law to be just must attempt to prevent a crime as well as to punish it, and this required laws that made detection of abortion likely and punishment of abortion "more certain." Detection would be strongly assisted by improved registration laws that required a physician to certify the cause of death, both in infants and mothers, and by laws against concealment of births and secret burials. Detection of abortion also would be facilitated by requiring that coroners be medical men "skilled in all that pertains to obstetric jurisprudence."[79]

Following this discussion of indirect means for controlling abortion, Horatio returned to the need to improve the abortion laws themselves. They should reflect the fact that the criminal intent is against the child. They should only require proof of the attempt at abortion, not its consummation. There was no need to prove intent to destroy the child or to consider how the abortion was attempted. There should be no exemption of the mother from penalty, given that she is nearly "always 'an assessory before the fact,' or the principal." In addition, he recommended that punishment should be increased, since most was so minimal that it did not deter. Finally, he argued that standards for when abortion *is* justified should be "fixed by law."[80] Horatio closed the chapter with a draft abortion statute that was nearly identical to that in the May 1857 report to the Suffolk District Medical Society.[81]

Horatio's final installment was "The Duty of the Profession," and Horatio wrote:

> We have seen that unjustifiable abortion, alike as concerns the infant and society, is a crime second to none; that it abounds, and is frightfully on the increase; and that on medical grounds alone, mistaken and exploded, a misconception of the time at which man becomes a living being, the law fails to afford to infants and to society that protection which they have an absolute right to receive at its hands, and for the absence of which every individual who has, or can exert, any influence in the matter, is rendered so far responsible.[82]

"Under these circumstances, therefore," Horatio continued, "it becomes the medical profession to look to it, lest the *whole* guilt of this crime rest upon themselves." He was referring to two things. The mistaken notions about "intra-uterine vitality" had come from early medical literature. The second basis for physician guilt was their current "apathy and silence" on the subject, despite the fact that "thousands and hundreds of thousand of lives are thus directly at stake, and are annually sacrificed." The explanations offered for physician "apathy and silence" were "either that we do not yet really believe in the existence of foetal life, though professing to do so, or that we are too timid or slothful to affirm and defend it." "It is my aim," he continued, "while setting forth a deliberate and carefully prepared opinion upon this point, to inspire, if possible, in my fellow-practitioners throughout the land, somewhat of the holy enthusiasm sure in a good cause to succeed despite every obstacle, and an earnest, uncompromising hostility to this result of combined error and injustice, the permitted increase of criminal abortion."

Horatio then took on the critics who argued against such speaking out:

But it is asked, is our silence wrong? Is there not danger otherwise of increasing the crime? These are the questions not of wisdom, or prudence, or philanthropy, but of an arrant pusillanimity. Vice and crime, if kept concealed, but grow apace. They should be stripped of such protection, and their apologists, thereby their accomplices, condemned. Answers, however, are ready at hand to the questions proposed.[83]

He then provided a dozen quotes from various editorials, articles, and books, which echoed his call for the medical profession "to urge upon individuals the truth regarding this crime." He continued:

it is equally their duty to urge it upon the law, by whose doctrines the people are bound; and upon that people, the community, by whose action the laws are made. And this should be done by us, if we would succeed in suppressing the crime, not by separate action alone, but conjointly, as the profession, grandly representing its highest claim,—the saving of human life.[84]

Horatio also provided a brief history of the American Medical Association Committee on Criminal Abortion, the acceptance of its Report by the Association with "high encomiums" and "without a single drawback," and the Association's unanimous adoption of the Resolutions appended to the Report. Horatio gratefully acknowledged this support of the members of the Association in the final paragraph of his nine articles:

In behalf of the committee, of whom he had the honor to be chairman, the writer cannot close this portion of his labors without thanking the physicians of the land, represented as they are by the Association, for their hearty and noble response to the appeal that had been made them. He would express, were it possible, the gratitude not of individuals, but society; for by this act the profession was again true to "its mighty and responsible office of shutting the great gates of human death."[85]

The nine articles of Horatio were published in 1860 as a book entitled *On Criminal Abortion in America*.[86] The book's publication was the occasion for the new editors of the *Boston Medical and Surgical Journal*, Dr. F.E. Oliver and Dr. Calvin Ellis, to write a strong antiabortion editorial.[87] They described the new book as coming "from the pen of one of our most painstaking and careful investigators, Dr. H.R. Storer." "This paper contains much interesting information," they continued, "and if it do as much for poor humanity as might be fairly expected, from the ability and good intentions of the author, he will have much reason for pleasant reflection."[88]

Oliver and Ellis reproduced much of Horatio's data that indicated the large increase of criminal abortion, particularly in Massachusetts. They indicated their "fear" that "little can be accomplished by legislation" to remedy what "is fast becoming, if it has not already become, 'an established custom,' not confined to the unfortunate, but resorted to by the màrried of all ranks and classes of society, for the purpose of ridding themselves of what they have learned to regard as burden too heavy to be borne." The editors offered the following alternatives to legislation:

> The physician may do much by warning his patients against the dangers and guilt of this awful crime, and using the "greater vigilance lest he become its innocent and unintentional abettor"; and the moralist may do more by the inculcation of those principles in the young, that shall lead them to regard with abhorrence such a violation of the positive laws of God, involving, as it does, the guilt of murder, and a total indifference to the most sacred privileges with which woman is endowed.[89]

David Francis Condie also provided a review of Horatio's book.[90] After discussing the original publication of the papers in the *North-American Medico-Chirurgical Review* and the evidence these papers provided for the conclusions of the 1859 American Medical Association Report on Criminal Abortion, Condie wrote:

> The investigation into which Dr. Storer ... has entered, is full, able, and satisfactory, and well worthy the serious consideration not only of every member of the medical profession who has a just appreciation of the important mission he has undertaken, but of every legislator, every expounder and administrator of the laws—of every individual member of the community, in fine, who, while he defends his own individual rights, would extend an equal defense to the rights of others, even the humblest and most insignificant of the human family, from the moment of conception until the period when they are called, by that fiat within whose scope we all are included, to leave this for another state of existence.
>
> Dr. Storer has established most conclusively, and upon data the validity and sufficiency of which will scarcely be denied, the extreme criminality of abortion in every case in which it is procured intentionally and for the sole object of destroying the life of the foetus—without such destruction being necessitated by a due regard for the safety of the mother, or by any other equally imperative cause—and in cases where, had not the product of conception been thus prematurely got rid of, it would doubtless have survived to the termination of the full period of utero-gestation, and been then born alive.[91]

Condie continued with three full pages summarizing the chapters of Horatio's book, often quoting whole paragraphs. Much stress in the review was laid on the question of whether or not the practice of criminal abortion could be "entirely, or in any degree, restrained by law." Condie stated Storer's optimistic predictions for this and included Storer's recommendations for achieving this goal. Condie noted that foremost in Storer's recommendations was improved legislation that eliminated existing distinctions between stages of pregnancy; punished the attempt at abortion even if the woman prove not to be pregnant; punished women for seeking abortions; fixed a uniform standard for when abortion is justified; and made it a crime to encourage "criminal abortion by any publication, lecture, advertisement, or announcement, or by the sale or circulation of any such publication."[92]

Condie reproduced four of Horatio's paragraphs to conclude the review. The final being:

> "We should as a profession, openly and with one accord appeal to the community in words of earnest warning, setting forth the deplorable consequences of criminal abortion—the actual and independent existence, from the moment of conception, of foetal life. And that the effort should not be one of words merely; we should, as a profession, recommend to the legislative bodies of the land the revision and subsequent enforcement of all laws, statutory or otherwise, pertaining to this crime, that the present slaughter of the innocents may to some extent, at least, be made to cease. For it is 'a thing deserving all hate and detestation, that a man in his very originall, whiles he is formed, whiles he is enlived, should be put to death under the very hands[, and] in the shop[,] of nature.'"[93]

Horatio must have been tremendously pleased to have such a supportive and complementary review of his first book in the country's premier medical journal.

CHAPTER 8
AMA MEMORIALS, GARDNER'S POPULAR ARTICLE, HALE'S HOW-TO-MANUAL

Storer's "the writer cannot close this portion of his labors," implied another and this was writing the "Memorial" that the American Medical Association sent to the "several legislative assemblies of the Union" and writing the "Address" the Association sent to the "various State medical societies" requesting them to also press their legislatures on this issue. The Memorial began: *"To the Governor and Legislature of the State of _____ the Memorial of the American Medical Association, an Organization representing the Medical Profession of the United States."*[1] The Memorial then indicated that criminal abortion was "the intentional destruction of a child within its parent; and physicians are now agreed, from actual and various proof, that the child is *alive* from the moment of conception." It described the high and increasing rate of criminal abortion that led to the deaths of "hundreds of thousands" and "the serious injury thereby inflicted upon the public morals." In case these were not enough to influence state legislators to take measures to suppress abortion, Horatio described the "decided and detrimental influence ... upon the rate of increase of the nation and upon its material prosperity." "Public sentiment and the natural sense of duty instinctive to parents proving insufficient to check the crime," the Memorial continued, "it would seem that an appeal should be made to the law and to its framers." The various problems with existing statutes were then briefly described including the inconsistency of the Common Law that "fails to recognize the unborn child as criminally affected, whilst its existence for all civil purposes is nevertheless fully acknowledged." The Memorial then referred to the "duty of the American Medical Association ... publicly to enter an earnest and solemn protest against such unwarrantable destruction of human life." "The duty would be but half fulfilled," the Memorial continued, "did we not call upon those who alone can check and control the crime, early to give this matter their serious attention." It concluded:

> The Association would in no wise transcend its office, but that office is here so plain that it has full confidence in the result. We therefore enter its earnest prayer, that the subject of Criminal Abortion in the state of _____, and the laws in force on the subject in said State may be referred to an appropriate Committee, with directions to report what legislative action may be necessary in the premises.

The Memorial was signed by the Association President Henry Miller and Secretaries S.M. Bemiss and S.G. Hubbard. There was no mention of the Chairman of the Committee who authored it. It included as an enclosure, Horatio's series of articles published in the *North-American Medico-Chirurgical Review*. Horatio himself requested the publisher of the journal to send "extra copies you have printed" to the President of the American Medical Association.[2]

The Address to the State Medical Societies consisted of the three Resolutions on Criminal Abortion adopted by the Association in May 1859 plus the following:

> In pursuance of our instructions, a memorial, of which a copy is here-with enclosed, has been transmitted to the Governor and Legislature of the State of _____, and it now has become our duty ear-nestly to request of the body you represent, such early and hearty action in furtherance of the memorial of the Association, as may insure its full success against the common, though unnatural crime it aims to check.

It too was signed by Miller, Bemiss, and Hubbard and made no mention of its au-thor. This Address reached the New York State Medical Society sometime before early February 1860 when, at its Annual Meeting, the following Resolutions were provided by the Committee that had previously been appointed to consider the recommendations of the American Medical Association:

> "*Resolved*, That this Society cordially approves of the action of the American Medical Association in its efforts to exhibit the extent of the evils resulting from the procuring of Criminal Abortions, and of the means which are adopted to prevent its commission, and cheerfully comply with the request to a 'zealous co-operation' for furtherance of more stringent legislation in regard to this most destructive and revolt-ing crime, committed almost with impunity, and with appalling fre-quency.
>
> "*Resolved*, That a committee of three be appointed to present the memorial of the President and Secretaries of the American Medical As-sociation, which has been read, to the Legislature of this State at its pre-sent session."[3]

As will be seen, other state medical societies similarly responded to the Address.

The American Medical Association held its 1860 Annual Meeting in New Haven, Connecticut during the first week of June and there was a large contingent of physicians from nearby Massachusetts, including David Humphreys Storer. Horatio was not among the delegates, although a Permanent Member and eligible to attend. It is unfortunate that he did not hear the Presidential Address of Henry Miller, much of which was devoted to the work of the Committee on Criminal Abortion and particularly generous in its praise of its Chairman. Miller first dis-cussed the American Medical Association Committee and its Report. He described the Resolutions adopted by the Association and the resultant memorials to legisla-tures and state medical societies. He continued:

> I am happy to acknowledge my obligations to the able Chairman for his valuable assistance, not only in furnishing the documents referred to,

but in the preparation of the Memorial as well as of the Address directed to the various State Medical Societies, requesting their co-operation with the Association, in pressing this important subject on the attention of the legislatures of their respective States. The memorial, with the accompanying documents, was transmitted in January last to the President of the United States and the Governor of each of the States and Territories of the Union, the legislatures of several of them being at the time in session. ... [T]he hope may be reasonably indulged that their Excellencies have submitted them to the National, State, and Territorial legislatures, or will embrace the earliest opportunity of doing so.[4]

Miller also described the challenges that remained for physicians and claimed "obstructions will be thrown in this path of your benevolent operations, which it may require years of ceaseless vigilance and unremitting effort to overcome." He described the major task of enlightening "popular ignorance on this subject" and the need to withstand "the jeers of the flippant, the superficial, and the unthinking in your own ranks." He then gave a primer on fetal development, recognizing that there was still physician ignorance as well as "popular ignorance." Miller then moved to the Association's effort to change state statutes on abortion.

It is difficult for legislation in a free country, where the people are the source of all political power, to rise higher than popular sentiment and intelligence; but is it not the duty of all wise legislators, in questions which can only be elucidated by the science of medical jurisprudence, to endeavor rather to elevate popular sentiment and enlighten popular ignorance than to degrade themselves to their low level? And how can lawmakers better give expression to their estimate of the crime of abortionism than by sedulously providing against its commission? The necessity of more stringent legislation has been clearly pointed out by the Chairman of the Committee, in the papers already referred to, and valuable suggestions, to aid in the enactment of a suitable statute, have been offered by him. May we not hope that our appeal to the different legislative bodies of the Union will not be in vain?[5]

While the Association was meeting in New Haven, it received a request from the Judiciary Committee of the Connecticut Legislature to "frame a suitable bill to serve as a guide for their action" in compliance with the Association's Memorial. Dr. Worthington Hooker and Dr. David L. Daggett from Connecticut and Horatio's father were appointed to provide this assistance.[6] Had Horatio been in attendance, this duty probably would have fallen on his shoulders, and one suspects that he assisted his father in preparing the result, which was a unique piece of legislation that combined "into a single forceful act the denial of the quickening doctrine, the notion of women's liability, and anti-advertising principles."[7] It was the forerunner of similar legislation that would be passed in almost every state and territory in the next two decades.

The Councillors of the Massachusetts Medical Society also took under consideration the Address from the Association. The Minutes included:

> A communication was read from the Committee of the American Medical Association requesting the aid of the Councillors in furtherance of the Memorial of the Association which has been sent to the Legislature of Massachusetts on the subject of the increased frequency of criminal abortion.
>   **Voted**, "To refer the communication to a Special Committee."
>   The Chair nominated Drs. C.G. Putnam, N.B. Shurtleff and H.R. Storer.
>   And they were appointed.[8]

This Committee reported back to the Councillors on October 3, recommending that the Society present the American Medical Association Memorial to the Massachusetts Legislature.[9] Horatio must have been gratified that his efforts had finally enabled him to meet the objective of having physician recommendations for abortion statutes presented to the Massachusetts Legislature. On the other hand, Horatio remained unhappy with the Massachusetts' statutes. Apparently the lawmakers did not heed or fully heed these recommendations.

Although the *National Police Gazette* had reported on Madame Restell and other abortionists with input from Gunning S. Bedford (much of his "Vaginal Hystereotomy," was copied in the *Gazette*),[10] popular literature describing and condemning the abortion epidemic had a major boost from a January 1860 article, "Physical Decline of American Women," in the *Knickerbocker*, a popular New York literary magazine with national circulation.[11] The article was written by the New York physician, Augustus Kinsley Gardner. Gardner was originally from Massachusetts and obtained his M.D. from the Harvard Medical School in 1844. Gardner worked in some capacity at the Tremont Street Medical School where David Humphreys Storer was one of the professors. After other jobs in Boston, Gardner studied in Europe for about a year and then settled in New York where he became professor of midwifery in the New York Medical College.[12]

Gardner's article on women's physical decline dealt with the bad effects women experienced from lack of exercise, late hours, improper clothing, and "sins against one's own self," i.e., masturbation. Gardner then moved to criminal abortion, noting that it was "not foreign to the theme of this paper, for it is not only a moral evil, but a physical wrong." However, Gardner could not hold back this discussion of the *moral* aspects of unnecessary abortion:

> This is a theme from which we would gladly shrink, both from the delicacy of the subject and from conscious inability to treat it as it deserves; to bring before you the most horrid social enormity of this age, this city,

and this world, and to hold it up to you in such a light as to make you all feel it, in its craven cowardice, its consequent bodily, mental and moral degeneracy, its soul-destroying wickedness. We look with a shudder upon the poor ignorant Hindoo woman, who from the very love of her child, agonizes her mother's heart, when in the fervor of her religious enthusiasm she sacrifices her beloved offspring at the feet of Juggernaut or in the turbid waves of the sacred Ganges, yet we have not a pang, nor even a word of reprobation, for the human sacrifices of the unborn thousands annually immolated in the city of New-York before the blood-worshipped Moloch of fashion. From no excess of religious faith in even a false, idolatrous god, are such hecatombs of human beings slain, but our women, from a devotion to dress and vain pride of outward show, become murderesses of their own children, and do literally in their own bodies become whitened sepulchres, pallid, with the diseases consequent upon such unrighteous acts, and sepulchral in thought and tone of voice from the remorse which always follows a guilty action.[13]

"We take the liberty of speaking freely and plainly," Gardner continued, upon a topic which the pulpit shirks and the community winks at." He listed a number of reasons that women were limiting their families and even avoiding children altogether, including expense, "care of children is such a slavery," and planned trips to Europe. He continued:

These are the excuses for not pro-creating children, and the right so not to do we will not discuss now; but are these good reasons for *murder?* … No, not murder, you say, for 'there has not been any life in the child.' Do not attempt to evade to man a crime which cannot be hidden from the All-seeing. The poor mother has not herself felt the life of the child perhaps, but that is a quibble only of the laws of man, founded indeed upon the view, now universally recognized as incorrect, that the child's life began when its movements were first strong enough to be perceptible. There is, in fact, no moment after conception when it can be said that the child has not life, and the crime of destroying human life is as heinous and as sure before the period of 'quickening' has been attained as afterward.[14]

Gardner followed with paragraphs detailing the frequency of criminal abortion and its frequent adverse maternal consequences, noting "this is not exaggerated, for we cannot recall to mind an individual who has been guilty of this crime, (for it must be called a crime, under every aspect,) but who has suffered for many years afterward in consequence."[15]

Gardner's condemnation of frequent criminal abortion summarized several of the points made by Horatio Storer in the recently published series of articles and it is probable that Gardner read and was influenced by them. However, Gardner's denunciations of married women seeking abortion are too strong not to represent his own long-standing opinions and beliefs about the frequency of abortion among the married and about its gross criminality, at least in the eyes of "the All-seeing."

A few years later, Gardner consulted with a homeopathic physician and this led to a rupture with the New York Academy of Medicine and his resignation.[16] The homeopaths were a significant factor in medicine in the middle of the nineteenth century. They prescribed medicines to increase the symptoms of a disease in the belief that symptoms were the body's means of curing itself. Although more-or-less despised by the regular physicians whom the homeopaths called "allopaths," the homeopaths largely shared the aversion to induced abortion of the regular physicians.

One homeopathic physician, Edwin Moses Hale, wrote extensively on the topic of abortion, beginning in 1860. In this respect, Hale might be thought of as a homeopathic equivalent of Horatio Storer. However, a major emphasis for Hale was the presentation of abortion techniques, and Storer never did this.

Hale was born in 1829 in Newport, New Hampshire. His family moved to Ohio and Edwin learned printing, journalism, and law as a youth and young man. A homoeopathic physician successfully treated Hale for a serious case of pneumonia and this stimulated Hale's interest in homeopathy. Hale attended the Western College of Homeopathic Medicine in Cleveland and "graduated from that celebrated institution with distinguished honor." He began practice in 1852 in Jonesville, Michigan and in 1862 took the chair of Materia Medica in the Hahnemann Medical College of Chicago.[17]

In May, 1860, Hale published "Abortion: Its Prevention and Treatment" in the *North American Journal of Homoeopathy*.[18] This was republished as a separate 22-page pamphlet, *On the Homoeopathic Treatment of Abortion*.[19] Hale indicated that abortion was now more common than at any time in history and implied that intentional abortion was inflating the numbers. He described the change in attitude toward large families, favorable in "all times previous to this century," now mothers "deem themselves lucky if they bear children few and far between." He continued:

> From my own experience, and the observations of others with whom I have conversed, I am satisfied that it can be safely asserted that there is *not one married female in ten, who has not had an abortion, or at least attempted one!* For not only have the generally enumerated causes become more prevalent, but the *intentional* production of abortion is especially noticeable. Now-a-days, if a married woman happens to go a few days beyond the menstrual period, she either swallows some domestic emmenagogue at that time, or with the recurrence of [at] the next menstrual period, procures some of the many nostrums so shamelessly advertised as "warranted to regulate the menses," with the especial caution that it "must not be taken during the first three months of pregnancy, as it will invariably produce miscarriage." Or what is worse still, resort is had to the use

of some one of the many instruments which are sold for the purpose
of mechanically inducing abortion.[20]

Hale continued the discussion of the prevalence of abortion, claiming that
he knew "women who have had respectively, eight, ten and thirteen children,
and *as many abortions!*" He indicated he had "attended over 300 cases of
abortion" and that none of these patients had died. "Under judicious treatment,"
Hale wrote, "I consider abortion to be attended with but little danger."[21]

One would expect that Hale's "over 300 cases" were accidental or
spontaneous abortions. However, nine years later, another homoeopathic
physician, Nicholas Francis Cooke, would refer to Hale without specifically
naming him as the "hero of three hundred abortions," and Cooke apparently
believed that Hale had induced 300 abortions, not treated 300 patients who had
undergone abortions from other causes (See below). Hale contributed to such an
interpretation of his "over 300 cases" when he provided explicit details in this
1860 pamphlet on how "to induce the premature expulsion of the ovum by
artificial means."[22] The pamphlet may well have become a guidebook for the
professional abortionist, although Hale's book, *A Systematic Treatise on
Abortion*, probably took that dubious honor when it was published in 1866.[23]

According to Hale, "premature expulsion" was only to occur, for "the
ultimate safety of the mother." He then claimed that these indications for inducing
abortion were increasing and "every practitioner should fully inform himself of the
most safe, efficient, and least objectionable manner of performing this
operation."[24] This was Hale's cue for providing four abortion techniques. He first
described introduction of the uterine sound, a thin metal probe that was
legitimately used to diagnose uterine disease. "This must be carried up nearly to
the fundus," Hale wrote, "then gently turned round two or three times." This he
recommended up to the end of the third month of pregnancy as the easiest and
safest method and, "if properly done, no second operation is necessary."[25]

Hale's second method was to use the "Colpeurynter," a device that was
inserted into the vagina and distended by filling it with warm water. After some
period the uterus would contract and expel its contents. He described an India
rubber bladder substitute that served the same function. He indicated: "Since this
paper was begun, I have several times used this simple instrument with the best
success."[26]

Hale also "for nearly six years" had injected water into the uterus with
syringes to separate the membranes from the uterine surface. Once detached,
"expulsive contractions set in, and the foetus with the placenta attached, is
expelled with little or no hemorrhage." Hale's final method was to puncture the
membranes and this was recommended after the fourth month of pregnancy, when
other methods had failed.[27]

Hale's reports of use of these various methods "several times" "[s]ince this
paper was begun," and "for nearly six years" do lead to the conclusion that he had
induced a score or more of abortions if not "over 300." Despite this apparently
substantial number of abortions induced by Hale, he would claim in an 1867
pamphlet, *The Great Crime of the Nineteenth Century*, that he had been "obliged

to cause the destruction of the fetus but *four* times, and in each instance it was *done to save the life of the mother.*"[28] Cooke in his 1869 book, *Satan in Society: By a Physician*, mentioned the "hero of three hundred abortions" and then made this distorted reference to Hale's 1867 claim of four induced abortions:

> In a subsequent work the same writer admits that he only found abortion necessary to save the life of the mother in four instances, thus publicly confessing that in an immense number of cases he has performed the operation on other grounds; and yet, in the face of all this self-accusation, several attempts at his expulsion from his county medical society have been defeated, and he is accounted "a brother in good standing" of several learned bodies, and holds an enviable position in a fashionable Church and fashionable society.[29]

Cooke would not be the only physician criticizing Edwin Moses Hale for his views and practices related to abortion. Much of this followed Hale's publication of *A Systematic Treatise on Abortion* in 1866 where he advocated induced abortion for the sake of the woman's "health." Hale would retract these statements and he may have written his 1867 pamphlet to deflect criticism that he was not sufficiently opposed to the taking of fetal life. Hale's 1866 book and 1867 pamphlet are discussed in Chapter 10.

The New York medical professor, Gunning S. Bedford, published a major treatise, *The Principles and Practice of Obstetrics*, in 1861. It included his strong objections to craniotomy and his call for the Caesarean section when the pelvis was too narrow to allow a normal birth. He made the following comments on when the induction of abortion was justified:

> It is manifest that the moral part of the question turns upon the simple interrogatory—is the embryo in the earlier states of its existence a living being? All correct physiology demonstrates that it becomes in truth, at the very moment of fecundation, imbued with vitality—the contact of the sperm cell and germ cell constituting the *act of the breathing of life*. Jorg, of Leipsic, I believe, alone claims the doubtful merit of describing the human foetus as "only a higher species of intestinal worm, not endowed with a human soul, nor entitled to human attributes." With his infidel notions on this point he might have added—*nor is the shedding of its blood of any more moment than the slaughtering of the calf!*
>
> Besides the proofs of physiology, we have the testimony of the early fathers of the Catholic church; that church has always maintained, with an unwavering consistency, so characteristic of its canons, that the destruction of the foetus in the womb of its parent, at any period from the moment of conception, is a crime equal in turpitude to *murder*.[30]

Bedford followed by indicating that when the pelvis would not allow passage of a viable fetus the Caesarean section was the proper choice over destruction of the unborn child for the "conscientious accoucheur, who is not actuated by a thirst for innocent blood, but who is most anxious to discharge with fidelity the sacred obligations which his profession imposes upon him."[31] On the other hand, when death was otherwise inevitable for a woman with a fetus that had not reached the age of viability, the Roman Catholic Bedford had no compunctions about preventing two deaths by inducing an abortion.[32] In a footnote to the section, he wrote:

> It is not of course intended here to discuss the general question of *criminal abortion*, which has become, both at home and abroad, a monstrous crime, owing in great measure to the laxity with which the laws on the subject are enforced. I may refer the reader to an instructive paper entitled *"Criminal Abortion in America,"* by Horatio R. Storer, M.D., 1860.[33]

As a result of this mention of Storer by Bedford, Storer would finally make reference to Bedford (See below).

Medical journal articles and editorials dealing with criminal abortion declined in the early 1860s and this no doubt was due to the Civil War. Horatio Storer's prolific output of articles on abortion and other medical topics stopped from 1860 through 1862. He resumed medical publication early in 1863 with an article dealing with *unintentional* abortion.[34] He began the article by discussing his earlier articles on criminal abortion and their "practical result."

> The general interest then evinced in his labors by the profession both at home and abroad, the approbation and encouragement received, and above all, the practical result of the whole matter (which has proved precisely that aimed at in the outset), namely, the awakening of the public mind as to the value of foetal life and the vindication of the character of the profession on this point alike in its own sight, that of the law and of the community, by the unanimous voice of the medical press,* are all convincing evidence of the importance and legitimacy of the investigation.[35]

His footnote read:

> *In verification of this statement, I refer to the current files of every medical journal, to the published Transactions of the National and minor Medical Associations, to many medical addresses, as that by Dr. Miller of Louisville at New Haven in 1860, and to nearly every general obstetric work of any importance issued in this country since that date—Bedford's Principles and Practice of Obstetrics, for instance.

CHAPTER 9

STORER'S PRIZE-WINNING ESSAY

The *Boston Medical and Surgical Journal* provided an August 1864 editorial that referred to recent highly publicized notices of child desertion, rarer "instances of unmistakable violence to new-born infants," and prevalent criminal abortion. "In point of morality we see no difference in these three varieties of crime," Editors Abbott and White continued, "but undoubtedly many a tender-hearted wife exclaims against the wickedness of the poor girl who thus leaves her offspring to the chance mercies of the passer-by to screen herself from a life-long infamy, and yet does not hesitate to destroy the fruit of her own womb before it has seen the light, if nature insists upon her becoming a mother more frequently than she desires."[1]

They described the "real surprise" women felt when "told of the sinfulness of an act which they seem to regard as of no moral importance whatever." They continued:

> Society needs a thorough awakening upon this subject, and it should be brought home to every woman and man in its true light. It should be taught in every school book of physiology, and every public print should reiterate it, that the child is alive from the moment of conception, and that every interference with its being is as much a sin at one period of its existence as at another.[2]

Their editorial may have been a second to a Resolution calling for enlightenment of women on the subject of criminal abortion that was made three months earlier at the Annual Meeting of the American Medical Association in New York. Michigan delegates proposed that the Association "offer a premium for the best *short and comprehensive tract* calculated for circulation among females, and designed to enlighten them upon the criminality and physical evils of forced abortion."[3] Their Resolution was approved and referred to the new Committee on Prize Essays.[4] Since the 1865 Association meeting would be in Boston, this Committee was made up of Boston physicians. Two of these, J. Mason Warren and John H. Dix, were close friends of Horatio. The third member and Chairman of the Committee was Horatio's father.[5]

The second day of the June 1865 Boston meeting was a particularly big day for Horatio. The Minutes included:

> "The Committee on Prize Essays beg leave to report that they have received a dissertation 'On the Surgical Treatment of Morbid Growths within the Larynx,' bearing the motto '*Quod vidi, scripsi*,' which they would unanimously recommend as worthy the usual prize of the Association.

"They would also award the premium offered at the last annual meeting of the Association for 'the best short and comprehensive tract calculated for circulation among females, and designed to enlighten them upon the criminality and physical evils of abortion' to an essay with the motto '*Casta placent superis, castâ cum mente venito, et manibus puris sumito fontis aquam.*'

"In the preface to which the writer very modestly remarks: 'If it be considered by the Committee worthy its end, they will please adjudge it no fee, nor measure it by any pecuniary recompense. Were the finances of the Association such as to warrant it in more than the most absolutely necessary expenditures, yet would the approbation of the Committee and of the profession at large be more grateful to the writer than any tangible, and therefore, trivial reward.'

D. Humphreys Storer,

J. Mason Warren,

H. I. Bowditch,

John H. Dix."

The seals were then broken, and Dr. Louis Elsberg, of New York, proved to be the successful competitor for the first of the prizes mentioned, and Dr. Horatio R. Storer, of Massachusetts, the author of the Essay on Criminal Abortion.[6]

There was no mention in the Minutes of the number of entries submitted for the regular or for the special prize. A May 10, 1865 entry in Jonathon Mason Warren's journal had included, "Returned Dissertation on *Abortion* to Dr Storer."[7] Warren's handwriting is poor, but it is almost certainly "dissertation" and not "dissertation*s*." However, if there had been other entries, Horatio's investigation of abortion, described by Condie as "full, able, and satisfactory," gave him a unique perspective on the subject that made his essay highly likely to capture the prize.[8]

Horatio attempted to hide his identity to the Prize Committee by referring in his essay to the author of his own published papers in the third person. For example:

I am constrained to acknowledge my indebtedness to the various publications of the writer from whom I have quoted, for much of the evidence I shall now present upon the subject of forced abortions. I trust that thus offered it may lose none of its freshness, point, and force. My frequent extracts from one who has given more thought to the subject than probably any other person in the country, will I am sure need no excuse.[9]

Horatio no doubt believed that anyone else making reference to his publications would have used such favorable terms.

"The writer," Horatio began his Prefatory Remarks, "who knew nothing of the project to elicit a direct and effective appeal to women upon the subject of criminal abortion, until after it had been decided at the New York meeting, has long been a member of the Association."[10] One might suspect that Horatio had planted the idea for such a Horatio-serving essay contest in the Michigan physicians who made the Resolution the year before. What is more, Horatio had been visiting insane asylums in Michigan in late 1863 or early 1864 as a member of the Massachusetts Commission on Insanity.[11] Perhaps he did plant the idea, but did not know it sprouted and bore fruit "until after it had been decided at the New York meeting."

"If the essay prove successful," Horatio continued, "its author only asks that the seal which covers his identity may not be broken until the announcement is made upon the platform of the convention, pledging himself that this is but a whim of his own, and that he is well, and he trusts favorably, known by many of the best men of the Association throughout the Union." An associated footnote in the *published* paper read: "Now that the decision of the Prize Committee has been made, the purpose of the above stipulation becomes evident. The committee consisted of Drs. D. Humphreys Storer, Henry I. Bowditch, J. Mason Warren, and John H. Dix, of Boston; the chairman of the committee being the writer's father."[12]

The breaking of the seal on the platform, at least partially removed the onus of favoritism in awarding the prize to Horatio, since it could be argued that no one knew the author of the essay until the seal was broken. However, one can hardly imagine that any member of the committee, and particularly its chairman, was totally surprised to see Horatio's name under the seal. Yet that is exactly what one physician was to note in a letter to Horatio a few months after the event. "Nothing pleased me so much as the gratification so pleasantly expressed by your good father," wrote his Philadelphia friend, "as he so unexpectedly found his son to be the essayist. For that reason, I am much pleased that you requested, 'for a whim,' to have the seals broken upon the platform."[13]

Some uncertainty *may* have existed in the minds of Prize Committee members, even that of David Humphreys Storer, as to the author of the Prize Essay. Horatio demonstrated his capability of concealing authorship in a later prize competition when he had his entry mailed from Pittsburgh to reduce the likelihood that the Boston judges would identify its source.[14] Horatio may have had this 1865 essay sent from some other city and he may have had the essay copied by another person to eliminate the cue of his distinctive handwriting. The "gratification so pleasantly expressed" by David "as he so unexpectedly found his son to be the essayist" *may* have been an expression of surprise, but more likely was one appropriate for confirmation of an expectation. On the other hand, David may have been a good actor.

Horatio began the actual essay by testifying to its importance. He noted that this may have been the first occasion when the profession had chosen to "directly address itself to the judgment and to the hearts of women upon a question vital to themselves and to the nation." He enumerated the various bearings of the essay on women's discretion, conscience, moral character, peace of mind, sanity, domestic happiness, and self-respect. He presented his plan for showing in the essay that induced abortions were "a crime against life, the child being always alive," as well as crimes against the mother, nature, public interest, and morality. Horatio then noted that even if one disregarded the ethical aspects of induced abortions, "they are so dangerous to the woman's health, her own physical and domestic best interests, that their induction, permittal, or solicitation by one cognizant of their true character, should almost be looked upon as proof of actual insanity."[15]

Horatio then provided a historical account of the medical profession's long silence on abortion; the efforts of Hodge and two Storers to break that silence; the American Medical Association's outstanding performance in the campaign; and the fine support to the campaign provided by medical journalists and textbook writers. He decried the popular belief that reputable physicians ever performed abortions for reasons other than to save the mother, but did admit that physicians sometimes appeared to devalue human life when the child at birth was destroyed for the sake of saving the mother, and in cases where abortions were inappropriately performed to remedy otherwise treatable conditions. He indicated that no abortion should ever be performed by a physician without concurrence of a second physician and called for laws making this a requirement:

> How much more requisite is it that in the question we are now considering, to one mode of deciding which the physician may be prompted by pity, by personal sympathy, the entreaties of a favorite patient, and not seldom by the direct offer of comparatively enormous pecuniary compensation, the law should offer him its protecting shield, saving him even from himself, and helping him to see that the fee for an unnecessarily induced or allowed abortion is in reality the price of blood.[16]

The next section of the Essay discussed inappropriate intentional abortions. "Physicians have now arrived at the unanimous opinion," he wrote, "that the foetus in utero is *alive* from the very moment of conception." "The law, whose judgments are arrived at so deliberately, and usually so safely, has come to the same conclusion," he continued, "and though in some of its decisions it has lost sight of this fundamental truth, it has averred, in most pithy and emphatic language, that 'quick with child, is having conceived.'" "By that higher than human law, which, though scoffed at by many a tongue, is yet acknowledged by every conscience," Horatio continued, then quoted himself, "'the wilful killing of a human being, at any stage of its existence, is murder.'"[17]

Horatio then became a biology teacher, noting that before the egg leaves the ovary and is impregnated "it may perhaps be considered as a part and parcel of herself, but not afterwards." He compared the temporary attachment of the fertilized egg to the womb to the attachment of the born child to the breast, throwing in the interesting and somewhat intermediate case of the tiny kangaroo fetus "born into the world at an extremely early stage of development" and placed by its mother in the external pouch to spend weeks attached to a teat therein before "in reality to be born." He continued: "Many women suppose that the child is not alive till quickening has occurred, others that it is practically dead till it has breathed. As well one of these suppositions as the other; they are both of them erroneous."[18]

He then pointed out that quickening was but a sensation of the mother and that movement of the fetus occurred much earlier. "These motions must be allowed to prove life," Horatio continued, "and independent life." He then asked: "In what does this life really differ from that of the child five minutes in the world?" Horatio's own answer is implicit in the following:

> In the majority of instances of forced abortion, the act is committed prior to the usual period of quickening. There are other women, who have confessed to me that they have destroyed their children long after they have felt them leap within their womb. There are others still, whom I have known to wilfully suffocate them during birth, or to prevent the air from reaching them under the bedclothes; and there are others, who have wilfully killed their wholly separated and breathing offspring, by strangling them or drowning them, or throwing them into a noisome vault. Wherein among all these criminals does there in reality exist any difference in guilt?[19]

Although much of this essay was taken verbatim from his earlier articles written for physicians, the following new paragraph was written for his female audience *and* for physicians:

> I would gladly arrive at, and avow any other conviction than that I have now presented, were it possible in the light of fact and of science, for I know it must carry grief and remorse to many an otherwise innocent bosom. The truth is, that our silence has rendered all of us accessory to the crime, and now that the time has come to strip down the veil, and apply the searching caustic or knife to this foul sore in the body politic, the physician needs courage as well as his patient, and may well overflow with regretful sympathy.[20]

Horatio next discussed "The Inherent Dangers of Abortion to a Woman's Health and to her Life." Much of the material was taken from the article, "Its Victims," of the 1859 series, including a direct quote several pages in length. Horatio described the short-term, medium-term, and long-term consequences of induced abortion, including the very real possibility of death. The non-fatal problems were judged due to premature interruption of the numerous preparations of the woman's body for birth and nursing, to incomplete abortion, and to damage of tissues during invasion of the womb. Horatio then noted that should the woman avoid physical impairment, there still was the potential mental problem:

> Add to this that even though the occurrence of any such feeling may be denied, there is probably always a certain measure of compunction for the deed in the woman's heart—a touch of pity for the little being about to be sacrificed—a trace of regret for the child that, if born, would have proved so dear—a trace of shame at casting from her the pledge of a husband's or lover's affection—a trace of remorse for what she knows to be a wrong, no matter to what small extent, or how justifiable it may seem to herself, and we have an explanation of the additional element

in these intentional abortions, which increases the evil effect upon the mother, not as regards her bodily health alone, but in some sad cases to the extent even of utterly overthrowing her reason.[21]

Horatio's next section was "The Frequency of Forced Abortions, even among the Married." Horatio summarized the statistics that comprised much of his earliest writing on abortion. He noted the sharp differences in abortion rates between Protestant and Catholic women, probably hoping to utilize the anti-Catholic sentiment of his primarily Protestant women readers and induce them thereby to bear their children. He claimed that abortion was more frequent among the married, and indicated that one reason was that the married woman was more apt to recognize a pregnancy at the early stage when most abortions took place. Horatio then claimed the frequency of abortion was still increasing and followed with this strict admonition taken largely from his earlier writing for physicians:

But not only is abortion of excessively frequent occurrence; the nefarious practice is yearly extending, as does every vice that custom and habit have rendered familiar. It is foolish to trust that a change for the better may be spontaneously effected. "Longer silence and waiting by the profession would be criminal. If these wretched women, these married, lawful mothers, ay, and these Christian husbands, are thus murdering their children by thousands, through ignorance, they must be taught the truth; but if, as there is reason to believe is too often the case, they have been influenced to do so by fashion, extravagance of living, or lust, no language of condemnation can be too strong."[22]

Next was "The Excuses and Pretexts that are given for the Act." This section discussed ignorance, ill health, fear of childbed, and effects on living children, using many of the same paragraphs of Horatio's earlier article, "Its Frequency, and the Causes Thereof." The final section was "Alternatives, Public and Private, and Measures of Relief." The initial paragraph dealt with women's "most valid excuse for the crime." This was the effect of the state of gestation on the woman's mind, and Horatio put in a plug for "the authority I have so freely drawn from," who, he claimed, also had provided the most thorough investigation of such gestation-mind effects. He was referring to his own American Medical Association Committee on Insanity Report presented at the same 1865 meeting in Boston and to his other articles claiming uterine factors as determinants of female insanity.[23] This factor made the woman "liable to thoughts, convictions even, that at other times she would turn from in disgust or dismay."[24] Horatio had cited this as the reason that women committing murder during pregnancy, or shortly thereafter, should not be executed.[25] Its inclusion in the Prize Essay perhaps reflected Horatio's hope that by telling women that such thoughts and convictions during pregnancy were crazy, the woman would eliminate them or at least would not act on them.

Horatio asked, "Is there no alternative but for women, when married and prone to conception to occasionally bear children?" His answer was that this was certainly in their best interests "for length of days and immunity from disease." He indicated that both prevention of pregnancy by artificial means and termination of pregnancy were "disastrous to a woman's mental, moral, and physical well-being."[26]

Horatio indicated the need for foundling hospitals. Not only would they prevent infanticide and abortion by the unwed mother, "they would save her from one element of the self-condemnation and hatred which so often hurries the victim of seduction downward to the life of the brothel." Horatio continued:

> But for the married, who have not this strong stimulus of necessity, and the excuse of having been led astray or deceived, there need be no public channel provided, through which to purchase safety for their children. Is it not, indeed, inconceivable that the very women who, when their darlings of a month old or a year are snatched from them by disease, find the parting attended with so acute a pang, can so deliberately provide for and congratulate themselves, and each other, upon a willful abortion? Here words fail us.[27]

This was the cue for Horatio to quote his "Of the mother, ... we leave those to speak who can" statement, which had ended his first 1859 article.

Instead of stopping with this powerful ending, Horatio continued with a final section where he included a series of quotes from his earlier work and elsewhere which recapitulated what had been presented in the essay. He also mentioned his strong interest in "the great territories of the far West," and asked "shall it be filled by our own children or by those of aliens?" "Aliens" were the recent immigrants who were not restricting their families. "This is a question that our own women must answer," Horatio continued; "upon their loins depends the future destiny of the nation."[28]

In conclusion, Horatio wrote:

> In the hope that the present appeal may do somewhat to stem the tide of fashion and depraved public opinion; that it may tend to persuade our women that forced abortions are alike unchristian, immoral, and physically detrimental; that it may dissipate the ignorance concerning the existence of foetal life that so extensively prevails, and be the means of promoting the ratio of increase of our national population, so unnaturally kept down, the National Medical Association addresses itself to all American mothers; for thus, in the closing words of the essay from which I have so frequently and so freely drawn, would "the profession again be true to its mighty and responsible office of shutting the great gates of human death."[29]

One of the last pieces of business of the Boston meeting was a request for the Committee of Publication, of which Horatio was a member, "to adopt such appropriate measures as will insure a speedy and general circulation of the Prize Essay on Abortion, provided this can be done without expense to the Association."[30] This request to do something in a hurry without spending any money was the authorization of Horatio to publish the Essay himself. The controversial title Horatio selected was *Why Not? A Book for Every Woman*.[31] The title gave no indication of the topic of the book, and a reader who did learn from some source that the topic was induced abortion, might expect from the *question*, *"Why Not?"*, a justification of induced abortion. Perhaps Horatio was hoping to attract as readers women seeking justification to end an unwanted pregnancy, expecting that his book would convince them to have their children instead.

The book went into four editions, 1866, 1867, 1868, and 1871. In 1897, when Horatio reviewed his antiabortion efforts he indicated that because of the book "hundreds of women acknowledged that they were ... induced to permit their pregnancy to accomplish its full period."[32] As will be seen, Stewart Morse told physicians to have the book "always at hand" as "the means of instruction and warning to his patients," and Henry D. Holton, of Vermont, reported *in 1907* that he routinely provided the little book to Protestant patients who requested unnecessary abortions (he sent Catholics to talk to their priests). At the American Medical Association Annual meeting in 1866, the same Henry D. Holton proposed a Resolution thanking Horatio for declining the $100 prize for his prize-winning essay.[33] One suspects that over four decades of Dr. Holton's practice many Vermont applicants for abortion got to read Storer's *Why Not?*

CHAPTER 10
HALE'S *TREATISE* AND "GREAT CRIME"

In April 1866, Edwin Moses Hale published *A Systematic Treatise on Abortion*. The dominant feature of the book was a long Section, "Obstetric Abortion," where he provided instructions on several methods for inducing abortion at each of the different stages of pregnancy. These were far more detailed than those provided in his 1860 pamphlet.[1] He also identified an instrument used by physician abortionists:

> It consists of four "claws," which are sheathed in a tube during its introduction, and are made to protrude and open when in the interior of the uterus. The instrument is pushed upward to the fundus uteri, to the position the ovum is supposed to occupy, when the "claws" are closed upon the embryo, if reached, and the whole forcibly extracted. This instrument is the one most generally employed by those villains who disgrace the medical profession and humanity by practising the vile trade of producing criminal abortion.[2]

Hale listed indications for "producing an abortion during the first third of pregnancy."

> Extreme contraction of the pelvis; voluminous, immoveable, and nonoperable tumors of the excavation; extreme dropsy of the amnion; irreducible displacements of the womb; haemorrhages which have resisted the employment of the most rational measures; eclampsia, mania; chorea, and obstinate, dangerous vomiting. If any of these indications obtain, the sooner after conception the embryo is destroyed, the better for the health and safety of the patient.[3]

Hale denied that there was a substantial risk of maternal death even when abortion was "necessarily induced by the skillful physician in early pregnancy." "My observation and experience in this matter have been quite extensive," he continued, "and I have been led to the conclusion that, if the operation is skillfully performed, the fatal results need not exceed one in a thousand."[4] Hale's "quite extensive" "observation and experience in this matter" of skillful induction of abortion, and other such references in his book, suggest many more instances where he was "obliged to cause the destruction of the foetus" than four in "nearly sixteen years" of practice (See below).

A sharp departure from typical recommendations to do everything possible to prevent a threatened abortion appeared when Hale discussed victims of seduction:

In such cases it is difficult to decide what should be the conduct of a physician in one respect: namely, should he attempt to arrest the abortion, and thereby bring the mother to inevitable shame and save the life of an illegitimate child, whose unnatural parentage will be a disgrace all through life? Probably the best and most consistent conduct for the physician to adopt, should be to simply let outraged nature take her own course, and only interfere by warding off those symptoms which threaten the life of the mother.[5]

In a section dealing with the jurisprudence of abortion, Hale reproduced a December 1864 lecture, "Criminal Abortion," by Alvin Edmund Small, Hale's "venerable friend and colleague, who lately occupied the chair of Medical Jurisprudence in Hahnemann Medical College." Professor Small had reproduced in his lecture substantial portions of Horatio Storer's first article in the *North-American Medico-Chirurgical Review*. When the quotes of Storer ended, Small continued with paraphrases of Storer's writing, including a terribly cumbersome adaptation of Horatio's "Of the mother ..." sentence.[6]

Hale followed Small's 1864 lecture with:

I cordially and sincerely subscribe to most of the views above set forth, so far as relates to the destruction of the ovum, without good and sufficient cause. I differ, however, with some of my professional brethren, in relation to the propriety of inducing abortion or premature labor when certain diseases and conditions exist.

I hold that in no instance should the life, or even *health* of the mother be sacrificed to save that of an impregnated ovum, before the date of its "viability."

The dogma that the embryo, before that date, is of the same importance as after, is yet debatable. I can not, therefore, look upon the destruction of the ovum before that period as *murder*.[7]

Hale's unwillingness to jeopardize the "*health* of the mother" for the sake of the "impregnated ovum," and his refusal to view "destruction of the ovum" as murder, caused a number of his homeopathic colleagues to criticize him for advocating abortion when the life of the mother was *not* at stake. One was the prominent homeopathic physician, William Henry Holcombe, who provided a review of Hale's book in July 1866.[8] Holcombe praised portions of Hale's book and noted that it was an important supplement to a very weak homeopathic medical literature. Holcombe followed this praise with criticism of Hale's medicines and his chemistry. These, however, were not Holcombe's major concern:

There is another subject upon which our criticism must pass into positive censure: viz., the failure of Dr. Hale to rise to the true scientific and moral position on the nature and permissibility of obstetric abortion.

The true scientific position is this: from the moment of conception, when the spermatozoa coalesces with the cell-wall of the ovule, the ovum is a distinct human being, with a human soul, simply attached to the other for the obtainment of nutritive material, but growing, living, organizing, by forces and powers entirely its own, and derived through nature from God.

The true moral position is this: The destruction of this ovum is always homicide, justifiable, perhaps, under a few extraordinary and painful conditions, after the failure of all reasonable medical and surgical means, and then imposing such solemn and fearful moral responsibilities that it should only be accomplished after the mature deliberation and concurrent advice of several respectable members of the profession.[9]

Holcombe noted how Hale had reinforced these proper scientific and moral positions by quoting Small's "admirable lecture." "It is after citing these beautiful paragraphs from Dr. Small, and giving them a partial approval," Holcombe continued, "that Dr. Hale states his own position—a position that is calculated to be, in turn, both cause and effect of a degenerate moral sentiment on this momentous subject."[10]

Holcombe then quoted Hale's statements of his differences from his "professional brethren." After Hale's "even *health* of the mother," Holcombe wrote in parentheses, "What a vast latitude is here given to criminal practices!" After Hale's mention that he did not view destroying the embryo as murder before "the date of its 'viability,'" Holcombe parenthesized, "six months, mind you!"

Holcombe also called attention to Hale's quandary about whether or not to attempt to save an unborn illegitimate child after the unmarried woman had suffered an attempt at abortion. "In our opinion," Holcombe wrote, "he might as well stand idly by, and see a wicked mother murder her little child on the street."[11] This led to a discussion of Hale's "apparently large experience in the induction of abortion."

He speaks, with a nonchalance perfectly frightful to us, of his "frequent use" of such and such an instrument, his repeated trial of such and such a measure, his "favorite method" in such and such cases. Embracing views fundamentally different, we have never had occasion, in our lives, to induce abortion, and there are very, very few professional men in this part of the Union, whose experience or opinions differ from ours. The shameful laxity of principle and practice on the subject of abortion prevailing in some communities, will never be rebuked or corrected by gentlemen who think with Dr. Hale, however sincere may be their convictions, however conscientious their practice, and however much they may deprecate the debauched public sentiment, to which they thus unconsciously contribute.[12]

Holcombe was not the only critic. At its meeting in December 1866, the Central Homoeopathic Medical Association of Maine also criticized Hale's "*health* of the mother" abortion exception and "Resolved, That the said language inculcates a direct violation of all moral law, of the sentiment of the whole Medical Profession, and of the statute law of all the States, and that we hereby express our strongest disapproval of the same."[13]

Hale reacted to the criticism by having the publisher of the *Treatise* paste a page with a revision of his health statement over the offensive passages on page 319 in the remaining unsold copies. This pasted sheet included many more words than the original, including:

> I hold that in no instance should the *life* of the mother be *sacrificed* to save that of an impregnated ovum, at any period of pregnancy. ... Both medical and legal authorities still differ as to the relative importance of the embryo, before and after the date of "quickening," and before and after the date of "viability." In the present advanced state of physiological knowledge, however, we can not believe otherwise than that the *impregnated ovum at any date is a human being.*
>
> Viewing the matter in this light, we can not do otherwise than designate the necessary or unnecessary destruction of the embryo at any date after conception as *murder.*

Hale also mailed this revision to homeopathic medical journals whose editors published it, typically including praise of Hale for correcting his errors.

Hale published a second edition of the *Treatise* in 1868 with a new title, *A Systematic Treatise on Abortion and Sterility*. He totally dropped the chapter that had provided detailed instructions on inducing abortion and added a long chapter on sterility. He explained these changes in his "Preface to the Second Edition."

> The omission of Part V., or Obstetric Abortion, was prompted by conscientious motives. It was written for physicians—for pure-minded and honorable men—but the information therein contained has probably been prostituted to bad purposes by immoral physicians. It must be admitted, however, that correct information relative to the induction of premature labor is often of incalculable value to the physician, as a means of saving life. In this respect the omission made will be a real loss. I prefer, however, that the profession shall repair this loss by consulting the works of such obstetric authors as Simpson, Caxeaux, Gardner, Barnes, allopathic; or Guernsey, Ludlam, and other obstetric writers of the homoeopathic school.[14]

Hale's reader interested in "repair[ing] this loss," would probably be more apt to locate a copy of Hale's 1866 *Treatise* than the "works of" the authors he listed.

Another prominent homeopath, Reuben Ludlam, Professor of Obstetrics and Diseases of Women and Children at the Hahnemann Medical College in Chicago, delivered a lecture, "Criminal Abortion," on February 4, 1867.[15] Ludlam referred to the statistics that Storer presented in 1859 showing the large prevalence of the crime in Massachusetts and New York, and to "a greater or less degree" in "every other State." He then singled out Chicago:

> Of the three hundred physicians who pretend to a legitimate practice of medicine in this city, not more than one-fourth gain their subsistence by an honest and conscientious discharge of the physician's duties. The remainder constitute a floating, fickle, unprincipled and unscrupulous class, which thrives upon the crimes and misfortunes of the ignorant and the wicked, whose improvidences and lack of conscience make them their prey.[16]

Ludlam called on the medical students to use their future weighty influence as physicians to "counteract and disprove the shallow sophistry upon which the practice of criminal abortion was founded." He claimed they would be faced with requests for abortion regardless of where they set up medical practice. They also would find themselves competing with "crafty and designing men, who, for a consideration, will not hesitate to discover the most plausible reasons why they should yield to the importunities of those who insist that this abominable work must be done at any cost, and even at the risk of their own lives."

Ludlam then cited three classes of "argument against the perpetuation of this crime," "the Physiological, the Moral, and the Politic." Of the first he described erroneous beliefs fostered by "physicians who have little principle" that the embryo was not alive prior to quickening. He discussed the process of fertilization and indicated that following this first step in the reproductive process, "whatever imperils the integrity of that germ, implicates life; and whoever intentionally intercepts the wonderful changes incident thereto, is a veritable murderer—no more and no less!"[17] He followed by indicating that quickening was "not a reliable criterion of the viability of the embryo."

Also under the physiological heading were the dangers to the woman undergoing abortion. "There are numerous avenues through which the murder may leak out," Ludlam wrote, "and means by which it may carry off the mother, as well as the child."[18] He cited various causes of death and followed with a long list of diseases incident to criminal abortion when death did not occur. "If this array of the more than possible consequences of foeticide does not deter you from its commission," he continued, "there certainly is nothing in the study of physiology and pathology that will."[19] He claimed that these dangers to health alone required the physician to persuade the woman requesting abortion to continue her pregnancy.

Ludlam then discussed the "Moral" arguments against abortion. The culmination of these for Ludlam was the commandment, "Thou shalt not kill!" He found the "intrauterine murder in civilized communities" no less "revolting and sinful" than the killing of newborns by the Chinese. He compared the casting of infants into the Ganges to the "equally deliberate sacrifice of the unborn, in Christian lands, to the Moloch of Fashion and Selfishness." He continued:

When I hear persons criticising [sic] the morality and propriety of this or that amusement and diversion, of this style of dress and equipage, or that class of books or companions, I ask myself, are they guiltless in greater matters? What myriads of little innocents have never had a name, or left either a memoir or a monument! What hosts of martyrs have gone up to the great white throne with no earthly record of their sacrifice![20]

Ludlam noted that the physician abortionists could not be ennobled or dignified by the "proudest position in their profession, in church, or in state." "They are worse than a pestilence in any community," he continued, "and there is some thing really contagious and contaminating about them." He warned his medical student audience to "keep aloof from all such characters."[21]

Ludlam refused to instruct his audience on means for inducing abortion. "I would not have you become more familiar with the tools than with the thoughts of the man-slayer," he wrote, "for it is a law of our nature that the practice of one iniquity begets a predisposition to others."[22] This refusal to instruct his audience on means for inducing abortion undoubtedly was a criticism of Edwin Moses Hale. Perhaps Ludlam even had Hale in mind when he warned his medical student audience to "keep aloof from all such characters."

Edwin Moses Hale probably was listening when Ludlam gave his lecture on February 4, 1867. Hale published a brief review of Ludlam's lecture that claimed to identify its faults and deficiencies.[23] He claimed that Ludlam and others in "similar pamphlets and articles" had failed "in explaining and defining the exact nature of the crime." They also failed to "expose the flimsiness of the subterfuges which are resorted to, as excuse for its commission," and "none fearlessly inform the public who the real criminals are, how they may and can be detected, and how they should be punished." It surely is no coincidence that these various weaknesses of Ludlam and others, were subject headings in Hale's soon to be published pamphlet with the full title, *The Great Crime of the Nineteenth Century, Why Is It Committed? Who Are the Criminals? How Shall They Be Detected? How Shall They Be Punished?*[24] Hale's *Great Crime* may have already been written when Hale wrote his Ludlam review.

Hale agreed with Ludlam's assertion that only one-fourth of Chicago physicians honestly and conscientiously "discharged their duties." Hale praised Ludlam's treatment of the "impregnated embryo" and for his "discard" of the "old theory of 'quickening.'" Hale also agreed that destruction of the embryo from the moment of impregnation was "doubtless 'murder,'" but: "Whether *human* justice will ever be educated up to the point of visiting capital punishment upon the person who destroys foetal life at either extreme of gestation remains to be shown by the progress of events."

Hale concluded:

We recommend this pamphlet to physicians as a good thing to circulate in the community in which they practice. It does not come up to our ideas of what the scope and depth of such a work should be, but is capable, nevertheless, of doing much good. The thorough expose of criminal abortion is yet to be written. Whoever shall write a treatise on this subject which shall fully arouse the people, as well as the members of the medical and legal profession, until they shall unite in demanding some special legislation which shall check this great crime, will be esteemed the benefactor of his race.[25]

His concluding sentence no doubt described the response he expected to receive from "his race" for his own soon-to-be published "treatise on the subject."

Hale began *The Great Crime of the Nineteenth Century* by indicating that he was not going to "treat of the statistics ... of abortion," these having been "fully considered" in his 1866 book. However, he then claimed "*two-thirds* of the number of conceptions occurring in the United States, and many other civilized countries, are destroyed *criminally*."[26] This probably represents the high-water mark of physician estimates of the frequency of criminal abortion in the nineteenth and twentieth century, but, according to Hale, this "would not be overrating the extent and prevalence of this fearful crime." Hale's willingness to listen to (and probably accept) requests for abortion and to treat the results of criminal abortion no doubt was well known by women in his community and he very well may have encountered a class of patients that led him to the "*two-thirds*" figure. These abortion-savvy women may have provided Hale with the unique information about city and country abortionists that is discussed below.

Hale next postulated that criminal abortion was a crime against the State or country, against physiology, against morality, and against the law. It was a crime against the State because it "lessens the population of a State or country, in an appalling degree," and the number of "Americans left on American soil," would be left "few and far between." Horatio Storer's December 1858 paper, "On the Decrease of the Rate of Increase," was finally published in March 1867, and Hale made reference to it to support this.[27]

Two sentences handled the crime against Physiology: "It arrests the normal course of the functions of physical life. Pregnancy is a natural condition which cannot be arrested without the most calamitous results, not only to the local condition of the reproductive organs, but to the general physiological functions of the whole system."[28]

It was a crime against morality because "the *soul* exists in the impregnated ovum from the date of conception." This was restated in five slightly different ways, including one that destroyed "quickening" as of any "real importance in its physiological relation."[29]

Hale's "crime against the law" occupied the bulk of the pamphlet. He first answered the question: "Why is It Committed?" He cited poverty, ill health, moral and physical cowardice, loss of beauty, love of fashionable life, adultery, seduction, prostitution, rape, and disgrace of maternity.[30] Storer was quoted in Hale's refutation of "Ill Health." "No plea could be more false," he wrote, "for, to quote the language of Dr. Storer, 'there is not a conceivable case where an abortion will not make it worse.'"[31] For Hale, an early and strong defender of "justifiable abortion," to mention this, was a little surprising.

"Loss of Beauty" was the fear of women who believed childbearing caused the changes in appearance of their contemporaries. Hale claimed that it was not the childbearing that produced the loss of beauty and: "Even should these results follow, how much more beautiful and attractive is a maternity unsullied by crime, than all the physical beauty possible, if stained by the sin of child-murder!"[32]

Hale indicated the married not infrequently let their "Love of Fashionable Life" cause them to end a pregnancy that interfered with balls, operas, vacations, etc. Hale then claimed the resulting disease often prevented attendance or travel and the woman who delayed pregnancy with an abortion not infrequently was unable to bear a child when it was not only convenient, but highly desired, because the abortion produced sterility.

Seduction and desertion were the plight of young women who often chose criminal abortion to hide their shame. Sometimes the woman and her lover simply wished to delay or avoid marriage and criminal abortion was chosen to save both from disgrace. Hale continued:

> When the crime is committed to save the victim of seduction and desertion from shame, the world is apt to view the act as justifiable, or at least wink at is [sic] commission. But the deed is none the less criminal in the one instance than in the other. The act is none the less murder, even if it be done to save the mother from disgrace. We are not justified in taking life for any other reason than that of saving a life of greater importance.[33]

Pregnancy resulting from rape was seen as the most plausible excuse for induction of criminal abortion by Hale. He continued:

> It is asked—would you not destroy the embryo or fetus in your own daughter, violated by a brutal Negro, Indian or white? This kind of argument, however, will not stand against the Divine injunction, "Thou shall not kill."
>
> Evidently the only proper procedure in such cases as the above, is to allow the child to be born alive. It will then be perfectly proper to remove it from the presence of the mother before she has looked upon the hateful object, and place it in the care of some charitable institution, where it will be forever hid from her eyes, forever ignorant of its own disgraceful origin, and where, perhaps, it may be reared with such care for its soul's welfare, that it may serve some use in the economy of Divine Providence.[34]

Hale's next reason for criminal abortion was "The Disgrace of Maternity!!" He contrasted former attitudes where "maternity was once considered a crown of honor" among the best and noblest people of all countries. Hale made reference to claims in the March 13, 1867 *Northwestern Christian Advocate*, editorial, "Criminal Abortion" (Discussed in Chapter 13), that these married women seeking and receiving criminal abortions were from the "most respectable classes" and were "even of high *religious* standing!"[35] However, Hale quickly moved to the problem of the physician losing his business to the less scrupulous physician who met the abortion requests of such prominent families.

> But these gentlemen omit or neglect to mention a fact of which they must have been cognizant, namely: *that the honorable physician who refuses to accede to the wishes of such patrons, is often obliged to see their patronage transferred to other and less scrupulous persons.*
>
> My colleagues will bear me out in the assertion, that such transfer of patronage is a growing evil which needs to be abated by some influence—moral, religious, or legal—which is not now in operation.[36]

Chicago physicians in 1888 would imply that Hale was such a "less scrupulous physician" who stole their patients by providing criminal abortions. Hale's "My colleagues will bear me out in the assertion, that such transfer of patronage is a growing evil," takes on an expanded meaning in light of these charges.

Hale next moved to "Who Are the Criminals?" Foremost among the "principals" was the mother. Only rarely if ever was the abortion done on the woman against her will. Hale noted that the law typically did not reflect this fact, but focused "only on the person who destroys the child." "In fact, she is often more guilty than the person inducing the abortion," He continued, "for she may, by various improper means, as bribes, threats, and other inducements, influence the physician or other person to commit the crime, when his better judgment and principle would revolt against it."

The other "principal" in the crime was "The Abortionist." This "class of creatures" was compared to "the Thugs of India, and murderers everywhere." Their chief business was "to destroy, for money, or worse inducements, the innocent unborn child." (The reader was left to guess what were "worse inducements.") It was in the "great cities" where "these vampires most abound," and the men took various titles including "Accoucher," "Astrologist," and "one who treats 'secret diseases,' or attends to 'private matters.'" "Female Abortionists, assume the name of 'Midwives,' 'Nurses,' 'Fortune-tellers,' 'Madam _____, Female Physician,' *et cetera*," Hale continued, "and under these apparently harmless avocations, ply their murderous trade." He indicated that the business was managed differently in the country: "Hundreds of persons of both sexes, are constantly perambulating the country, stopping in the smaller towns and villages, who have for their chief means of subsistence, no other means of support than the induction of criminal abortion." He indicated they called themselves "'Professors,' 'Doctors,' 'Lecturers,' etc."[37]

Family members too were among the "chief criminals." The "husband, seducer, or unlawful companion" had been known to administer the potion, wield the instrument, or use physical force to "destroy his unborn offspring." Even the mother of the pregnant woman had been known, from "undoubted evidence," to be responsible for the instrument-induced or drug-induced "death of the foetus."

From principals, Hale moved to "accessories before the fact." The "unnatural father of the child, be he husband, seducer, or unlawful companion," fit this category since he typically arranged or otherwise sanctioned the crime. Hale indicated he should be "considered guilty, and should be tried for his participation in the crime, and punished severely."[38]

"Next in venality" were the manufacturers and sellers of "nostrums" extensively used "for criminal purposes." He called for laws punishing the manufacture of these "nostrums." Other accessories before the fact were the "venal publishers of newspapers and periodicals" who published advertisements for the products.

Like Storer, Hale was for making it a crime to advise women to have abortions. He mentioned female friends, "venal nurses," and unprincipled physicians, and called for bringing them to justice "if possible, and a requisite punishment meted out to them."[39] Hale next accused as "accessories before the fact" physicians who failed to treat conditions such as "inflammation and ulceration of the neck of the uterus" that he indicated were a prime cause of spontaneous abortions. These were "sins of omission" and Hale recognized that no law could "at present be framed" to reach these perpetrators. They included the mother and father who were aware of the problem and purposely failed to seek treatment since they preferred the associated miscarriages.[40] Hale appears to be the only physician who considered incriminating physicians and others who did not take available means to prevent spontaneous abortions.

Hale's pamphlet continued by discussing "Accessories To the Fact," i.e., the rare witnesses to the abortion, and "Accessories After the Fact," including the doctors who failed to inform authorities about a criminal abortion when they became aware of it. Following this he discussed "How Shall They be Detected?" and "How Shall They be Punished?" with "They" primarily referring to the principles, i.e., the person or persons requesting the abortion and the person providing it.[41]

Hale then proposed punishments for these principles. He acknowledged his earlier discussion that pregnancy stage was irrelevant, but "until the popular sentiment is educated up to the proper point," he proposed different punishments at different stages. For "embryocide," committing or attempting the crime from conception to the end of the third month, he called for a minimum of seven years imprisonment. For "foeticide," committing or attempting the crime from the end of the third to the end of the sixth month, the penalty would be a minimum of 14 years imprisonment. After the sixth month he referred to the crime as "infanticide" and proposed a minimum 21-year sentence.[42]

Hale ended with an Appendix that included a proposed law written by the prominent Chicago lawyer, Charles Carroll Bonney. Bonney drafted the law after reading Hale's *Great Crime* and it closely followed the pamphlet in specifying the crimes of principals and accessories and outlining punishments for these. Hale praised Bonney's effort and called for passage of a "similar to, or identical" law at the next session of the Legislature.[43]

The "Appendix" included "Testimony Related to Justifiable Foeticide." Hale wrote to current "Professors of Obstetrics and Diseases of Women, in our Medical Colleges," and others with similar experience. The 11 respondents reported that they had rarely been in situations that required destruction of the fetus to save the life of the mother. The few cases typically were craniotomy at full term.[44]

Finally, Hale described his own experience: "In a quite large obstetric practice, extending through nearly sixteen years, I have been obliged to cause the destruction of the foetus but four times, and in each instance it was done *to save the life of the mother.*"[45] As noted earlier, Nicholas Cooke would latch on to this claim of four *necessary* abortions by Hale and indicate that the many other inductions of abortion Hale had described in his 1860 pamphlet must have been *unnecessary*.

The Great Crime was read by Cooke and probably other homeopaths. However, unlike Storer's popular books, Hale's pamphlet appears to have received little distribution. Still, it is possible that it helped make physicians, the public, and legislators aware of *The Great Crime of the Nineteenth Century*. It also probably helped restore Hale to the good graces of those homeopaths that had vilified him for his 1866 *Treatise* blunders. However, it hardly qualified as the "treatise on this subject which shall fully arouse the people, as well as the members of the medical and legal profession, until they shall unite in demanding some special legislation which shall check this great crime" and it did not make him the "esteemed" "benefactor of his race" that Hale forecast as the fate of the author of such a treatise.[46]

CHAPTER 11
BUTLER'S "INFANTIPHOBIA," FALLOUT FROM *WHY NOT?*

The editor of the Philadelphia-based *Medical and Surgical Reporter* was Samuel Worcester Butler, a native of Georgia who obtained his M.D. from the University of Pennsylvania in 1850.[1] Butler's editorials related to criminal abortion increased sharply after Horatio's 1865 Prize Essay was published and this may not have been a coincidence. The first discussed the conviction of a New York abortionist, Charles Cobell, whose attempt to induce abortion resulted in the woman's death. Butler included: "Suffice it to say that the evidence in the case was as shocking as it was conclusive against the prisoner. But the great point to which we wish to call attention, in connection with this case, is the utter inadequacy of the law, as it stands at present, to properly punish these murderers." After details of the case, including Cobell's "light punishment" of two years in prison, Butler wrote:

> We hope that our legislatures will remedy the defects in our present laws regarding child-murder, or criminal abortion. To this end no class of men can contribute more than physicians. Let every influence be exerted to place abortion among the catalogue of the highest criminal offences, with the most severe punishment. Nothing short of this will stop a wide-spread and constantly growing social evil.[2]

Three months later, Butler wrote "A Social Evil—Infantiphobia." It began:

> There is to be found among a numerous class of American women, ... a perversion of the moral instincts of human and *womanly* nature, which it is difficult to account for, and which, unfortunately, finding practical application in the relations of woman, as *wife* and *mother*, has given rise to a social evil, which is daily growing, and threatens to assume almost the character of a national vice. We allude to what may be expressed in one word, coined for the occasion—INFANTIPHOBIA.[3]

Butler discussed the traditional restrictions on women's activities compared to men, then pointed out "there is *one sphere*, at least, in which, if she chooses, she can display without danger of restraint, her full powers and her greatest genius." He continued:

> Or, can the audacity of the so-called *"progressive ideas"* of this century go really so far as to claim that the raising, bringing up, and

educating of children, which was from times immemorial, even among the ancient heathen, considered a sacred one among the duties of the womanly sphere, is entitled to no more consideration than any of the common accidents of life? Can indifference regarding the highest moral obligations of man exercise a more baneful influence than just here, where it undermines the very foundation of society, and saps the roots upon which depends the healthy growth of the *family-life?*[4]

Butler saw only one remedy, "a radical change in female education," which would change current emphases on "ancient and modern poets" that left girls unable

> to take care of themselves, their husbands or their children. And as the latter are of some trouble to the *best* of mothers, no wonder if these poor miseducated girls fall into the traps of abortionists, and become firmly converted to INFANTIPHOBIA.
>
> This is plain talk, but it is needed. The influence of physicians is great in directing family sentiment and education; and it is our duty to counteract with all our might this rapidly growing evil.[5]

A follow-up editorial, "Infantiphobia and Infanticide," described the higher rates of abortion for married women and for those among the higher social classes.[6] Butler again blamed "*misdirected, perverse female education.*"

> We know that it is very fashionable now-a days to talk of the rights of woman. But of what benefit will all legislative protection to secure woman work and proper wages be, if you continue to educate her in the belief that *idleness is her destiny*; that the first duty of the girl is to become a young lady, and get married; that no woman can be a lady who does her own household work, and unless she has a squad of servants about her? *There* is the bottom of the evil, plainly. We must knock out the bottom, if it is to be abolished. Educate girls to consider household work a duty and a pleasure, and to look upon married life as something else than hours of idleness, and you will find happier homes, merrier firesides, and fewer victims of criminal abortion and infanticide.[7]

One physician who responded to the "Infantiphobia" series was "Dr. H. A. Spencer, of Erie, Pa.," who strongly agreed with Butler. Spencer noted the "fearful" extent to which it was carried out and that it was "much more prevalent among married women."[8] He was "surprised that so little is said and published upon a matter of so much importance." He "long desired that our medical journals would give this subject proper attention." He also believed that there were some physicians who "instead of sharply rebuking this practice, tolerate it, under their own eyes, and in many instances even help it on."

Butler did not agree that regular physicians induced abortion unnecessarily:

> The profession, as a whole, has in this matter been true to itself. But there are black sheep in every community, and in every profession, and one of the objects, which we have had in view in opening this discussion, is to arouse the profession to the importance of dealing summarily with such men, and in exerting their influence in favor of stricter legislation regarding the crimes of infanticide and abortion.[9]

"An esteemed correspondent from Washington, D.C." questioned whether married women were seeking abortions to the extent that Butler had described. He indicated that in his forty years he had occasionally had a married woman request an abortion, but had succeeded in discouraging such intentions by pointing out to the woman "the moral and physical objections to such a course."[10] As will be seen, many other physicians would describe their successful persuasion of women to continue pregnancies.

A Brooklyn physician thanked Butler "for your denunciation of the very prevalent practice of abortion among married women."[11] The bulk of his letter dealt with the advertising strategies of the abortionists and sellers of drugs that women used in attempts to induce abortion. Like Flint, Christian, and others, this physician believed that these "noxious drugs" were having the effect of encouraging abortion. He described books published by "villainous quacks" that advised "the process of abortion by one method or another" and advertising the "medicines or instruments of their nefarious trade." "One of them, I learn from the printer," he continued, "has been sold to the extent of over 400,000 copies, and most of the others to the amount of 100,000, or over."[12] The 400,000-copy book probably was *The Married Woman's Private Medical Companion* discussed earlier. It is available for sale today by many used book dealers and a substantial number of libraries own it.

Butler, his *Reporter*, and Storer's Prize Essay were praised by the Zanesville, Ohio physician, Thaddeus A. Reamy, in Reamy's 1866 "Report on Obstetrics" to the Ohio State Medical Society.[13] Reamy indicated that he had encountered much reluctance by physicians to discuss the "delicate subject." "But from a very large verbal and written correspondence in this and other States, together with personal investigation and facts accumulated," he continued, "I am convinced that we have become a nation of murderers."[14] Reamy's "nation of murderers" statement would soon be quoted in the *Northwestern Christian Advocate*.

Reamy noted that physicians were repeatedly consulted about how to end a pregnancy "with as much coolness and businesslike composure ... as would characterize a consultation with a gardener as to plucking weeds from among flowers." He continued:

> If a physician informs them ... that he can not consent to such a thing, that it is murder, he will quite likely be informed that, if he will not, some other will; and it is to be greatly feared others do. ... And the

practice is not confined to the first three of four months of pregnancy. So intent are they often that if success has not attended their efforts sooner, when quickening occurs, instead of having a mother's sympathy aroused, and solicitude for the welfare of her offspring, she is only reminded that she must be prompt in dispatching it before it is larger to give her trouble.[15]

After describing the killing of infants by the Egyptian Pharaoh, the destruction of offspring in the Roman Empire, and the current sacrifices of Hindu and Chinese infants, Reamy wrote:

> But in Christendom, yea, in our own beautiful Ohio, there prattle around the hearthstones of cottages and palaces, children who have dead infant brothers and sisters hidden and unnamed, who were murdered by their parents' hand. What mockery for the voice of evening and morning prayer to be heard, asking God to bless and protect "Willie" and "Ellie," while from the same heart from which goes out the prayer went out the determination to destroy an unborn child! In many instances the pages of the sacred volume are turned for the reading of the morning lesson by the very hand that so recently directed the weapon for destruction. Can God hear with favor the prayer that goes up incensed with the blood of murdered innocence?[16]

Reamy discussed the effects of criminal abortion on women's health, including how it was "filling our cemeteries." He also claimed it was rapidly "prostituting woman from the noble and God-given embodiment of virtue, innocence and affection, which has, and always should, make her an object of adoration and tender care, to a cruel monster whose level is far below the brute."[17]

Reamy was somewhat optimistic that things could change and noted that if women were counseled properly about their fallacious belief that before quickening abortion "did not amount to much," "they will generally desist" in seeking abortion. He called on physicians to avoid being "party to this atrocity" and "to bring to justice and condign punishment any and every medical man in his community who degrades himself to such an office." He concluded:

> Much has been said, and well said, by the editor of the Medical and Surgical Reporter, Philadelphia, against the evils I have been trying to portray. This Journal, an excellent one, should have our warmest commendations for its outspoken fearlessness in condemning this business.[18]

Reamy appended a letter to the Report from John G. Kyle, a Xenia, Ohio physician. It included general obstetric information plus the following on the partakers of criminal abortion:

They, the abortions, occur most frequently among those who are known as the *better class;* amongst church members, and those generally who pretend to be the most polite, virtuous, moral and religious. A venal press—a demoralized clergy—the prevalence of charlatanism, and the reception of the new axiom in morals that, "whatever you may do to gratify the *senses,* or *natural passions* is right, provided, you do not bring *scandal by being found out*," are the principal causes of the fearful increase of the abominable crime of *procuring criminal abortions.*[19]

Kyle's indictment also would be quoted in the *Northwestern Christian Advocate.*

The concerns of Ohio physicians about criminal abortion were communicated to their Legislature and in February 1867 the Ohio Senate passed a bill strengthening the state's abortion law. The special committee that generated the new legislation provided a Report that was included in the Senate Journal and 200 extra copies were printed at the request of another Senator. The Report first mentioned the epidemic of criminal abortion "in one of the Eastern States" and speculated that, if statistics were available, "Ohio would not show a much better state of things." The Report included:

We are happy to say that regular physicians are not responsible for the state of things described. The American Medical Association, composed of delegates from all the States and Medical Colleges, appointed a committee to report upon this evil, and at its annual meeting in Boston, in June 1865, awarded a gold medal to Prof. Horatio Robinson Storer, for an able essay upon this subject. From this essay we have drawn many of the facts presented in this report. The Ohio Medical Society also, at its last meeting, made an appeal to this Legislature to enact more stringent laws upon the subject.[20]

Storer was the only physician mentioned in the Report, but Reamy and Kyle likely were involved in their Society's appeal. The *Northwestern Christian Advocate,* would shortly note how "the statute laws of Ohio, Massachusetts, New York, Virginia, Michigan, Wisconsin and other states now conform to the remodeled theory of gestation." By 1880 nearly all would do so and some of these efforts, like Ohio's, probably were supported by the most readily available antiabortion literature, *Why Not? A Book for Every Woman.*

The Maine Medical Association formed a Committee on the Production of Abortion that was chaired by Dr. Israel Thorndike Dana, Professor of Theory and Practice of Medicine at the Medical School of Maine. Dana's Report included quotes of Percival, Beck, Storer, and others to make the case that a human being existed from conception and that its unnecessary destruction was a form of murder.[21] Dana provided a hypothetical example to emphasize this:

A woman conceives and soon after conception has occurred her husband dies. The child he had begotten is, by the common law, his father's heir. The father may have been the King of England or the Czar of all the Russias. Some interested party desires to divert the inheritance into another channel, and assumes the responsibility of destroying this young life.

Who will pretend that the moral character of the act is materially changed whether that life is destroyed at three months or at ten months after conception? It is only a question of "intra-uterine murder", or extra-uterine murder.[22]

Dana also had some unique words about the immense pressure to procure an unnecessary abortion that a physician experienced from his regular patients. He discussed the situation when an illegitimate pregnancy threatened a family's good name:

"Out of pity, Doctor:" "For the love of God." These are some of the appeals that most move the generous heart, and *tempt* the mind to look about for some pretext to interfere and save this private grief and shame, already too terrible to bear, from all the further agony of rude exposure to the public gaze. But what can he do? *Nothing but pity*. It is evident that natural sympathy, though entirely proper and amiable in itself, is no reason to justify the physician in committing a second and at least equal crime, to conceal the one already perpetrated. If another has been guilty of breaking the seventh commandment, he may not on that account transgress the sixth.[23]

However, these disgraces on an honorable family, "a thousand times worse than death," were not the main cause of criminal abortion. "[T]he most remarkable and appalling feature of the case," he wrote, "is that it prevails chiefly amongst married and otherwise respectable women." Dana identified the "one great reason" for the prevalence of criminal abortion: "Undoubtedly many women still believe, and many more try hard to believe, that there is no sin in it if the thing is done at an early date of pregnancy."[24] Other factors he cited as promoting criminal abortion were the availability of abortionists, the makers and sellers of abortifacients; the authors of books promoting abortion; the newspaper publishers who advertised the drugs and books; lawyers and judges who protected abortionists when they came to trial; Governors who pardon the few convicted; and "all those members of society both male and female, who solicit, consent to, or in any way encourage the use of any of the means of procuring miscarriage." Dana then warned his physician audience that of all the factors promoting the "perverted sentiment and practice" of criminal abortion, "no one else can possibly do so much harm, or incur so fearful a load of guilt as a physician in regular and reputable standing, provided he lends himself to the practice."[25]

In his 1871 Presidential Address to the American Association of Medical Editors, Horatio Storer would comment on how few physicians read medical journals.[26] Probably only a few physicians attended medical society meetings such as the meeting where Dana presented his Report. The physician most willing to "lend himself to the practice" may have been the physician least likely to hear or read Dana's words implicating him as doing the most harm.

Horatio's Prize Essay was published in April 1866 as *Why Not? A Book for Every Woman* with no changes other than a few unplanned omissions of quotation marks and footnotes. Horatio did add to the "Prefatory Remarks" and added an "Appendix" where he discussed his views on anesthetics during labor and noted that these were not universally held by physicians of the American Medical Association.[27] This disclaimer was prompted by his unidentified Philadelphia friend who requested that Horatio drop the recommendations in the essay for "use of anaesthesia in all cases of labor."

Why Not? was reviewed by Butler's *Medical and Surgical Reporter* in July1866.[28] This review was generally favorable and included the recommendation: "we wish and hope for it an extended circulation and many readers." However, Butler regretted "that in a few instances the earnestness of the author leads him to speak in a tone almost of exaggeration, which in this, as in *every* case, must so far weaken the cause upheld." One instance Butler cited was Horatio's claim that some means for preventing pregnancy led to the "'evils and dangers, mental and physical, of self-abuse.'"

The *Boston Medical and Surgical Journal* did not get around to their mention and brief review of *Why Not?* until the end of August.[29] This three-month delay no doubt was related to some lingering animosity of the editors who had condemned Horatio in late April for an article in the *Medical Record* accusing the Boston physician, Calvin Ellis, of "vivisection" during an autopsy.[30] Their review was generally positive, although they questioned whether criminal abortion "be so general as some, whose special practice is the most likely to bring them into cognizance of it, are led to believe." They also indicated that the title would better have made some actual reference to the subject of the book. "It will be likely to excite curiosity," they concluded, "among those who are too young to need to have the subject presented to their minds; and who, in our estimation, had better not know anything of such things until maturity of years or the marriage relation has drawn aside the veil with which we should prefer to keep them enshrouded."[31]

The *New Orleans Medical and Surgical Journal* presented a highly critical review of *Why Not?* a year after the book's publication. One illustrative paragraph read:

> While we admit the general incumbency upon writers for a medical journal to avoid all disparaging personal allusions to authors whose works are being reviewed, our sense of duty leads us, in this instance, to a different course. We honestly believe that, if we can, by truthful statements or well-sustained suspicions disparaging to this book or its author, counteract its general circulation, we shall thereby subserve the cause of virtue and morality.[32]

The following indicates some of the writer's objections:

The title of the book is, in itself, such an offence against public decorum and good manners, that it justifies a relentless crusade for its expulsion from general marts of literature. It presents obtrusive and immodest claims for general notice; it is not a book for some women, for certain women, for those women whom it may concern, but it is "a book for *every* woman" (so-called). No lady can enter a book store which tolerates such literature upon its shelves, without danger of being victimized by the Yankee ingenuity of the title, so prettily printed in gilt letters upon the cover.[33]

Horatio quickly became aware of this diatribe against him and his book, and even against New England and the North. Horatio recommended it "to all lovers of truly scientific criticism" in an article on masturbation in women published a month after the scathing review appeared.[34]

On June 5, 1866, Mrs. Caroline Dall, of Boston, "a lady of great intellectual and moral worth, well known indeed throughout the country" (as Horatio described her in his next book), wrote a highly complementary letter to Horatio related to *Why Not?* which she had just "laid down." Her letter included: "But the book needs a counterpart addressed to *men*. Till *they* are willing to spend as freely for wife and children as for the mistress, hidden but a few doors off, women will hardly be free agents in this matter. No woman dreads her travail, as she dreads the loss of what she calls, in her unhappy ignorance and blindness, her husband's love."[35]

Horatio responded:

My dear Madam,

 Want of a moment's leisure has prevented me from acknowledging your kind note till now. Your comments are very just, & I may take occasion to print them, in part or in whole, in case my publishers think best to issue another edition of "Why Not?" & you do not object. Were you to send a terse & Dallian notice of the book to one of our Journals, say to the Atlantic, I doubt not it would aid greatly in its circulation.

 As for myself, my time is now so wholly engrossed that I am unable to look after the welfare of any such fledgling once launched from the nest.

Yrs sincerely
Horatio R. Storer[36]

One could argue that his request for a "terse & Dallian notice of the book" represented very much a "look after the welfare" of his "fledgling" *Why Not?*

The *Boston Medical and Surgical Journal* was to make two more references to *Why Not?*. One was a long letter published November 1, 1866 entitled, "'Why Not? A Book for Every Woman.' A Woman's View."[37] A footnote of the editors indicated that the author was "the wife of a Christian physician," from "one of our most distant New England towns" and not from Massachusetts. The editors hoped her expression of "the universal feeling of her sex" on the subject "might find its

way, in some more popular form than our pages afford, to the eyes of every husband in the land." The thrust of the lady's letter was that many women were victims of husbands who forced sex on them indiscriminately, preventing the timing
of intercourse that could prevent unwanted pregnancy. These inconsiderate husbands were apt to blame the woman for her condition when she became pregnant.
It was understandable that some women would opt for measures to prevent birth,
particularly if they believed that they were not taking a life when the abortion was
induced early in pregnancy. She claimed that abortion was not a consideration of
women with sympathetic husbands. For the "worthy husband," "careful for her
comfort and her preferences," "be she ever so slight and fragile, ever so much adverse to motherhood," "she will bear it all, even to the end, cheerfully."[38] "If Dr.
Storer will perform as noble service for our brothers and husbands, as for ourselves," she concluded, "and send the two books out hand in hand, they will bring
him back a rich harvest of gratitude, and amendment in morals."[39]

The woman's letter so closely mimicked Horatio's views on use of chloro-
form during childbirth; the high and increasing frequency of criminal abortion; the
agony of childbirth, "akin to nothing else on earth;" and the unspeakable vice of
holding fashion as god that it could have been written by Horatio himself.
However, Horatio would later expressly deny any knowledge of who wrote it
when he called attention to it in *Is It I?*

A few weeks later, the *Boston Medical and Surgical Journal* published a
letter praising the letter providing "A Woman's View." It too is a little incredible,
but Horatio later also indicated no knowledge of the author of the following:

> Messrs. Editors,—I cannot refrain from expressing my feelings of
> thankfulness at your publication of "A Woman's View," in a late num-
> ber of your Journal, relative to abortion. Dr. Storer's work had already
> been brought to my attention with—as must be the result to every right-
> minded man—approval; but the addenda, or rather complement, of his
> valuable little book, lies in that "nutshell of pertinence," the article re-
> ferred to. I lit upon your Journal by the merest chance. I am on the eve
> of marriage myself, and though not a whit more sensual than most men,
> cannot be too grateful for having thus forcibly brought to my mind a
> view which I for one had doubtless scarce otherwise considered. I
> would to God that it might meet and claim the serious consideration of
> every man born of woman's agony.
> Yours very truly,
> A Fighter for the Right Against Wrong.[40]

Many coincidences were required to produce this letter. The author, though
male, had read and approved *Why Not? A Book for Every Woman*; though apparently not involved in medicine, he had read the issue of the *Boston Medical and
Surgical Journal* with the lady's "view;" and though single, he was unusually
aware of woman's agony during childbirth. Not the least coincidence was the remarkable pertinence of "A Fighter's" letter for another book that would communicate "to every man" "A Woman's View." Still, there is another plausible explana-

tion for the letter from "A Fighter" and for "A Woman's View" other than Horatio lying about not being the writer. Despite Horatio's problems with the medical powers of Boston and Harvard, we know that Henry Orlando Marcy and other students at the Harvard Medical School strongly supported him in his battles with the establishment. Marcy in 1910 referred to his "ardent" early defense of Horatio in the following:

> There is no doubt that Dr. Storer was the "best-hated" member of the profession in Massachusetts. A long and dangerous illness removed him from the active arena and years were spent in Europe in quest of health, unfortunately never fully restored. He gave brilliant promise of being the leader of gynecology in America, notwithstanding the vituperative abuse unsparingly showered on him by men who should have known better. A generous share of this attention was bestowed on me as his ardent defender. I have somewhere a letter of his, written at the time, containing a touching appeal to forget him and his service to suffering humanity lest it work my ruin. He is a man of strong magnetic power, quick of thought and action, fluent of speech, equally ready to attack his enemies and to defend himself; and there are yet many who hold his service in grateful remembrance.[41]

It may have been a pair of these strong supporters who provided to the *Boston Medical and Surgical Journal* these letters that were so very favorable to Horatio, to some of his most controversial ideas, and to his new supplemental career as an author of popular books on criminal abortion.

CHAPTER 12
STORER'S AND OTHERS' ADDRESSES

Horatio Storer read a paper, "The Abetment of Criminal Abortion by Medical Men," at the May 30, 1866 annual meeting of the Massachusetts Medical Society.[1] Horatio referred to his 1859 "abetment" article and its theme that "by any apparent disregard of the existence or sanctity of foetal life, however evinced, we in reality increased its disregard by the community." He provided a new example of physician abetment of criminal abortion that involved the Councillors of the group he was addressing. This was the 1858 decision of the Massachusetts Medical Society Committee on Abortion "that 'the laws of the commonwealth are already sufficiently stringent, provided they are executed.'" Horatio noted that his "earnest protest" against the Committee's action in his absence "seems never to have been acted upon." Horatio named each of the six other members of the 1857-1858 Committee and then spread the blame to the rest of the Councillors who had approved the 1858 Resolutions that omitted the recommendation to address the legislature. Horatio cited this as another instance "where the profession become directly accountable for the increased frequency of the crime."

Horatio went on to discuss other physician actions that abetted abortion, including the frequent resort to unnecessary craniotomy when "turning," long forceps, or prematurely induced labor would allow the survival of the child. Most serious, however, in his list of physician "abetments" was the induction of abortion for medical reasons, other than for saving the life of child or mother.

Horatio quoted the paragraph from his 1859 "Its Perpetrators" that claimed abortion was almost never performed by regular physicians. He then waffled on this point:

> On the other hand, it is no uncommon thing for women of good position to assert to me that abortion has been induced for them by gentlemen of excellent standing in the profession, especially among the older men, and I am constantly conferred with by other physicians to whom similar charges have been made. Allowing, as I cheerfully do, that many, perhaps the majority, of such allegations must be false, still there is in a certain number of cases a foundation in truth.[2]

No doubt some of these women would have also identified their abortionist. When Horatio strongly suggested that some of "the older men" might have been abortionists it is possible that he was aiming a barb at specific members of his audience who had been so identified by these women. However, this time he did not name names.

The Minutes of that Massachusetts Medical Society meeting indicated:

Dr H. R. Storer read a paper on "The Abetment of Criminal Abortion by Medical Men."

Dr Hartwell (of Southboro') moved a vote of thanks, & also that Dr Storer's Essay be published by the Society. An Amendment was offered that it be submitted to the Committee on Publications. Dr Ordway spoke against the Amendment. The Amendment was carried; and the original motion withdrawn.[3]

Horatio apparently did not even receive the "vote of thanks" portion of Hartwell's motion. The Committee on Publications turned the paper down and Horatio published it in the *New York Medical Journal*.

A new journal, *The Medical Record*, was published in New York beginning in 1866. The editor was George F. Shrady, a New York City physician who had served as a surgeon during the Civil War. Shrady would later come into prominence when he attended Ulysses S. Grant during Grant's last illness. One of Shrady's first references to criminal abortion was published in July 1866:

At the twenty-sixth annual meeting of the Hampden County Massachusetts District Medical Society recently held, the following resolutions relative to the alarming increase of the crime of abortion were unanimously adopted:—

Whereas criminal abortion has become an alarming evil by its frequency in society; and

Whereas many suppose it to be a crime of little magnitude,

Resolved, That we deem it our duty to society, to publicly express our opinion of its nature and criminality, and also the detestation in which we hold all who may in any way abet the crime.

Resolved, That we regard the unwarrantable taking of life of the unborn foetus at any time after conception in a moral sense, as much the crime of murder as to destroy the infant at full term.[4]

Their resolution to hold in detestation "all who may in any way abet the crime," may have been stimulated by Horatio's recent paper condemning such physician abetment. Horatio may have provided these Resolutions of his probable Massachusetts' supporters to Shrady, since Horatio published a letter in the same July 16 *Medical Record* that dealt with his definite Massachusetts' detractors.[5]

Edmund Potts Christian again claimed criminal abortion was the taking of a human life in a paper read before the Wayne County Medical Society.[6] Christian noted that abortion was justified "only when the safety of the mother is depending upon it." He indicated this followed from the "dangers, both immediate and remote," associated with abortions and miscarriages regardless of cause, "but the profession plants itself on even higher ground, and champions the rights of 'the unborn being, whose destruction is thereby accomplished."[7]

Christian discussed how women openly approached physicians with requests for abortion and blamed this on the public's "mistaken estimate of the standard of morality in the medical profession, as it regards this subject."[8] He blamed the public's "mistaken estimate" on men with low moral standards who falsely called themselves physicians and on the "glaring advertisements" in daily newspapers for "such things as should be named only in the lecture room, or in the *confessional* between patient and physician."[9]

Christian called on physicians to aggressively educate the public to the physicians' standard of morality on the issue. He claimed that physicians alone were in position to "properly expose, and successfully oppose" the wrongs and errors that were contributing to the crime. "We are missionaries," he concluded, "having a dispensation of Divine wisdom and goodness, as revealed in the gospel of human physiology, to preach and make its application to those wrongs and sins which cannot be reached from the pulpit."[10]

A Vermont physician, William McCollom, made reference to another way that physicians abetted abortion:

> I fear that there are too many physicians who understand well their professional obligations and duties, and possess a correct moral sense of right and wrong, who come near being unintentional abettors of the crime by failing to reject with indignity and warning, applications made to them to commit an act in flagrant violation of human and divine law. For fear of offending, the applicants are turned away with a recommendation to do this, or that, the physician knowing it will do no good, or harm.[11]

Other physicians would mention the problem associated with giving a "recommendation" or placebo "that will do no good or harm" and thus leaving the applicant for abortion with the belief that the physician did not view abortion as a crime. One of these also was named William McCollom, whose 1896 address was "Brooklyn, N. Y." (See Chapter 24).

We have speculated that Horatio was a stimulus for the antiabortion editorials of Samuel Worcester Butler. Horatio and his Prize Essay may also have stimulated a paper by the prominent Detroit physician, Morse Stewart.[12] Stewart began:

> The subject of criminal abortion has been so fully discussed by Dr. H. R. Storer of Boston, in a paper published in the *Boston Medical and Surgical Journal* of February 5th, 1863; as also in a prize essay, read before the American Medical Association at its sixteenth annual meeting held in June, 1865; and since published, in a popular form for general distribution, as to leave but little further to be said in relation to it. The essay, while it treats of the subject in a clear and succinct manner, is sufficiently comprehensive—and must, if anything can do so, carry to the mind of the reader conviction of the author's conclusions. It should be in the library of every physician, not only for his own profit, but also that, he may have always at hand the means of instruction and warning to his patients; and through its appeals to *selfish* interests, where higher considerations fail, to restrain in them any previously

formed purpose to evil.[13]

Stewart indicated that abortion "has from time immemorial been regarded by the profession, as a crime; and for any of its members to be guilty of it, is derogatory to the whole body." "The legitimate cause which furnished the only exception, is and can only be, a necessity growing out of conditions, from which the life of the mother, or child, or both is in jeopardy;" he continued, "and even on this point—so sensitive has the mind of the profession ever been upon the propriety of sacrificing the foetus *in utero*—that some of its members have always opposed it.[14]

After a long state-of-the-science discussion of fertilization of the ovum and its separate existence, Stewart wrote that the fertilized ovum

> certainly is a new existence; and she from whom it springs, has no more right to destroy and cast from her the minute organic living atom, than she has to turn from and leave to perish in its helplessness, the newborn babe, given to her at the fullness of mature gestation. This is now the conclusion of the medical world, whoever causes intentionally the destruction of the impregnated ovum is guilty of taking life, and that the life of a human being. This is nothing less than murder.[15]

Stewart was aware that some physicians were willing to procure abortions for their patients. He wrote:

> [W]hat language can express the utter baseness of that man, whose education has been that of a *physician*, whose *standing in society* is that of a *physician*, (a word, which should be held by every man in the profession as synonymous with honor, honesty, integrity, and an earnest, single hearted purpose to preserve human life) what shall we say of such a man, dishonoring his profession, making it a stench in the nostrils of society, debasing his own conscience, by becoming a *murderer*? Stimulated to murder by no hot and fiery passion, he breaks the sixth commandment, for what? For greed! He sells his own soul; he demoralizes all with whom he comes in contact; he sells that boon which no wealth can buy, for thirty beggarly bits of silver. May the doom of the arch traitor fall upon him! "Let his days be few, and let another take his office,—Let his posterity be cut off; and in the generation following let their name be blotted out."[16]

Stewart concluded with discussion of the popular study of physiology. He was convinced this "has already accomplished as much or more towards the present fearful prevalence of induced abortion, as any known cause of this great wickedness."[17]

In 1867, a Catholic physician, Edward P. LeProhon, published a "short essay," the object of which was to show: "Feticide, or voluntary abortion, is a crime of the most odious character, impeaching the wisdom of the Creator, and degrading the nature of man."[18] To show "the extent of this criminal habit amongst American ladies," LeProhon quoted Storer's comments about "the wretch" "heaviest with guilt" who "too often becomes a heroine."[19]

LeProhon claimed that "immoral and criminal advertisements in daily journals" were responsible for "a large proportion of the increase of abortion among married women."[20] "As a drop of water, constantly falling will wear away even the solid rock," he wrote, "so the habitual reading of such advertisements must make a fatal impression upon the minds of females who read them."[21] He called for "serious attention of legislators, who could soon put a stop to the scandalous advertisements of quack doctors," and chided Massachusetts legislators for severely punishing the sale of liquors instead of looking "out for the morals of wives and daughters!"[22]

LeProhon noted from his experience in "communities where both Catholics and Protestants are mixed up," that criminal abortion was "mostly" among the Protestants. He claimed Roman Catholicism was the only means to "reach the evil."[23] As will be seen, the Episcopal Bishop of Western New York would take issue with LeProhon's thesis of Protestant incapability of dealing with criminal abortion and even with LeProhon's claim that Catholics were less guilty of the crime.

LeProhon praised "some of the most distinguished members of the American Medical Association" for their "able papers" on abortion "since 1859." However, "very little good, if any, has been effected by their united efforts, and I fear that something more than their good advice will be required to check the increase of abortion in the United States."[24]

If Horatio Storer became aware of LeProhon's claims that physicians' "united efforts" had produced "very little good," he surely disagreed. However, abortion rates may not have been dropping as a result of Storer's crusade. In a March 1867 editorial, George F. Shrady claimed that abortion was *increasing*. He noted:

> So prevalent is the belief that criminal abortion is extensively practiced, that arguments are unnecessary to further establish it. During many years past the subject has claimed the attention of medical men in every country; resolutions condemnatory of the crime have been passed by medical bodies everywhere; papers almost without number have been written about it; legislation, religion, morality, and physical well-being, have all been in turn appealed to; but all efforts to arrest its progress have not only proven futile, but worse than this, we have undeniable assurances that it is on the increase.[25]

"We do not propose to remark upon the general subject of abortion," Shrady continued, "as it has long since been worn threadbare; in fact, we should consider ourselves as having no excuse to allude to its general prevalence and increase, were it not that some new facts have lately transpired which invest it with no little interest."[26] The "new facts" were from the Lowell, Massachusetts physician, Nathan Allen, whose research showed a sharp reduction of children in the current families of English immigrants in Massachusetts compared to previous generations. Allen also reported fewer children in the current families of these "natives" compared to the families of recent immigrants. Allen's initial article, "Vital Statistics of Massachusetts," was published in the October 4, 1866 *New York Observer*.[27] Allen actually did not mention criminal abortion, only "the settled determination among a large portion of them in married life *to have no children, or a very limited number*."[28] Shrady probably read Allen's article when it was republished in a *Boston Medical and Surgical Journal* editorial that referred to criminal abortion as "the chief causes [sic] of this deplorable condition of society."[29] Shrady feared that the same result was true in New York and other states and he called for further investigations, since he believed the drop in births of the "natives" was a major cause for alarm.[30]

It is puzzling that only ten years after Horatio started the physicians' crusade, Shrady viewed the "general subject of abortion" as having "long since been worn threadbare" and that "papers almost without number have been written about it." Some physicians, like "Dr. H. A. Spencer, of Erie, Pa.," were "surprised that so little is said and published upon a matter of so much importance," and "long desired that our medical journals would give this subject proper attention." Spencer had published his letter in the *Medical and Surgical Reporter* in response to Butler's "Infantiphobia" editorials. Shrady may have been finding fault with the abundance of material dealing with criminal abortion in that competing journal when he described the subject as "long since been worn threadbare." As will be shown, this "general subject of abortion" would continue to be discussed and almost unanimously condemned in medical articles for decades. What is more, many of these articles would be published in Shrady's *Medical Record*.

CHAPTER 13

PROTESTANT EFFORTS AGAINST ABORTION

Several references have been made to the editorial, "Criminal Abortion," published on March 13, 1867 in the Chicago-based *Northwestern Christian Advocate*, a popular Methodist newspaper.[1] This rare discussion of criminal abortion by a non-Catholic religious authority received considerable attention from the medical press and may have been a powerful influence on the general public. The Editor of the *Advocate* was Rev. Thomas Mears Eddy and the Associate Editor was Rev. Arthur Edwards. They described their article in a second editorial as "our Report," "our recent article," and as "an utterance of our solemn convictions."[2] It began:

Nine years ago, at the bedside of a repenting, dying woman, reputed a Christian, we received the first shuddering glimpse of an evil which, as we expect to show, is fearfully wide-spread and a suicidal crime. The suspicion there and then startled into existence has, by years of observation, some medical reading and abundance of professional testimony, been shocked into the resistless conviction which prompts this article. That dying woman was a type of thousands who by attacks upon foetal life, involve the added responsibility of suicide. Clad in darkness we were powerless to dispel, she was descending into a valley darker than David's, and, where a papal priest must have refused absolution, we could only thankfully remember that "with God all things are possible."[3]

The editors noted their present "duty" was "not pleasant," their efforts might "prove thankless," and some readers would be shocked and offended. They continued:

We expect to show that a species of Infanticide is fearfully prevalent in American society—that the practice is murder—that it is a prolific and almost exclusive source of American female diseases—that it eclipses in iniquity, and is promotive of nearly all other social crimes, and that, therefore, the prevalent toleration and excuses for the practice are outrages against decency, humanity, and high Heaven.[4]

The editors then honored the medical profession for its contributions, but noted that its efforts only reached "a tithe of the people" and were "powerless to create that correct Christian sentiment which will throttle the monster abuse and socially outlaw the unnatural sinner against God." "Those two mighty movers of moral reform, the Pulpit and Religious Press," they continued, "must at once come to the rescue." They further complimented the physicians:

> We are, however, very glad to have in advance the example of accomplished authors, the expressed wishes of eminent physicians of Chicago and elsewhere, and a file of letters pleading for discussion of the subject in these columns where it will reach more of the people of this country than have ever before been reached by the theme.[5]

The editors mentioned a "private note from Dr. Storer of Boston" and Horatio surely was among those "pleading for discussion." The Storer contact also may explain another comment that there had been "ten years" of discussion of the problem by the medical profession. Storer had initiated his crusade exactly ten years earlier.

The editors quoted Thaddeus Reamy, Hugh Lenox Hodge, Morse Stewart, and Horatio Storer to document the prevalence of criminal abortion and described "one little village of one thousand," of which one or both apparently had direct knowledge:

> Miscarriages are frequent and certain uninstructed or embruted feminine circles have their centers where the means employed and successes attained are topics of exchangeable information. For instance, we could to [sic] prove that in one little village of one thousand inhabitants, prominent women have been guilty of what we will presently show to be *murder*. And, sadder still, half of these are members of Christ's Church. Yet here, and elsewhere, where fifteen per cent of wives have the criminal hardihood to practice this black art, there is a still larger and additional per cent who endorse and defend it. One of the worst features of the case is the fact that if a young, pure and inexperienced wife is shocked by revelations made by hardened abortionists, she is straightway ridiculed into silence, or argued into acquiescence. The very worst feature, however, is that young girls, too young to marry, are initiated into these mysteries of massacre, thoroughly imbued with a dislike of children, especially their future own, and are thus prepared to perpetuate this horrid villiany [sic] when; their more aged instructors are gone up before God.[6]

Their "little village" would find its way into several medical articles, editorials, and books.

They discussed how "gangs of scoundrels" sent "vile circulars promising immunity from offspring to all newly married couples" and decried the newspapers "whose satanic advertisements of quack nostrums and quack doctors further this fearful Evil." They reluctantly admitted that criminal abortion was sometimes endorsed and even resorted to by "not only the pews but the pulpit," and quoted Dr. Kyle's claim that criminal abortion occurred "most frequently" "amongst church members and those generally who pretend to be the most polite, virtuous, moral and religious."

As evidence of criminal abortion's prevalence the editors reported Horatio's fetal death statistics from Massachusetts and New York. They noted that registration systems were not operating in the "younger states" "or we might be similarly overwhelmed with unwelcome truth." "It is sufficient to know that Doctors Storer, Hodge, Stewart, Byford, Davis, Jewell, Roler and others," they continued, "believe that the persistent system of foetal extermination has been increasing in prevalence and success since the years upon which published statistics are based." The last four, William Heath Byford, Nathan Smith Davis, James Stewart Jewell, and Edward O. Roler were prominent Chicago physicians and medical professors. Davis had been the major impetus for founding of the American Medical Association. We earlier noted his disagreement with Brainard about the dangers of induced abortion (See Chapter 5) and he was a major player in a Chicago expose of physician abortionists in 1888 (See Chapter 22).

The editors next provided proofs that procured abortion was in some degree murder. They cited John Brodhead Beck to show that life existed from conception and Storer to show that quickening was irrelevant to the magnitude of the crime. The editors then summarized recent appropriate law changes:

Ancient authorities and decisions and laws were based upon absurd theories, but the legislation of later years is more in harmony with more recent medical science, hence the statute laws of Ohio, Massachusetts, New York, Virginia, Michigan, Wisconsin and other states now conform to the remodeled theory of gestation. A private note from Dr. Storer, of Boston, informs us that vigorous measures are being taken to so change the laws of a few remaining states that statutes may secure the punishment which is escaped under certain constructions of the common law.[7]

The editors described the fine record of the early Christian Church in defending the unborn and contrasted it to present day Protestantism, which they claimed was "blackly stained by this crime of child-murder." They noted that "among the many errors of the Papal Church, foeticide does not appear," and claimed this could lead to Catholic dominance in the population. "We neglect the commandment," they began, "kill the children, enervate and finally kill the mother, and involve the possible murder of our Protestant dominance on this continent."

The editors then discussed "the fearful throng of diseases resulting from foeticide." They presented Storer's claim that abortion was "a greater tax upon a woman's health and more surely followed by uterine disease" than giving birth. Quotes from Byford and Davis provided similar conclusions. A long list of "calamitous results" for the woman who aborted followed. One was uterine displacement, and the editors claimed that this was so rare in England "that good treatment must be sought in Edinburgh."[8] They indicated that "here that pest is omnipresent, as one of God's penalties for child murder." Storer probably provided the information about the different frequency of uterine displacements in the two countries and probably also recommended his Edinburgh mentor, Simpson, as the source of "good treatment."

Criminal abortion was seen as a source of "weak, stunted, diseased, deformed, idiotic or insane" children. This they claimed applied to the child surviving a failed attempt at abortion and to children born in pregnancies occurring after a criminal abortion. "An equally common and more just result" was sterility, and Storer was cited as a source on this along with an unnamed physician who claimed 50 of his patients were sterile because of their abortions.

The editors criticized various excuses given for abortion. These included poverty, ill health, "demands of fashion," and unwillingness "to perpetuate malignant disease or hereditary insanity." For the latter, they indicated the couple never should have married, but having done so, should "[l]eave the little ones to God's mercy and save the parents' souls from an ineffaceable stain of guilt."[9]

Their final section was "Foeticide Promotes Other Crimes." They believed that there was an increase of infanticide as a result, and that homicides were increased as well, since both were now being treated leniently in the courts following the model of lenient treatment of criminal abortion. They also saw the child, born after an unsuccessful abortion attempt, imprinted with the mother's "intense emotion" of "*meditated murder.*" The child was a likely candidate to "some day appear in court as a murderer."[10] They did not identify any physician or other authority for this notion that would be repeated by John Harvey Kellogg a few years later and by other physicians even into the twentieth century.

More justifiable was their hypothesis that criminal abortion increased divorce: "One parent's natural love for little children may be brought into direct antagonism with the foeticidal dislike of the other and from this disturbance of the very design of the marriage relation, discord must result—and divorce is made easy."

The editors briefly touched on ways to correct the problem. Their recommendation that abortionists be "purified by fire" in the following would be quoted by several physicians in their articles condemning abortion and abortionists:

> The primary causes of, and the proper measures for correcting this national tendency to Foeticide are important topics which must be reserved from this article. We cannot, however, refrain from indicating and condemning a potent agency—a[ny] newspaper whose satanic advertisements of quack nostrums and quack doctors further this fearful Evil, should be treated as a social Enemy, and its unscrupulous publishers be socially outlawed.
>
> Quack Doctors, Irregular Practitioners and the whole race of vagrant female hyenas who will take foetal life for fifty dollars and gratuitously kill or ruin the credulous wife or "unfortunate," should be treated as pests to be "purified by fire," if necessary. The odor of such a burnt offering would be more grateful than their offenses which smell to Heaven.
>
> Don't fear chaste, open discussion, even with such young persons as you are entitled to instruct. The plain, vital truth of a delicate but in-

evitable subject is far more pure than the uninstructed devices of the human heart. "The Truth shall make you free" of the evil which is working such calamitous results.

The Methodist Church may, or may not, be involved—but her past agency in breasting all waves of iniquity is a matter of history and that future agency will be equally sure. Pulpit and Press must echo the cry until the cry is heeded. We would be glad to soon see a small, compact, inexpensive tract upon the topic come from our presses and be distributed by multiplied thousands for the instruction of our Methodist millions.

We gratefully acknowledge our obligations to Doctors W. H. Byford, N. S. Davis, J. S. Jewell and E. O. F. Roler and others of Chicago, and to Doctors H. R. Storer, of Boston, T. A. Reamy, of Zanesville, Morse Stewart, of Detroit, and others. The kind words or letters of encouragement, and the documents furnished us have proved vitally important to this extended paper. "Why Not?" by Dr. Storer, we especially commend.[11]

Almost all of Horatio's papers dealing with abortion were mentioned in the article. They probably were enclosures to the "private note from Dr. Storer, of Boston."

A follow-up discussion of their editorial two weeks later included only a fraction of the letters they received from ministers and physicians praising their effort. "The article revised, enlarged and strengthened at all points," they concluded, "will be speedly [sic] issued in *very* cheap form, and will go out on its errand, at cost price. We wish we had money enough to give away a million copies."[12] Efforts to locate this revised article have been unsuccessful.

The *Boston Medical and Surgical Journal* called attention to the *Advocate's* "most timely, able and judicious" article in their issue of March 21, 1867.

We welcome this effort as one in the right direction, from the right source—a religious journal; for the newspaper obviously reaches the very readers who now need to be influenced in this matter—the non-professional public; and we are sure that to put a stop to the wholesale "massacre of the innocents," which is bringing shame to American civilization and *Protestantism* (for the Romanists are not guilty of it), it is only needed that the religious conscience of American women should be enlightened and aroused. From a late number of a Western medical journal the cry of "murder" has been sounded, and an almost heart-rending appeal gone forth to all Christian mothers in the land to stay the hand of assassination of their unborn offspring.[13]

The "cry" from "a late number of a Western medical journal" probably was the article by Morse Stewart. Detroit was still "Western" in 1867.

Shrady's *Medical Record* also made reference to the *Advocate* article, calling it "a well written, elaborate, and truthful article, [that] fearlessly commences the discussion of this subject." Shrady indicated it was the first time that "a religious paper has dared to give the theme a fair and full notice." He hoped other such periodicals would follow this example, "as by the proper presentation of the ample facts in the case it will undoubtedly be productive of great good."[14]

The *Buffalo Medical And Surgical Journal* referred to the *Advocate* article as "the first public discussion of the subject we have ever known."[15] They obviously were unaware of Gardner's January 1860 article in the *Knickerbocker*. The editors reproduced several paragraphs from the article including the four objectives and the claim that both medical writing on criminal abortion and the large increase in prevalence of criminal abortion were ten years old. Other excerpts included the Protestant Church "blackly stained" by criminal abortion, and "one little village of one thousand inhabitants" where half the women obtaining criminal abortions "are members of Christ's Church."

The editors added the following footnote after stating that the *Advocate* article was "the first public discussion of the subject."

> Since the above article was written, we have received *The Congregationalist*, containing an article from Rev. John Todd, D.D., upon this subject. He says: "I appeal to New England women—the daughters of an ancestry who never were spotted with the blood of innocents, who never stifled the natural longings of a mother's heart and never quenched life immortal for the sake of ease or fashion and ask them if it is so, that they are so degenerated that they cannot meet the holiest position and duties ever imposed on woman? We can show that France, with all her atheism, that Paris, with all her license, is not so guilty in this respect, as is staid New England, at the present hour." He has treated the subject in his unsurpassed style, and his article cannot but impress the thousand murderesses of New England churches and fashionable circles, with a sense of guilt and shame, with an idea that the curtain of secrecy has been lifted, and that the eye not of God only, but of the world, which they much more dread and fear, is upon them.[16]

Todd was a Congregationalist minister from Pittsfield, Massachusetts. His article was republished as a pamphlet entitled *Serpents in the Dove's Nest*. It noted, in part, that:

> As a class, the medical profession have taken a noble stand. The desolutions have become so fearful, that, as the guardians of human life, they were compelled to do so; and society owes a debt of gratitude to Dr. H. R. Storer, of Boston, especially, for his powerful arguments, lucid arrangement of facts, patient investigations, and earnest and eloquent remonstrances. Among his writings on this subject, the little work entitled "Why Not?" is a "book for every woman." and I wish every woman might carefully read it.[17]

Horatio was a professor at the Berkshire Medical College at Pittsfield when Todd wrote his article. A few years later, Horatio referred to "our old friend, the

Rev. Dr. John Todd, of Pittsfield,"[18] and Horatio may have prompted Todd's effort as he almost certainly prompted or helped prompt the efforts of the *Northwestern Christian Advocate*,.

We have discussed the references to Horatio by Revs. Eddy and Todd in their antiabortion articles. A few months later, in a paper on female masturbation, he acknowledged their work:

> Of late, the clergy, in the matter of arresting the spread of criminal abortion, and the correlative evil of preventing pregnancy in the married, have taken a manly stand in aid of the efforts of our profession. The writings of the Rev. Drs. Todd, of Massachusetts, and Eddy of Chicago, have been pioneer to a mass of literature upon the subject.[19]

The *Boston Medical and Surgical Journal* published the Report of the June meeting of the Vermont Medical Society on July 11, 1867. It referred to a pair of presentations dealing with criminal abortion. One was by Henry D. Holton, Vice President of the Society, who a year earlier at the American Medical Association Annual Meeting introduced the Resolution thanking Horatio Storer for declining the $100 prize for his prize-winning essay.[20] Holton described the "alarming prevalence" of criminal abortion and "its dangerous consequences and effect on population." Holton also introduced medical education and insanity in women as topics "for contemplation." However, the reported discussion dealt entirely with criminal abortion:

> An interesting discussion followed, during which Dr. Warner, of New Haven, President of the Society, entered the Hall and took the chair. Dr. Hyde, of Hardwick, thought the portion of the address relating to abortion should be circulated throughout Vermont. There is great ignorance on the subject of the danger and wrong of the practice. Every physician has such applications to him, nine tenths of them from married women. The profession has a duty in building up a wholesome public sentiment on the subject.
>
> Dr. Fassett, of St. Albans, thought a committee should be appointed to memorialize the Legislature on the subject, especially for preventing the circulation of the advertisements of abortionists and their medicines in the newspapers.
>
> Dr. Stiles thought that if the profession was kept within bounds it would help much towards the object in view. The idea that the world would be peopled faster if the proper ends of marriage were more generally regarded, was a very good one; but on looking around him, he noticed as few children among the medical profession as out of it. He thought in this matter "Charity should begin at home."
>
> Dr. Warner said his absence hitherto had been owing to attendance on a dangerous case resulting from the practice in question. He was glad to find the subject under discussion. No woman ever came

to him but once to procure abortion. He always endeavored to show
them the danger and wrong of such interference with nature, and in
some cases had threatened exposure if he should discover that they
had applied to other parties for the same end.

The discussion was further continued by Drs. Perkins, Keith and
Harding, in the same general line of remark.[21]

Lucius Castle Butler made the other presentation and it was published in
full by the *Boston Medical and Surgical Journal*.[22] Butler first documented the
large drop in family size by "Americans" and contrasted this with the large
families of the "foreigners," i.e., the more recent immigrants. One cause he cited
for the avoidance of children by the former group was the large numbers of advertisements for various means of restoring menstruation in magazines. Another
was the changing role of women from mother and homemaker to "mingler" in
public affairs, answerer of the "demands of sociability," and occupier of "public
pursuits and offices hitherto held exclusively by man." Also mentioned was
women's typical belief that life did not exist until three months of pregnancy.[23]

Butler then presented what he called the Catholic Church's "edict" upon
abortion. This was a large portion of the November 14, 1858 letter that the
Catholic Bishop of Boston had provided Horatio Storer and which Storer reproduced in his third 1859 article, "Its Victims." This included stern prohibitions
against interfering with pregnancy at any stage, condemnation of anyone "who
deals an exterminating blow to the incipient man," discussion of the double guilt
of the young woman who hides with abortion "the honor she has forfeited," and
discussion of the worse sin of those "who, finding themselves lawfully mothers,
prefer to devastate with poison or with steel their wombs rather than bear the
discomforts attached to the privilege of maternity, rather than forego the gaieties
of a winter's balls, parties and plays, or the pleasure of a summer's trips and
amusement." Butler contrasted this "correct" Roman Catholic position to the
absence of "guides to a right or wrong decision" in Protestant churches.[24]

Butler provided four suggestions for remedying the "decadence of the
American race." The first was to affect "a more determined and uniform moral
sentiment among medical men." He also called for uniformity of opinion among
physicians regarding the period when life begins. Current diversity in this area "is
seized upon by the abortionist to promote the circulation of his nefarious opinions
and nostrums," and was a cause of "the prevailing sentiment among women, that
miscarriage at three months is an innocent affair."[25]

His next "suggestion" was a call for a mighty public relations effort by physicians:

The moral sentiments must be cultivated. The conscience must be
aroused. The deep and damning guilt of destroying the life of a human
being at any stage of its existence must be portrayed. The consequences
of the act, in the feebleness of future life, in the prostration of the vital
powers, in the fearful result of remorse, shame, utter sterility as the

curse of Heaven upon the guilty, and sometimes insanity, must be presented with all the earnestness and eloquence of truth.[26]

Butler's third suggestion was to involve the press. On the one hand, the editors needed to eliminate the advertisements that were "the most shameless violations of decency and propriety." On the other hand, these editors needed to use their enormous power to foster "virtue and morality" and to "aid us in arresting the evil they have contributed to inflict upon us."[27]

Suggestion Four was another call for an awakening of moral and religious sentiment.

The church and the christian [sic] community have slept, while the evil has been growing and strengthening, widening and deepening its flow. It will need strong arms and determined effort to stay its progress and turn the tide in another direction. But the salvation of a race, imperiled by its continuance, demands that the effort shall be made. We rejoice to see any signs of awakening. Through the columns of a widely circulated religious journal, Rev. Dr. Todd, of Pittsfield, Mass., has uttered the bold, plain, eloquent language of a christian heart awakened to a keen sense of the sin and danger of the increasing evil. Public attention is arrested and startled by the array of facts presented. The voice from the East has found an echo in the West, and the press informs us that a recent Western Congregational convention adopted resolutions denouncing the practice of destroying unborn children as inhuman, unchristian and immoral, and to urge as a solemn duty on ministers, christians, and friends of virtue, to strive in all judicious ways to awaken the pubic conscience, and form a healthful public sentiment against the enormous crime.

Let the same voice be echoed and re-echoed through the length and breadth of the whole land, till the sentiment becomes established among all classes, "that he or she is a *criminal* and *murderer*, who deals an exterminating blow to the incipient man," and destroys "a being to whom God designed to give a living body and an immortal soul."[28]

The Presbytery of Troy, New York also approved a pair of antiabortion Resolutions. One condemned the prevention and destruction of human life which were described as "common sins of our age" and the other was an appeal to the membership to "avoid patronizing and encouraging journals" that included "advertisements proposing to assist in committing such crimes."[29] The elder offering the resolutions was a physician, John Lambert, of Salem, New York.

Physicians like Lambert with key roles in religious organizations probably account for some of the other antiabortion efforts of congregations and their parent bodies. We earlier noted the key instigation and information roles that physicians played in the condemnations of abortion in the *Northwestern Christian Advocate*, and Todd's *Serpents in the Dove's Nest*. As will be seen, American physicians may also have had a key role two years later when Pope Pius IX made induction of abortion at any state of pregnancy a ground for excommunication.

CHAPTER 14
IS IT I?, PALLEN, ALLEN, AND OTHERS

Horatio Storer's next major effort was his treatise on criminal abortion written primarily for husbands.[1] We have already described possible etiologies of this companion book, including the letters from Caroline Dall, the "wife of a Christian physician," and "A Fighter for the Right Against Wrong." Another was described in a letter from Horatio to Thomas Addis Emmet, to whom he dedicated the book. Horatio claimed the publisher wanted a second book, given the high sales of the first.[2]

Is It I? A Book for Every Man went to press shortly after August 1, 1867, the date at the end of the "Publishers' Note" that preceded the text. This "Note" is a unique personal account of Storer during this most tempestuous and productive period of his life.[3] Horatio began the Prefatory Remarks by describing the history of the earlier *Why Not?*. He claimed the "propriety" of the American Medical Association's resolution to distribute the Prize Essay was shown by the huge demand for the book and the fact that every medical journal in the country had given it "kindly notice."[4] (The "unkindly" notice in the *New Orleans Medical and Surgical Journal* was yet to appear.) Horatio briefly summarized *Why Not?*, discussing the criminality of induced abortion and also its effects on the woman's health, her family, and society. "The nail upon which society is to hang its faith has been driven;" Horatio continued, referring to *Why Not?*, "to clinch it, and so to render its hold secure, another blow is needed. The necessity I proceed to show, and the stroke to give, only regretting that my feeble arm is not that of some one of the Association's stronger men, and my pen tipped with the flame which should cause these words to burn their way to the very hearts of those to whom they are addressed."[5]

Horatio mentioned the letters of the "wife of a Christian physician" and "A Fighter for the Right Against Wrong," which discussed men's large contribution to the problem of criminal abortion and the need for widespread education of men on the subject. He noted that both letters were "apparently made in the most perfectly good faith," and that he knew nothing of the "personal identity of their authors."

Horatio's first chapter was called "It is not Good to be Alone." The major subjects were the dangers for a youth associated with the premature excitation of his sexuality, the near impossibility of avoiding mistakes along these lines, and the admission of the near necessity of experiencing the consequences of such mistakes in order to learn the self-control needed for their future avoidance. Sexuality while "alone," i.e., masturbation was mentioned, but the primary subject was man's instinctual need for a mate.

"Marriage as a Sanitary Measure" was the second chapter and marriage, prostitution, the keeping of a mistress or mistresses, and masturbation were the major topics. Marriage was cited as the preferable means of satisfying the instinctive sexual urge. The dangers of prostitution were described, including that of venereal disease, and the man with a mistress was deluding himself if he thought he was safe from such infection. Horatio described the not infrequent tragic event where a married man contracted the disease from a prostitute or mistress, did not manifest the symptoms, transmitted it to his wife and then believed infidelity on her part was the source of the disease. Next came the dangers of masturbation. "It is customary," Horatio continued, "but still a grave error, to preserve silence upon this subject," "physiologically a worse crime against nature" than resorting to prostitution. The dangers were such that Horatio appeared to pledge to undertake a physicians' campaign against masturbation when he wrote: "If the subject is decided, as I believe will be the case, to be of the importance that is claimed by every philosophical physician who has looked into the matter, a voice will go out into every corner of the land, caught up and re-echoed by all the medical men thereof, that will cause those who care either for their souls or their bodies, to pause and tremble."[6]

After reiterating the various "sanitary" benefits of marriage, Horatio moved to "How Early in Life is Marriage to be Advised?" He mentioned recommendations of others that men wait until they were 25. However, Horatio (who married at 23) did not see this as important in an expanding country, where there was need for the increased children one would expect with earlier marriage. In line with this, he pronounced long engagements to be decidedly bad.

Horatio's next chapter finally impinged on the original reasons given for writing the book. It was called "The Rights of the Husband." Horatio noted that these rights "are usually considered total and indisputable. Till now they have seldom been challenged; certainly seldom of men by men." In the following, Horatio explained his atypical male defense of women's rights:

> What, then, do we [men] usually claim? All that the law, and still more tyrannical custom, grants to us, in our wives; all that they have, and all that they are, in person and in very life. And here let me say, that I intend no ultra ground; that I am neither a fanatic or professed philanthrope; and that in loosing, as I hope to do, some of woman's present chains, it is solely for professional purposes, to increase her health, prolong her life, extend the benefits she confers upon society—in a word, selfishly to enhance her value to ourselves; and yet there is somewhat in this effort, as I believe there is also in the hearts of all those who will peruse it, of gratitude to her for the love with which she has solaced us, as mother, and sister, and wife, and daughter,—all of which I have myself possessed; unhappy he who has not.[7]

Horatio's reference to his experience as father of a daughter must have been painful. Scotland-born Jessie Simpson Storer had died of whooping cough three months after her first birthday.

After discussing women's slave status in primitive times, the frequent killing of wives for disobedience or infidelity in "former days," and the possession of multiple wives "in by-gone times, and among heathen, as at present in a remote valley of our own great land," Horatio finally got around to abortion. He asked whether the slaughter of new-borns by the Spartans was less wicked than

> the pre-natal murders of the present day, daily in occurrence, fashionable even, and be-praised by professing Christians, repeated over and over again by the same married woman and mother? You will exclaim with horror that it is not! And yet, in a very large proportion of instances, this shocking and atrocious act is advised and abetted, if not compelled by the husband—by us men. Who enjoys asking now, "Is it I?"[8]

Horatio indicated that the woman had a "certain measure of excuse," but "For her husband none." He continued:

> This is a matter concerning which the public mind is now undergoing a radical change. Slow to set in motion, but every day gaining more rapidly in force, the world's revival proceeds. In "Why Not?" or "Why should women not commit this crime?" I have sounded almost a trump to wake the dead. Would, indeed, that it might arouse a better life in every man who reads these words: ...[9]

Then followed the "Of the mother, ... we leave those to speak who can" passage from his first *North-American Medico-Chirurgical Review* article.

After further discussion of abortion as a moral problem, Horatio mentioned the problems of increased "ill health of women" and "the gradual dying out of our native population."[10] He also indicated that insanity was sometimes caused by abortion, several cases observed by him, and his claim had also been recently backed by Dr. John Gray, the Utica, New York Asylum Superintendent.[11] Thus, as in *Why Not?*, Horatio recognized that moral persuasion would not work with at least some of his audience, and he appealed to self-interest as well.

Horatio's next chapter was "Are these Rights Absolute, or Reciprocal, with Duties?" The final paragraph gives the answer and the gist of the chapter:

> For these [conjugal] rights, of which I have been speaking, are, in reality, not absolute, but reciprocal with duties. How can we ourselves expect enjoyment, if perchance we are inflicting terrible suffering? How can we look for constant and untiring affection, if inconsiderate or brutal, we compel what would be withheld perhaps, however reluctantly, by ill health? Is it thus we would cherish? As we sow, even so must we reap. No true conjugal enjoyment can exist, unless it is mutual. We cannot be loved, unless we are respected. We cannot be respected, even by our wives, unless we respect them. The true rule should be to take only what is freely given; were this the case, far more freely would gifts be offered.[12]

Next was "Should mere Instinct, or Reason, be the Rule?" Horatio claimed that excessive sexuality was harmful to the health of the woman. Bearing of children was essential, but not too frequently. He recommended two-and-a-half or three years between births.[13] Breast-feeding was important for avoiding uterine disease. Pleasure was an appropriate reason for sex, but the wife must not be compelled to do anything "she herself does not freely assent to."[14] Forcing women to engage in sex was a major reason for women averting "impending maternity."

Horatio's next chapter on divorce called for less of it and certainly no change of statutes that would make divorce easier. Forgiveness of human errors was cited as the key to avoiding divorce. One notable passage was:

> Were divorces more common, or more readily obtained, the very foundation of all society and civil government would be uprooted. The stability of the state rests upon that of the element of which it is composed. When these return to chaos, or dissolve themselves into the thinnest air, the commonwealth itself must prove a bubble, collapsing as soon as pricked by circumstance.[15]

Horatio's final chapter, "A Plea for Woman," was basically a recapitulation of the book. Horatio stressed the frequent lack of consideration husbands showed for the complaints of their wives. Although "there almost always exists a physical cause for all the many peculiar woes that women suffer." Horatio claimed that many husbands, and even some physicians, passed these off as "vain imaginings of a distempered mind, or the restless chafing of a soured and impatient disposition," which it was best not to encourage. "Courteous to strangers," he added, "we should be still more so to our own, and so be most truly brave in fighting down and conquering ourselves." "Let each of my readers," he concluded, "before closing this book, again ask himself, 'Is It I?'"[16]

Is It I? went into two editions, 1867 and 1868, and at least three physicians would make reference to it. However, this contrasts with four editions of *Why Not?* and scores of references by physicians and others to the book.

The eminent New York physician and Bellevue Hospital Medical College professor, Benjamin Fordyce Barker, presented a paper on abortion at the February 3, 1868 meeting of the Medical Society of the County of New York. The topic was prevention and treatment of spontaneous abortion, but he also noted the great danger to the woman's health when abortion in the third and fourth month was "the result of irritating medicines or of puncturing the membranes in criminal abortion."[17] The discussion following Barker's paper included comments on criminal abortion by another eminent New York physician and Bellevue Hospital Medical College professor, Dr. George T. Elliot.

> He would allude to a topic not yet touched upon, the unfortunately wide-spread tendency to the procurement of criminal abortion, not only in illicit pregnancies, but among the married of the highest social standing, to prevent inconvenient increase in the size of their families. Ap-

peals with this object were constantly made, not only to the unscrupulous practitioner, but as well to the most honorable members of the profession who would scorn to aid or countenance the practice. ... Everywhere and at all times the tendency to this evil can be seen cropping out. The duty of the profession is clear and imperative.[18]

Elliot probably would have agreed with Hodge, Horatio, and numerous other physicians that one "clear and imperative" duty was to persuade patients requesting abortion to continue their pregnancies. The Peoria, Illinois physician, M.M. Eaton, provided a case history, "Four and a-Half Inches of Whalebone in the Uterus.—Abortion.—Narrow Escape from Death," to assist physicians in carrying out this duty.[19] Eaton was called to attend the case following the woman's attempted self-abortion. He described the woman's near death from blood loss, his successful strengthening of her pulse with rye whiskey and ice, and the arduous task of extracting "a very large whalebone" from her uterus. The woman eventually recovered from the ordeal. Eaton discussed how the case could serve as a warning to other women:

> I wish every woman in the land who is, or is tempted to be, guilty of the crime of producing abortion on themselves, or anyone else, could have seen this case. I am sure, if they could have done so, few would be willing to subject themselves to such danger. This is but one out of thousands, it is true, where women resort to some means to rid themselves of unborn children; but, it is one calculated to impress the thoughtful mind with the danger women subject themselves to, who sin in this way against God and man, and furnishes us with a case to cite, to persuade ladies never to be guilty of such an act.[20]

A controversial Missouri physician, Montrose Anderson Pallen, read a paper, "Foeticide, or Criminal Abortion," before the Missouri State Medical Association in April 1868.[21] Pallen was a professor of medicine at three medical schools in Missouri. During the Civil War, he had been a medical director for the Confederate Army and served on missions abroad and to Canada before being captured and held on parole in New York.[22]

Pallen began with a pessimistic description of the state of the nation noting how "national vices and national crime have crept upon us, and now flourish with a luxuriance of growth, which the skilled hands of Society's gardeners will find great difficulty to uproot and destroy." He continued:

> With many of these defects it is not our province as physicians directly to cope,—such is the duty of others who claim to be philanthropists, legislators and political economists,—yet we may indirectly assist and do much towards their eradication. With one of the loathsome heads of the hydra, we can and must accomplish Herculean efforts. Pandora's box has been reopened with newer additions: from it, *criminal abortion or foeticide* has been bestowed upon the American people. Of such

frequent occurrence is the deed, that it may be said to be one of the national crimes, and carries with it a disgrace so deep, and a shame so damning, that, lest we, as physicians, strive to stay its progress with all our might and main, we may be held accountable as *particeps criminis* in the sapping of our nation's life.[23]

Pallen indicated that it was the duty of the "clerical, legal, and medical" professions to "inveigh against" this frequent crime. He admitted that some physicians, "either from ignorance or willfulness," did not properly handle this duty, failing to point out to those requesting abortion that "foeticide is murder of an unborn being." He also had harsh words for the ministry:

> Our clergy, with some very few exceptions, have thus far hesitated to enter upon an open crusade against it. Fearful as are the numbers of criminal abortions among the rich as well as the poor, the married as well as the unmarried, open and shameless, secret and nefarious, we have yet to find the subject entertained by any one of the numerous conclaves of the religious men of our country who sit in high authority all over the land, and who pronounce upon topics political, religious and governmental.[24]

Pallen quoted extensively from Hodge's Introductory Lecture and from T. Gaillard Thomas' *Diseases of Women* to show that other physicians agreed to the frequency of the crime and agreed in condemning it. Thomas' concerns included the failure of the law to deal with abortionists or even their newspaper advertisements. Pallen indicated that the same problems existed in Missouri. He called on physicians to make up for these deficiencies of the legal system by "strenuously" acting "to manufacture a public opinion, which will force the police to arrest and prosecute, and which will shame any decent editor into an absolute refusal to publish the vulgar, obscene, and criminal advertisements." He continued:

> The men and women who professedly or secretly follow the loathsome trade of foetus-murder, are not all known, but very many are recognized as such, by those of us whose duty it is to snatch from the very jaws of death, the unfortunate victims of their vampire deeds. Among the medical fraternity there are villains who cast a foul stain upon the profession, and who are thought by the public to be upright, honorable men, and who are notorious abortionists.[25]

As will be seen, other physicians would note that the public often held a high opinion of the physicians who performed illegal abortions.

A unique feature of Pallen's paper was his discussion of the frequency of criminal abortion in various countries and in the different sections and cities of the United States. He indicated the United States led in the crime, England and

Scotland were next, and France and Prussia followed, somewhat ahead of Austria. On the other hand, the crime was rare in Ireland, Spain, and Italy. He continued:

> we of the United States stand foremost in the list, and bear off the disgraceful prize of having a national crime of abortion! This may not be absolutely true as regards the entirety of the country, but, were it not for foreign immigration, and the births arising therefrom, the States of Massachusetts, New Hampshire, Connecticut and Rhode Island, would in all probability be depopulated in less than a century. ... Traveling westwardly, we find New York, Pennsylvania and Ohio afflicted in the same way, but in a less degree, the nearer we approach the valleys of the Western rivers. But in the cities of New York, Baltimore, Buffalo, Cincinnati and Louisville we recognize the frequency of foeticide. Particularly do the first two rival, if they do not excel, the land of honest, honorable old Miles Standish! In the smaller towns, throughout the country proper of the Middle and Border States, we find that the crime exists, but nothing in proportion to that of the Eastern States. In Chicago, and Cincinnati, however, the scale seems to mount as high as does that of New York or Philadelphia, but it is perhaps not higher than that of St. Louis. In proportion to the densities of population, these five cities stand about on an equal footing.[26]

Pallen did not indicate his sources, but he was active in the American Medical Association and may have questioned Association members from around the country. It is questionable whether Baltimore was as bad as Pallen claimed. The Catholic Archbishop located in that city would shortly report that abortion had not "reached this latitude, at least to any great extent." Pallen's later comment about the highest abortion rates of "New York or Philadelphia" suggests that he earlier meant to write: "But in the cities of New York, Philadelphia, Buffalo, ..."

After a discussion of women's current abnormal preoccupation with voting and lawmaking instead of with the bearing and forming the character of offspring, Pallen concluded:

> we as medical men must labor to promote public hygiene; and criminal abortion has gotten to be so frequent, ... the diseases and dangers it engenders, are so numerous, ... we should call upon all good and honest citizens to assist us to stay its increase, and to check its frequency, lest it so affect the public hygiene and public weal, that it cannot be controlled for generations yet to come.[27]

Cincinnati physicians shared Pallen's view about frequent criminal abortions in their city. The Cincinnati Academy of Medicine adopted a series of Resolutions that decried the frequency of criminal abortions and claimed they were generally performed by irregulars and "female 'accoucheurs.'" The resolutions also condemned the advertisements for "abortionists and abortion drugs" and called for "all good citizens, and especially physicians, to discourage the circulation and patronage of the journals in which are published the advertisements of those who profess to produce abortion, or prevent impregnation."[28]

Two weeks later, the *Medical and Surgical Reporter* published a letter from "Wm. C. Todd M.D.," claiming high levels of criminal abortion among the married in Philadelphia, another city high on Pallen's list. Todd's source of data was the women whom he treated for the effects of criminal abortion. He asked one of these married women how she had come to seek an abortion and she responded:

> "My attention was drawn to the subject by reading advertisements in the *Sunday papers.* I did not want the trouble of children. I was three months gone. I went to Madam _____, No. ____ ____ street. I found quite a number waiting for the same purpose; they did not seem to make any secret about it. In turn I was taken in and operated on. It was done by piercing the womb. She charges fifteen dollars for the operation."[29]

Her account substantiates the claims of several physicians that the advertisements for abortion services and drugs were a major factor, if not the major factor, influencing women to seek abortion.

The *Reporter* published notes in January and April 1868 praising local medical societies in New Jersey[30] and Maine[31] for their efforts to suppress the crime and praising a Rhode Island jury for convicting an abortionist.[32] The latter article described how the Rhode Island abortionist compounded his crime by attempting to bribe the witnesses against him. "We are glad to see," the editor continued, "that some of the vampyres [sic] of society are likely to get a share of their just dues." Other correspondence in the same volume of the *Reporter* was from Massachusetts and Missouri. These letters, Reamy's praise of the *Reporter*, and many earlier and later letters to Editor Butler from distant physicians show that Butler's *Reporter* was widely circulated in the United States. It undoubtedly was an important factor helping physicians to resist the various pressures to perform abortions and inspiring them to counsel their women patients to continue unwanted pregnancies.

The *Reporter* obtained a co-editor in 1867, Daniel Garrison Brinton, who may not have fully shared Samuel Worcester Butler's concerns about abortion. Brinton's presence may explain the somewhat diminished concern about criminal abortion shown in an item in the "Notes and Comments" section for August 15, 1868.[33] It began: "Criminal Abortion. Two physicians were arrested in Hartford on the 3d inst. for doing that for a 'respectable married woman' which the Roman Catholic Church calls murder." The editor thus seems to be contradicting the almost universal claim by physicians in medical journal articles and editorials that abortion *was* murder. Butler had called criminal abortion "the *crime of murder*," in November 1865 and it is doubtful that he had changed his mind. Brinton probably wrote this particular "Comment."

We referred earlier to Nathan Allen's discussion in an October 4, 1866 *New York Observer* article on the sharply lower birth rate of New England women, compared to previous generations and compared to recent immigrants. Allen believed that the women of New England were in decline and had suffered a "radical change" in their organization due to their unbalanced emphasis on brain activities relative to activities associated with other organ systems. In the earlier article, Allen did not discuss criminal abortion as a factor in women's determination "*to have no children, or a very limited number.*" However, Allen did discuss criminal abortion in an article in *Harper's New Monthly Magazine*, where he claimed "wealth and fashion" were the goals people now held in life and children did not fit with these selfish goals. As a result, "worse expedients are resorted to, in order to effect certain ends, than were ever countenanced by the doctrines of Malthus." Allen continued:

> While it may be difficult to describe the full extent of this evil, or decide just how far it operates to prevent the increase of offspring, it is the opinion of some medical men who have carefully investigated the subject that it is, directly and indirectly, a powerful check on population, and, moreover, that the evil is constantly increasing. The various laws passed against it in different States afford comparatively no barriers to prevent or break it up; neither does public opinion, which on this point is very much perverted. It should be stated that believers in the Roman Catholic faith never resort to any such practices; the strictly Americans are almost alone guilty of this great crime.[34]

Allen attributed these conclusions about abortion to "some medical men who have carefully investigated the subject." Despite this, Allen would be selected as a scientific source by the 1871 AMA Committee on Criminal Abortion rather than Horatio Storer who almost certainly was Allen's primary source of information. Allen's criticisms of Malthus, his attack on the "quickening" distinction, and his denial that Catholics "resort to any such practices" strongly resemble Storer's discussions and conclusions.

Allen's condemnation of criminal abortion in this popular magazine may have had a substantial effect on the public. His *Harper's* discussion was quoted a month later by the Rev. Elijah Franklin Howe in a sermon, "Ante-Natal Infanticide," presented at his First Congregational Church of Terre Haute, Indiana.[35]

CHAPTER 15
STORER'S NEW BOOK AND NEW JOURNAL

The summer of 1868 marked a "new" book, *Criminal Abortion: Its Nature, Its Evidence, and Its Law*,[1] written by Horatio in conjunction with an eminent Boston lawyer and author, Franklin Fiske Heard. The "Preface" indicated that "Book I" was "rewritten from" the 1859 *North-American Medico-Chirurgical Review* articles. This "rewrite" involved relatively minor changes and only a small amount of new material. "Book II" aimed at exhausting the subject of the Criminal Law as it pertained to abortion.[2]

In 1859, Horatio had written in his first article in the series: "To ... his father, and to the journalists ... by whom the effort then made was so warmly and eloquently seconded, the writer acknowledges his indebtedness for the thought of the present undertaking." In the new book, "thought of the *present* undertaking," became, "thought of the undertaking, *which has culminated, he has reason to believe, in an agitation which is now shaking society, throughout our country, in its very centre.*"[3]

Horatio also added a long paragraph that described the large progress of the crusade since its inception. It summarized the efforts of himself, the American Medical Association, Rev. Todd, and others. Storer also noted that his own articles had "already affected the ruling of courts."[4]

In Horatio's second chapter, "Its Frequency, and the Causes Thereof," Horatio repeated the data originally presented in 1859 along with a few additional recent supporting statistics. He added a key footnote following the 1859 paragraph claiming that abortion's "frequency is rapidly increasing." It read: "Thus we wrote in 1859. Since then, though so great a flood of light has been poured upon the subject, the times seem little changed. Let us hope, however, that the apparent fact may be owing to the unveiling of what was formerly more frequently practised, but kept concealed."[5]

Also new was a six-page quote from a report by Nathan Allen that showed large differences in births between the "American" and "foreign" populations similar to those Horatio had described in 1859.[6] Horatio described Allen as "indefatigable in calling the attention of investigators to this important question." However, Allen would not have been fully pleased with Horatio's treatment. Horatio indicated that Allen's theory of a constitutional change in New England women was "not born out by facts." He claimed these women menstruated "as well as ever they did" and "if their husbands are potent" "women can conceive."[7]

An addition to a footnote in "Its Victims," expanded on the differences between Catholics and Protestants in the frequency of criminal abortion, noting that "several hundred" Protestant women had obtained abortions compared to seven

Catholic women. What is more, Horatio had learned "upon further inquiry, that all but two [Catholics] were only nominally so, not going to the confession."[8]

Considerable reshuffling of 1859 material occurred in the final chapters of the 1868 book, but almost all of it is there. The notable exceptions were the various state statutes on criminal abortion (or lack of same) and the analyses of these that Horatio had provided. These might have been expected to be covered in Book Two, which was produced by the lawyer, Franklin Fiske Heard. However, only a few statutes were mentioned, and Book Two seems a rather weak effort that Horatio may have been dissociating himself from when he wrote in the initial footnote of the book: "the latter half is wholly due to his accomplished colleague, Mr. Heard."[9]

Horatio closed his portion of the book with a new footnote including an optimistic view about the American Medical Association's Memorial that had been provided to governors and legislatures of the states and territories some nine years earlier. "There is good reason to believe," he concluded, "directly and indirectly, it was productive of a great deal of good."[10]

In January 1869, Horatio started the Gynaecological Society of Boston. Although the initial plan was to have the "Proceedings" published in established medical journals, Horatio quickly decided that there was a need for a new journal and the first number of the *Journal of the Gynaecological Society of Boston* appeared in July 1869.[11] Numerous published "Proceedings" of the Society and numerous "Editorial Notes" of the monthly *Journal* dealt with criminal abortion.[12] One of the first such mentions occurred at the April 6, 1869 meeting of the Society. Horatio exhibited the "pelvic viscera from a patient dead of criminal abortion, the case being one then in court." This exhibition was followed by discussion of medical testimony in criminal abortion trials. Horatio noted that "medical experts must be very careful, when put upon the stand, lest by turning counsel they let their zeal destroy the value of their testimony." Although he did not elaborate, it is not hard to imagine that Horatio himself was too zealous on some occasion. He then described "the reluctance of physicians to assist in bringing to justice these gross offenders who strike at man's life in the very citadel of its commencement." He also indicated that a physician in a nearby county was performing abortions, but was "still accredited as a member of the Massachusetts Medical Society, whose disgrace it was that it had not yet moved in the affair."[13]

At a meeting of the Society two weeks later, Horatio described the draft legislation related to criminal abortion, which the New York State Medical Society had prepared and recently sent to the State Legislature. Horatio discussed the etiology of this draft statute including the American Medical Association's Memorial to the State Medical Societies, the resolution of a Troy, New York physician urging compliance with the Memorial, and a series of resolutions submitted a year earlier by the New York State Medical Society to the State Assembly prior to their draft bill. After noting that he had had the honor of being consulted during the drafting of these resolutions, Horatio said: "How different from what has obtained in our own State! It was here that the advance was initiated, which has received the benediction of the whole country. Having given the key-note to other States, the courage of our brethren failed them,—Boston, which claims to control the opinions and actions of the rest of the State, first showing the white feather."[14]

The intense efforts of the New York State Medical Society that Storer referred to were discussed by James Mohr in his *Abortion in America*. Mohr reproduced a Resolution of the Society that read:

> "*Whereas*, from the first moment of conception, there is a living creature in process of development to full maturity; and whereas, any sufficient interruption to this living process always results in the destruction of life; and whereas, the intentional arrest of this living process, eventuating in the destruction of life (being an act with intention to kill), is consequently murder; therefore,...*Resolved*, That this society will hail with gratitude and pleasure, the adoption of any measures or influences that will, in part or entirely, arrest this flagrant corruption of morality among women, who ought to be and unquestionably are the conservators of morals and of virtue."[15]

The New York legislation that resulted totally eliminated the quickening doctrine, making killing of the fetus a crime of second-degree manslaughter at any stage of pregnancy. The law also made an attempt at abortion a misdemeanor even when the woman was not pregnant. Prosecutors therefore no longer had to prove pregnancy. The new law also allowed the woman obtaining the abortion to testify against her abortionist and granted her immunity for so doing.[16]

In Horatio's "Editorial Notes" for September 1869, he condemned many of the unsanitary practices in the area of Boston, including the environmental pollution by the Revere Copper Company. He added:

> In making these remarks we may perhaps wound the sensibilities of some; we are pretty sure to receive the condemnation of others. Better to do this, however, than by our silence become accessory to the continuance of public evils whose influence in causing disease and death is more than commensurate, oftentimes, with their age or apparent importance. Every life lost is not an isolated one; *every life saved is, as a general rule, the precursor of others that else would not have been called into existence.*[17]

Horatio surely recognized that many more lives were being saved by preventing abortions and that the "others" subsequently "called into existence" increased exponentially in succeeding generations. As discussed in Chapter 1, almost every North American reader of these words can credit the "physicians' crusade against abortion" for one or more of his or her ancestors.

A demonstration of Horatio's continuing fierce antipathy to criminal abortion followed:

> We desire to call its [the State Board of Health's] attention, and that of our professional brethren, to the fact, that in a neighboring city, not

more than ten miles distant from Boston, a member of the Massachusetts Medical Society, in regular standing, who bears the reputation, well earned, no doubt, of being an unblushing abortionist, resides, and practices his nefarious art without let or hindrance.

More than once has the law striven to vindicate its violated authority and failed of its object, being struck spellbound by the all-potent charms of Mammon. More than once have dying lips borne testimony to the blood-guiltiness of this monster in human form. ...

The wretched mothers who lose their lives in this mad attempt to set at defiance the laws of God and man, may be virtually suicides, but their educated accomplice is, in a far truer sense, a murderer.

There cannot be the slightest doubt in regard to the truth of the statements which we have made, and yet the members of the District Medical Society, and of the Medical Association in his own city, allow this man to go in his course, without a single vigorous effort to arrest the diabolical work which is demoralizing the community, and tarnishing their own good name. Shame on the profession which makes such high pretension, and tolerates such baseness! Shame on the manhood of those who retain in their fellowship, and admit, ay, to their very homes, and to a leading place in their councils, this professional Herod, whose garments are indelibly crimsoned with the blood of unborn innocence!! Dare any man who has virtually taken the solemn oath of Hippocrates, who has sworn to regulate his conduct by the noblest maxims of justice, purity, and benevolence, give countenance to the most cowardly of assassins, and even clasp his bloody fingers as those of a friend? If so, then farewell honor! farewell integrity! farewell all that is lofty and worthy of regard in human character![18]

Four months later, Horatio wrote that the same abortionist had recently been "charged with causing the death of a young woman from a distant town," but had never appeared for trial. "Report has it," he continued, "that three thousand dollars in greenbacks answered as a sufficient hypnotic for the conscience of the prosecuting attorney as well as anodyne for the agonized feeling of the fond parents." Storer continued:

It is clearly the duty of the County Medical Society to disown Dr._____, if guilty, and to make an emphatic public protest against his acts, whether it attempt to procure his conviction and punishment, or not. It should do this for its own sake, and that of the community. Right here, in professedly Christian Massachusetts, where the crime of induced abortion is perhaps more frequent than anywhere else in the world, and where public opinion, stringent on so many points of morality, is unaccountably lax on this, should the brave Christian work begin of stemming the torrent of evil, that it may not gain such strength and volume as to overflow and devastate the world. Why are philanthropists and good men so timid? Do they love their own ease and pecuniary interests more than they do the cause of virtue and righteousness in the earth? Do they forget that the career of the professed follower of Christ is to be one of continual warfare, and that he is not to regard even life itself in the service of his Master? Significant indeed is that passage in the Apocalypse which speaks of the "fearful," in company with the "unbelieving," and with "liars" and "murderers," as receiving the final punishment described under the dreadful image of a lake burning with fire and brimstone.[19]

Horatio invited two physicians with recent experience in criminal abortion prosecutions to the meeting of the Gynaecological Society on June 7, 1870, and an unusually frank discussion of the role of regular physicians in providing criminal abortions resulted. It began with a letter from a Lynn, Massachusetts physician, Joseph G. Pinkham, who wrote:

"I hope the Gynaecological Society will not fail to take immediate and decided action in regard to the 'Lynn Abortionist.' The prosecuting officers of the Commonwealth complain that public sentiment is against them in their efforts to procure the conviction of this class of criminals, and in a measure they are right, although their own timidity makes the matter seem worse than it is. The Society has it in its power to create, or control, public sentiment by bold action in a case like this. If it leads the van bravely in the good fight, scores will join its ranks who now stand aloof from sheer cowardice,—men whose consciences have long tormented them for their culpable inaction. Come out in the way that may seem best to you, but *come out by all means, and that at once.*"[20]

After the letter was read, Horatio "reminded" members that "many years ago" he had called on the Massachusetts Medical Society "to cease its notorious harborage of habitual abortionists" and had been frustrated "by the allegation that to do so would be but to 'stir a dunghill.'" "In consequence partly of this professional and most criminal apathy," he continued, "the public sentiment had become more and more blunted, until it was given as a reason by the public prosecuting officers that a jury could not be found in Boston to convict of this crime, even in the most flagrant and indisputable cases of maternal death."[21]

This was the first reference that has been found to Horatio's attempts to end the Massachusetts Medical Society's "notorious harborage of habitual abortionists." It may have occurred during his 1866 paper to the Society on physician abetment of abortion. However, his published paper did not include such charges and 1866 barely qualified as "many years ago" in June 1870. The New Bedford meeting of the Massachusetts Medical Society in 1857 is another possibility, although the minutes of that meeting did not mention any charge that the Society harbored "habitual abortionists." John Preston Leonard's "Quackery and Abortion" may have qualified as a call to eliminate "habitual abortionists" from the Massachusetts Medical Society, although Leonard only referred to "our medical societies." Medical student Horatio may have supported Leonard's attempt when it was published "many years" prior to June 1870, if he did not actually propose it to Leonard.

Horatio then introduced the visiting Drs. Whittier and Weston. Whittier "had zealously labored during the past year to bring some of these professional as well as unlicensed wretches to their deserts." Weston was coroner in a nearby county and "had lately placed evidence of the strongest character in the hands of the State constabulary, but without avail." A long discussion followed of the public's acceptance of abortion, the unwillingness of district attorneys to prosecute abortionists, the apathy of some physicians about the problem, and the actual conduct of abortions by some regular physicians. Various members cited regular physicians who performed abortions. One who was arrested had the case dropped when he told prosecutors "that he had several years ago attended the woman for syphilis, and that therefore he did not do wrong in destroying her offspring." Dr. Martin, "as evidence of the appalling state of public opinion and the recklessness with which this crime is committed," described the small five-dollar fee charged by the Lynn abortionist and "the peculiar nonchalance with which women apply for the procurement of abortion." After discussion of the need to purge the Massachusetts Medical Society of its abortionists, the following Resolutions were adopted:

> I. That the Gynaecological Society is ready to receive such evidence as may be sufficient to convict a Fellow of the Massachusetts Medical Society of criminal abortion, and to present the case and prosecute the same before the officers of that Society, with a view to his expulsion.
> II. That the Society address the Governor of the State, by memorial, setting forth the failure of his prosecuting officers to take cognizance of this crime, and requesting that he direct them to perform the duties of their office, or supply their place, if he can legally do so, by more competent men.[22]

This Society discussion belies Horatio's repeated insistence in his earlier writing that regular physicians almost never performed criminal abortions. Horatio in 1859 surely had been aware that some regular physicians were abortionists. He may have been defending the name of the graduates of legitimate medical schools, despite some being guilty. It is also probable that many regular physicians had commenced the practice after 1859.

The August 1870 "Editorial Notes" congratulated the physicians in the neighborhood of the Lynn abortionist for taking steps "to vindicate, so far as they are concerned, the good name of the profession."[23] Their actions apparently led to more than vindication. The Massachusetts Medical Society Councillors expelled the Lynn abortionist at their meeting of October 5, 1870. The Minutes indicated: "Dr. Asa T. Newhall, of Lynn, had been expelled by a Board of Trial, for alleged criminal abortion."[24]

In the October 1870 "Editorial Notes," Horatio discussed Newhall's expulsion and congratulated the Lynn physicians who "have done their duty tardily but well." He continued:

His expulsion has purged our ranks of one dishonorable name. Are there any others? Let us look well to it! A ball has been set in motion which should not cease rolling; a movement has been inaugurated which should not be arrested until it has overthrown the grim Moloch to whom our children are being yearly sacrificed in numbers that would seem incredible to one not familiar with the statistics of the abominable rite. Earnest, persistent labor is required, both inside and outside of the profession. In our keeping, fellow-physicians, lies the great issue. We can, in time, create a healthy public sentiment where it does not now exist. We can speak out boldly and let people know what we, who have had the best opportunities for investigating the subject, think of criminal abortion, both in its medical and legal aspects. In this way we can at least drive the harpy from the abodes of the virtuous and good, where it too often makes its foul nest, and banish it to regions inhabited by persons of no doubtful character.[25]

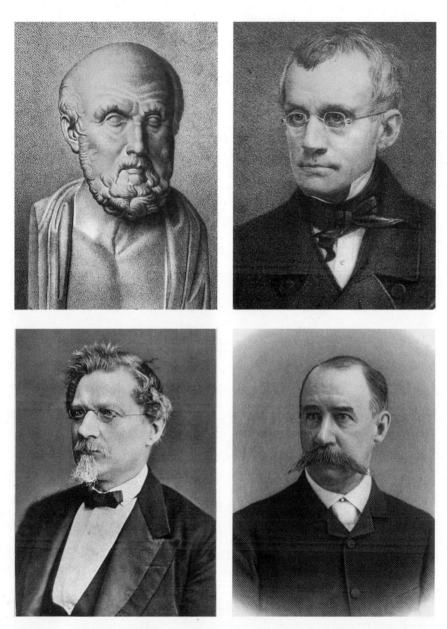

Figure 1 The Pioneer Antiabortion Crusaders. Clockwise from top left: Hippocrates, John Brodhead Beck, Gunning S. Bedford, Hugh Lenox Hodge. *Courtesy of the National Library of Medicine.*

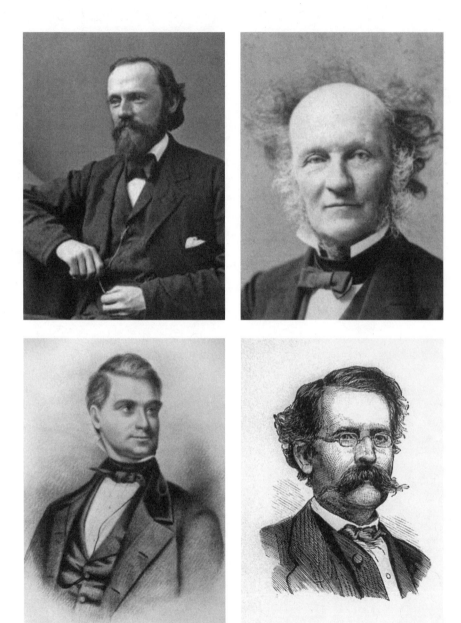

Figure 2 Early Crusaders. Clockwise from top left: Horatio Robinson Storer,
David Humphreys Storer, Augustus Kinsley Gardner, David Meredith Reese.
*Storer photographs courtesy of a great granddaughter of Horatio Robinson Storer.
Others courtesy of the National Library of Medicine.*

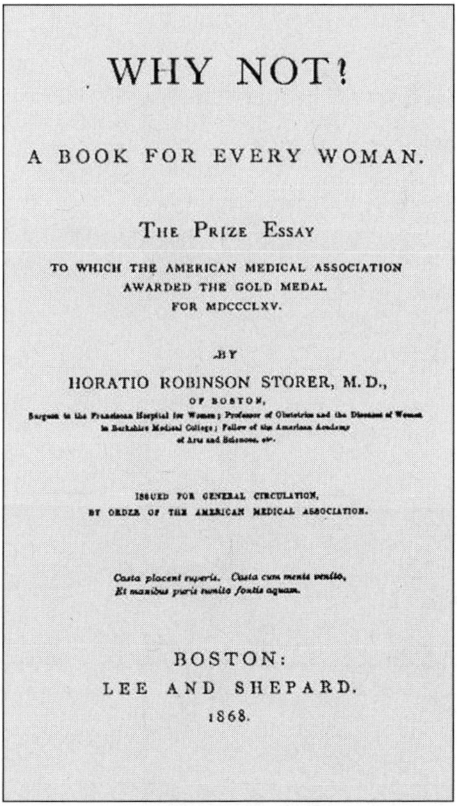

WHY NOT!

A BOOK FOR EVERY WOMAN.

THE PRIZE ESSAY

TO WHICH THE AMERICAN MEDICAL ASSOCIATION
AWARDED THE GOLD MEDAL
FOR MDCCCLXV.

BY

HORATIO ROBINSON STORER, M. D.,
OF BOSTON,

Surgeon to the Franciscan Hospital for Women; Professor of Obstetrics and the Diseases of Women
in Berkshire Medical College; Fellow of the American Academy
of Arts and Sciences, etc.

ISSUED FOR GENERAL CIRCULATION,
BY ORDER OF THE AMERICAN MEDICAL ASSOCIATION.

Casta placent superis. Casta cum mente venito,
Et manibus puris sumito fontis aquam.

BOSTON:
LEE AND SHEPARD.
1868.

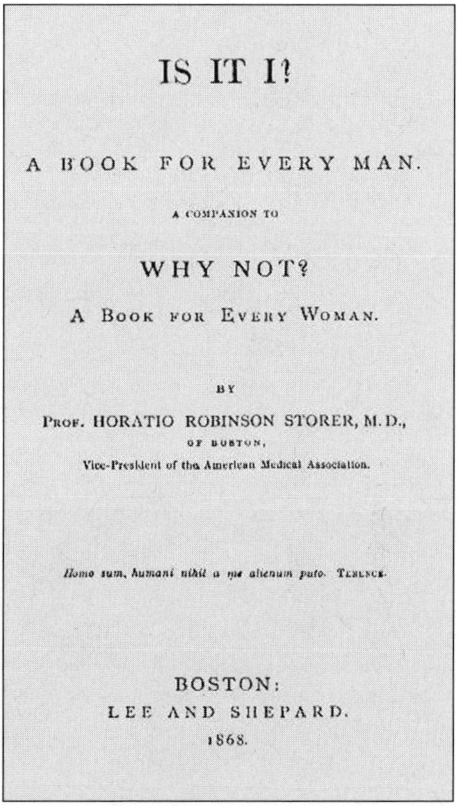

IS IT I!

A BOOK FOR EVERY MAN.

A COMPANION TO

WHY NOT?

A BOOK FOR EVERY WOMAN.

BY

PROF. HORATIO ROBINSON STORER, M. D.,
OF BOSTON,
Vice-President of the American Medical Association.

Homo sum, humani nihil a me alienum puto. TERENCE.

BOSTON:
LEE AND SHEPARD.
1868.

Figure 3 Horatio's books on abortion written for popular audiences.

THE JOURNAL

OF THE

GYNÆCOLOGICAL SOCIETY OF BOSTON:

A Monthly Journal

DEVOTED TO THE ADVANCEMENT OF THE KNOWLEDGE
OF THE DISEASES OF WOMEN.

EDITED BY

WINSLOW LEWIS, M.D., HORATIO R. STORER, M.D.,
GEORGE H. BIXBY, M.D.

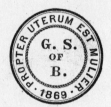

VOL. VII.

JULY TO DECEMBER,

1872.

BOSTON:
JAMES CAMPBELL, PUBLISHER,
18 TREMONT STREET, MUSEUM BUILDING.

Figure 4   Cover of Horatio Robinson Storer's *Journal of the
Gynaecological Society of Boston.*

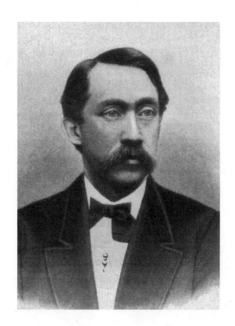

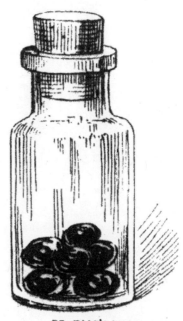

DR. HALE'S PILLS.

Figure 5 Edwin Moses Hale and the pills he provided the *Chicago Times* Girl
Reporter. *Photograph courtesy of the National Library of Medicine.*

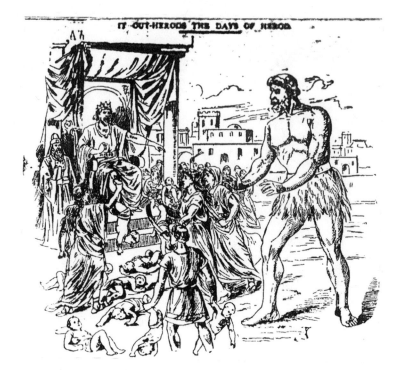

Figure 6   Cartoon from the 1888 *Chicago Times* exposé.

CHAPTER 16

BISHOP COXE, ARCHBISHOP SPALDING, AND HODGE'S ENCORE

The Episcopal Bishop of Western New York, Arthur Cleveland Coxe, provided a January 30, 1869 Pastoral Letter to the Diocese that warned of the "enormities of theatrical exhibitions, and the lasciviousness of dances too commonly tolerated in our times." These were "disgraceful to the age, and irreconcilable with the Gospel of Christ." However, his strongest admonitions were related to criminal abortion. He wrote:

> I have heretofore warned my flock against the blood-guiltiness of infanticide. If any doubt existed heretofore as to the propriety of my warnings on the subject, they must now disappear before the fact that the world itself is beginning to be terrified by the practical results of the sacrifices to Moloch which defile our land. There are scientific and statistical documents before the people which fully sustain my remonstrances.
>
> Again I warn you that they who do such things cannot inherit eternal life. If there be a special damnation for those who "shed innocent blood," what must be the portion of those who have no mercy upon their own flesh?[1]

The "scientific and statistical documents" probably were Storer's recent books and Nathan Allen's articles. Two months later, in an address Coxe elaborated on the physician writing:

> As to those crimes which I have likened to the sacrifices of Moloch, I am glad that our physicians are beginning to be preachers. They tell us of frightful retributions; of lunatic cells, and early graves as the consequences; of haggard and premature old age, unenlivened by the sweet society of sons and daughters, and terrified by the conscience as by the ghosts of murdered babes. ... If legislation sleeps, while such things are preying like a canker upon the very vitals of our Nation, surely the pulpit should be heard.[2]

In a later section of his address, Coxe provided a long quote from Thomas Fortescue Rochester, Professor of the Principles and Practice of Medicine and Clinical Medicine at the University of Buffalo. After introducing the "eminent physician," he copied the following from Rochester's February 24 "Address to the Graduates of the Medical Department of the University of Buffalo."

"Fashion in *morals!* Witness, the atrocious soul and body imperilment by the avoidance of the sacred duties of legitimate maternity, by practices both indelicate and immoral. This is called an American fashion: it is certainly a fashion, an immorality, a vice, but it *is not an original American fashion.* It is derived *from that people who are Fashion's chief votaries*—who dethroned the God of the Bible and made adoration of a day to a painted creature—miscalled reason. Medical men were the first to sound the alarm, both in its moral and physical aspects. Philosophers and statisticians re-echo it, in its national and generic relations. The religious and the secular press alike expose and denounce it—and the pulpit implores, persuades and fulminates against it. This usage is *not limited to any people, nor is it avoided, as has been stated, by those of any creed.* Medical men know this. It is one of the banes of civilization. That it finds more congenial soil in our country than elsewhere, cannot, alas! be denied. Poverty and inconvenience are urged in extenuation. These do not excuse infractions of human law, much less of divine—but even the excuse is false—the real culprits are fashion, frivolity, laziness, selfishness, and, *O tempora! O mores!*—national demoralization."[3]

Coxe used Rochester's *"nor is it avoided, as has been stated, by those of any creed,"* to counter the 1867 claim by LeProhon that criminal abortion was primarily a Protestant phenomenon. However, Rochester almost certainly was wrong about this. Most other medical writers had reported Catholics to be much less apt to purposely abort their children. As will be seen, the same claim that Catholics were largely abstaining from the crime would be made over the next several decades by other physicians. Some of these may have been parroting Storer, but many no doubt were reporting from their own experience.

The Catholic Church's longstanding opposition to abortion was reinforced in 1869, both in the United States and in Rome. On May 29, 1869, the following was published in the *Medical and Surgical Reporter*:

The Crime of Abortion.

Archbishop Spaulding [sic], the distinguished primate of the Roman Catholic Church in the country, in a pastoral letter at the close of a recent Council, speaks in these decided terms of a crime only too common in this generation.

"The abiding interest all feel in the preservation of the morals of our country, constrains us to raise our voice against the daily increasing practice of infanticide, especially before birth. The notoriety which this monstrous crime has obtained of late, and the hecatombs of infants that are annually sacrificed to Moloch, to gratify an unlawful passion, are a sufficient justification for our alluding to a painful and delicate subject, which should not even be mentioned among Christians. We may observe that *the crying sin of infanticide is most prevalent in those localities where the system of education without religion has been longest es-*

tablished, and been most successfully carried out. The inhuman crime might be compared to the murder of the 'Innocents,' except that the criminals in this case exceed in enormity the cruelty of Herod. If it is a sin to take away the life even of an enemy; if the crime of shedding innocent blood cries even to Heaven for vengeance, in what language can we characterize the double guilt of those whose souls are stained with the innocent blood of their own unborn, unregenerate offspring. The murder of an infant before its birth is, in the sight of God and of this Church, as great a crime as would be the killing of a child after birth, with this aggravating circumstance, that in the former case the unborn child dies deprived of the essential grace of baptism. No mother is allowed, under any circumstances, to permit the death of her unborn infant, not even for the sake of preserving her own life, because the end never justifies the means, and we must not do evil that good may come from it."[4]

This was Section III of the Pastoral Letter written by Bishop James Gibbons of North Carolina at the request of Archbishop Martin J. Spalding. It was released at the close of the Tenth Provincial Council of Baltimore on May 2, 1869 and was to be read in all the Catholic Churches of the Baltimore Province.[5] Other Sections dealt with avoiding round dancing, obscene theatricals, and other "dangerous amusements," providing religious education to children, and adopting "all measures" "for the religious improvement of" "Our Colored Brethren."

The *Reporter* copied Section III of the Letter from the May 15, 1869 *Philadelphia Catholic Standard*, but omitted a final paragraph that claimed that criminal abortion was not prevalent among Catholics. It began:

We confidently believe that you, Beloved Children in Christ, are strangers to this unnatural vice. Our words therefore are the language rather of warning than of reproof. Let these sins, dearly loved; be "not so much as named among you as it becometh Saints, ... for know ye this, that no one who doeth such things, hath any inheritance in the kingdom of Christ and of God."[6]

On October 12, 1869, less than six months after the Tenth Provincial Council of Baltimore ended, Pope Pius IX made induction of abortion at any stage of pregnancy a ground for excommunication.[7] It is possible Archbishop Spalding's May Pastoral Letter or other possible communications from the Archbishop about the problem of criminal abortion in the United States was a factor in this Papal action. The claim by Pallen, Rochester, and other physicians that unnecessary abortion was most prevalent in the United States suggests that this action by Pope Pius IX was stimulated by these frequent United States' abortions. Orson Squire Fowler would shortly write of criminal abortion: "The Catholic Bishop of Baltimore, and some others, have anathematized it, and turned St. Peter's keys against its perpetrators."[8] Fowler may have been guessing about this or may have read somewhere that Archbishop Spalding "and some others" had been advisors to the Pope on the problem of abortion in the United States.

Archbishop Spalding's awareness of the "hecatombs of infants that are annually sacrificed" surely stemmed from the medical and popular articles and books of Storer and other physicians or from the popular antiabortion writing of Todd, Eddy and Edwards, Coxe, and other Protestant clergy that definitely did stem from the antiabortion writing of physicians. The Archbishop's letter to Bishop Gibbons included: "You might hit again at round dancing, obscene theatricals, & perhaps [the] 'murder of the innocents' & the practice of some physicians to kill the child in order to save the mother."[9] The last phrase shows that Spalding was aware of craniotomy and it is possible that Dr. Gunning Bedford's views had been directly or indirectly communicated to him. Bedford was still alive, although outside Spalding's Province. Closer Catholic physicians were Joseph Meredith Toner and David Francis Condie, but none of these show up on the list of correspondents among the Archbishop's papers.[10] Horatio had repeatedly and extensively condemned craniotomy in his books and articles and Storer probably was Spalding's source.

Archbishop Spalding had made reference to criminal abortion three months earlier in his February 14, 1869 Lenten Sermon and this apparently was his first reference to the problem.[11] The actual Sermon was not preserved, but the *Catholic Mirror* of February 20, 1869 summarized it, first describing references by Spalding to obscene performances and immodest dancing. The *Mirror* then turned to his comments on abortion:

> Finally, the Most Rev. Orator said, that he could scarcely trust himself to refer to what was still behind and was far worse than all this; an abomination leading to the depopulation and desolation of the land; to excesses worse than the murder of the innocents by Herod, because committed not so much through sudden passion or the motive of cruel ambition, but with deliberately wicked purpose: a practice worse, probably, than any ever generally adopted even among heathens, but which, nevertheless, was becoming frightfully common in this enlightened age and country, and which was even occasionally defended as an evidence of growing enlightenment!! He would not refer more particularly to a turpitude too shocking to think of, one which should not even be named among Christians; but he deemed it a sacred and solemn duty to give this warning, in general and sufficiently intelligible language; as, though these horrible and unnatural excesses referred to were almost unknown among Catholics, and were not as yet, thank God, believed to have reached this latitude, at least to any great extent, they were fast approaching us, and threatening the ruin of our people, body and soul. He wished to put it on record, that the Catholic Church utterly abhors such abominations in every form and shape, and under whatsoever pretext they are practised, as an atrocious violation of the divine commandment—Thou Shalt not Kill.[12]

The references to abortion not having "reached this latitude, at least to any great extent," also suggests that Horatio or some other writer who had emphasized the New England abortion problem was the Archbishop's major source of information. Storer's claims that criminal abortion was virtually unknown among Roman Catholics and that abortionists were worse than Herod also were repeated in the Archbishop's sermon. Spalding may have read Storer's popular *Why Not?* or his recently published *Criminal Abortion: Its Nature, Its Evidence, and Its Law.*

Archbishop Spalding was not reluctant to communicate with the Vatican.[13] It does not seem far-fetched to claim that Pope Pius IX's October 1869 classification of unnecessary abortion at any stage of pregnancy as "an excommunicable offense" was stimulated by Spalding. If so, Pope Pius IX's landmark "Apostolicae Sedes" may have been another result of the "physicians' crusade against abortion," since American physicians directly or indirectly led the Archbishop to his concerns about criminal abortion.

Hugh Lenox Hodge republished his 1839/1854 Introductory Lecture sometime after May 29, 1869 when Archbishop Spalding's pastoral letter appeared in the *Medical and Surgical Reporter.*[14] Hodge mentioned the Archbishop's warning to "his flock" in his Preface to the republished lecture and followed the *Reporter* in misspelling "Spaulding."[15] It could be the Archbishop's attention to abortion and the editorial discussion of this by Butler of the Philadelphia-based *Reporter* were factors in the Philadelphia-based Hodge returning to the issue.

Hodge's Preface discussed the recent history of efforts by physicians, the clergy, and legislators to suppress the crime. It included:

"In 1856 Professor Storer of Harvard University, assisted by his son, Dr. Horatio R. Storer, so greatly interested the profession upon this subject that the American Medical Association in 1857 appointed a committee of leading physicians in different parts of the United States, to investigate the extent of this crime, and to report what legislative enactments were necessary for its repression."[16]

The actual date of David's Introductory Lecture was 1855, and, given this error, one must be particularly cautious in accepting Hodge's claim that Horatio assisted David in "greatly interesting" the profession in criminal abortion. Admittedly, we have already suggested that this may have been the case, based on other circumstantial evidence.

Hodge indicated he was republishing his lecture "to protect the health and welfare of individuals, and to promote the best interest of society." "A few additional observations will be added," his Preface included, "to contribute as far as possible to illuminate the minds of parents, guardians and all those intelligent and virtuous citizens who superintend the education of youth, or who, in any way, can contribute to form the character of the rising generation, or stay the progress of this alarming social evil."[17]

Hodge's "few additional observations" occupied eight pages. He described different strategies for convincing women seeking abortions to continue pregnancies. "Intellectual and moral appeals" would work with some women: "let his language be plain and urgent, and he will often have the satisfaction, not merely of preserving the life of the unconscious foetus, but also of contributing to the intellectual and moral welfare of his confiding patient." However, he claimed such appeals were certain to fail for the unmarried woman whose need "to preserve their reputation and escape degradation becomes the all-absorbing idea, and renders them perfectly insensible to all other considerations." Hodge cautioned the physician never to "swerve from the path of duty." He should "be kind, sympathetic, and charitable, and contribute in any possible way to diminish the anxiety and protect the character of his patient, short of sanctioning, either directly or indirectly, any injury to the intra-uterine being, which he and its unfortunate mother are solemnly bound to protect."[18] While "intellectual and moral appeals" would fail for the selfish woman, appeals to her "selfishness" could be effective. These should be based on the dangers to her health and life and Hodge presented a long list of fatal and nonfatal consequences of forced abortion.

The 73-year-old Hodge concluded his "few additional observations" with the following:

> The corollary or conclusion from this whole argument is that human life commences at the time of conception; that the embryo and foetus therefore should be protected during its intra-uterine life as sedulously as after birth. Hence, that all efforts, direct or indirect to disturb the progress of gestation, or to injure the product of conception, are criminal, alike violating the laws of nature and of God. That this crime, fatal to the foetus, is often destructive also to the mother's life, and in a large number of cases, where her life is not forfeited, she becomes prey to a long catalogue of physical and moral evils; injurious alike to the health of her body and mind.
>
> It results also that the best interests of society, and the prosperity of the nation, are deeply involved in this subject.
>
> Hence every citizen, every parent and guardian, every right-minded and virtuous individual should throw the weight of his influence and authority against this wide-spread crime, destructive alike to domestic happiness and to the national prosperity.[19]

Demand for Hodge's republished lecture was sufficient that editions were published in 1872 and 1876, the latter three years after Hodge's death. Physicians would continue to refer to the lecture for several decades.

The July 24, 1869 *Medical and Surgical Reporter* included the following brief note that could be interpreted as evidence that abortionists felt remorse, at least after conviction for the crime:

Conviction and Suicide of an Abortionist.

Dr. John Day, of Battle Creek, Michigan, was tried and convicted, June 1st, of committing abortion on the person of Mrs. Graves,
a married woman. When he learned of the verdict, he did not seem
much dejected, but that night he took morphia sufficient to destroy
him, and was found dead in the morning.[20]

However, it may be that this Michigan suicide was a result of the pain associated
with being falsely labeled an abortionist. In March 1889, the *Canada Lancet* provided an editorial claiming that false charges of abortion were not uncommon
against the physicians who only treated the aftereffects of criminal abortion. The
Editor indicated that "in more than one instance" the falsely charged physician had
committed suicide.[21]

Andrew Nebinger, M.D., the retiring President of the Philadelphia County
Medical Society, presented a paper condemning criminal abortion before that
Society on February 9, 1870.[22] It was a restatement of the data and conclusions
of Storer, Hodge, Gardner, and others related to the high prevalence of forced
abortion, particularly among educated married women. Nebinger called on
physicians to instruct women about the living being in their wombs that they
were so unconcernedly having destroyed. He also called on the Legislature, the
courts, and all legal instrumentalities to take up "the good work of crushing out
the accursed crime."[23]

Nebinger viewed condemnation of induced abortion by the clergy as
essential in any major reduction of the crime. He noted that Catholics and Jews
avoided criminal abortion and claimed that women of other faiths also could be
persuaded to allow their unborn children to be born. He called on the leaders of
religions to make "a well-concerted attack upon the front and flank of the
abomination." They should persist "until success shall have crowned their
efforts, and woman shall stand in glorious grandeur disenthralled from the great
vice of our day, the murder of unborn babies."[24] As will be seen, several other
physicians would echo Nebinger's call for clergy involvement in the crusade
against criminal abortion. However, even more physicians concluded that the
Protestant clergy was unwilling to address the issue.

CHAPTER 17
POPULAR BOOKS CONDEMNING ABORTION

Several books written by physicians appeared at the end of the decade that included long discussions of abortion. *The Science of a New Life* by John Cowan, first published in 1869, may have been the most widely read.[1] There were more than twenty printings with at least one for each of the years from 1869 to 1875. Its popularity occurred despite the fact (or perhaps because of the fact) that Cowan advised married couples to abstain from sexual intercourse except for the purpose of procreation. Cowan's chapter, "Foeticide," began with an explanation of why criminal abortion existed:

> Out of the licentiousness of the man and bondage of the woman there is developed the ever-present and ever-increasing great wrong and monstrous crime of an undesigned and undesired maternity—a wrong and crime, the perpetrators of which, rather than be thwarted in the exercise of the licentious of their nature, commit without thought of consequence here or hereafter, the crime of foeticide—the killing of the foetus while in the mother's womb—the murder of the unborn.[2]

The earlier "wrong and crime" of an unplanned and unwanted pregnancy that abortion compounded had been the subject of an 1858 book by Henry Clarke Wright.[3] Wright, an abolitionist who opposed the domination of women as well as slaves, preceded Cowan in describing criminal abortion as a frequent result of unplanned and unwanted pregnancies. Wright's awareness of abortion stemmed from his efforts as an investigator and advisor of couples with marriage problems.

Cowan claimed that there was a great deal of criminal abortion in the country and substantiated this with quotes from Allen, Reamy, and "Rev. Dr. Eddy," including Eddy's "'in one little village of one thousand inhabitants, …'"[4] Numerous authors would repeat Cowan's references to Allen, Reamy, and Eddy that Cowan himself clearly obtained from the March 1867 *Northwestern Christian Advocate*.

Cowan used the following to back his claim that life began at conception and to show the implications of purposely ending this new life:

> At no other possible time of pre-natal or ante-natal life can the soul and body of a new being be originated than at its conception; and the forcible removal of this being during its growth in the mother's womb causes its premature death, and therefore its [sic] MURDER, and the party or parties who do it, or are accessory to it, are MURDERERS.[5]

Cowan noted that married women were more likely to seek abortion than the unmarried. He made a distinction between married women who sought abortion because the offspring interfered "with their pleasures" and married women who sought abortion "because of poverty or sickness, or otherwise being unprepared to lovingly assume the burden of a desired maternity." Of the former group, he could say: "Not one good word in extenuation of their unholy lives and unlawful crimes. This class of women … is the most to be reprobated, and deserve in full measure the severe pains and penalties attached to their wrong-doings."[6]

However, he saw these "wrong-doers" as fewer in number than the married women seeking abortion "because of poverty or sickness, or otherwise being unprepared to lovingly assume the burden of a desired maternity." He blamed the husband's "unrestrained licentiousness" for causing these women to seek abortion.[7] However, should a woman reader believe a contemplated abortion was thus justified, Cowan followed with a list of forced abortion dangers that caused immediate death, death within hours, or death in from one to ten days. And should she escape death, there followed

> such an array of evil results as might well deter any woman from the commission of this great crime. Diseases of the pelvis—such as vesical and uterine fistula, adhesions of the os or vagina, etc., all of which are often incurable; uterine displacements, and all of their attendant miseries. Sterility sooner or later results, so that when the woman really desires offspring, her desires and prayers bring no echoing response. Should the woman succeed in bearing children, they will likely be puny, unhealthy, deformed and short-lived.[8]

Cowan also claimed that the woman who had an abortion faced an increased risk of "that fatal disease, cancer," when she reached menopause.

However, an even more effective ploy for discouraging criminal abortion may have been the threat he claimed it posed to her appearance. Cowan wrote: "The woman who produces abortion destroys the bloom of her ripe womanhood, hardens and deepens the face-lines, angularizes the hitherto rounded contours, the outward loving expression of the soul's interior presence is darkened, the rich maternal love-nature is lost, and premature old age comes on with galloping strides."[9]

He continued:

> And lastly, there is the ever-present remorse of conscience—the ever-present phantom of a great crime—a crime against humanity—a crime against the loving mercy and justice of God, ever asserting the individuality of its thought-nature, ever destroying all peace and happiness of the perpetrator. And well it may; for if murder will not do it, and especially the murder of one's own child, what will do it?—what can do it?[10]

Cowan claimed that it would be better to kill the child after birth, since this would be less dangerous in its effects on the mother.

"This," you may exclaim, "is horrible!" No doubt of it; but it does not differ in the least from the taking life during its existence in the mother's womb—and it has this to recommend it: that the murder of the child after birth would prevent all the serious after-consequences to the mother that attend its prenatal murder. Without doubt, the doing this would subject the perpetrator to arrest, imprisonment and trial for murder before a jury of her countrymen, yet this trial and punishment would be but an evanescent and trifling affair in comparison with the trial she will have to encounter at the Bar of Judgment, the throne of God, before the earth's assembled multitudes, and having as witnesses these undeveloped souls that she thoughtlessly and recklessly or knowingly and determinedly deprived of life before even they entered on their post-natal existence.[11]

Cowan ended his abortion chapter with recommendations to prevent its further increase. He believed that overcoming women's ignorance about the enormity of the crime would "forever banish all thoughts of murdering their unborn offspring." Men needed to be "educated into a right understanding of the use and abuse of amativeness," and this meant restriction of sexual intercourse to procreative efforts. Ministers and teachers needed to become better versed in human physiology so they could properly educate men and women. The wife whose husband was overly licentious needed to separate herself from her "licentious master," despite the hardships this might entail. It would not "cost as much as would her debasing slave-life with her so-called husband."[12]

The large sales of Cowan's book over more than 50 years and its dozens of favorable notices, including one from Elizabeth Cady Stanton who "made it my text-book in lectures," argue for its large influence on the public. Cowan no doubt prevented many of his women readers from seriously considering abortion as the solution to their *Undesigned and Undesired Maternity.*

Augustus Kinsley Gardner's 1860 article, "Physical Decline of American Women," was among the earliest popular articles condemning unnecessary abortion. Ten years later, Gardner published a popular book, *Conjugal Sins Against the Laws of Life and Health and Their Effects upon the Father, Mother and Child.*[13] Gardner noted in his Preface that the book was an extension of his earlier article and he included "Physical Decline" as an appendix to *Conjugal Sins.* His chapter, "Infanticide," began:

Of all the sins, physical and moral, against man and God, I know of none so utterly to be condemned as the very common one of the destruction of the child while yet in the womb of the mother. So utterly repugnant is it, that I can scarcely express the loathing with which I approach the subject. Murder! Murder in cold blood, without cause, of an unknown child; one's nearest relative; in fact, part of one's very being; actually having, not only one's own blood in its being, but that blood momentarily interchanging! Good God! Does it seem possible that such depravity can exist in a parent's breast—in a mother's heart! ...

We can forgive the poor, deluded girl,—seduced, betrayed, abandoned,—who, in her wild frenzy, destroys the mute evidence of her guilt. We have only sympathy and sorrow for her. But for the married shirk, who disregards her divinely-ordained duty, we have nothing but contempt, even if she be the lordly woman of fashion, clothed in purple and fine linen. If glittering gems adorn her person, within there is foulness and squalor.[14]

Gardner followed with long quotes describing abortion in past civilizations and quoted Ambrose Jardine, a French expert on medical law, who claimed that abortion was a regular business in the United States. He discussed the frequent deaths of women that resulted from criminal abortion and claimed that when they survived they often became diseased. However, he recognized that even these dire health consequences would not dissuade some women from attempting abortion and, like Andrew Nebinger, made a special plea to the clergy:

The pulpit of every denomination should make common cause and fulminate its anathemas against every abettor of this enormity. I know not why there should be such tenderness of speech on the part of the clergy, for there is no such modesty on the part of the actors concerned. Arrayed in gorgeous silks, satins and velvets, covered with flashing gems—mine is but the common story of every physician—I have had unknown women walk into my office, and inquire, "Are you the doctor?" and upon an affirmative reply without further preface, say, "I want you to produce an abortion for me," as coolly as if ordering a piece of beef for dinner.

Do the clergy consider this less a sin than lying, blaspheming or stealing? Do they sympathize with it? It is impossible for them to ignore it, for it is everywhere. Do they think it enough to publish, once a year, resolutions against it, which few men and no women ever see? Rev. John Todd has come out boldly and eloquently. Should not it be the subject of, at least, one sermon yearly by every clergyman in America and the world?

I have dedicated this volume to the clergy of America, because they are the great moral lever-power of the country. They can make this vice disgraceful; they can compel it to be kept dark; they can prevent its being the common boast of the women, "that they know too much to have babies."[15]

At least nine editions of *Conjugal Sins* were published with the ninth in the 1920s long after Gardner's death. *Conjugal Sins* also must be considered a factor in the prevention of many abortions, although it did not stimulate the widespread clergy response Gardner wanted.

Another popular book that dealt with criminal abortion came from the phrenologist, Orson Squire Fowler. In a section, "Abortion the commonest yet worst of crimes," Fowler indicated that abortion was "civilization's climax of abominations; and yet so alarmingly prevalent" that the medical profession "lately got up, indorsed, and published a prize essay, entitled, 'Why Not?,'" dealing with "its prevalence and evils. Read [it] and shudder at what it says of both."[16]

Fowler's statistics certainly bespoke "alarming prevalence." He claimed "thousands" of unmarried women "thus hide their shame," and "millions" of married women "deal death to the fruit of their own bodies!" Fowler also transmitted a bit of gossip: "A great statesman justly repudiated his new wife for its perpetration; he wanting issue, she to be the fashionable wife of a President."[17] He did not identify the "great statesman."

Fowler claimed that the crime was prevalent among church members and bolstered this with the following quote from a physician "in Washington Territory."

> "Going out from communion, a church communicant asked me to call on her professionally soon. I walked right home with her, into her parlor, when she insisted that I produce a miscarriage, then and there! Responding to another woman's call, I found her at family prayers.
>
> "Rising from her knees, she urged me to produce immediate abortion."[18]

Any Christian women who had purposely aborted must have winced at Fowler's repeated attacks:

> What thinks Christ of your killing His little lambs? Let Christian (?) civilization (?) take lessons of Chinese Heathenism, which lets them be born, then strangles, and casts them into the streets, to be picked up by morning scavengers, unless devoured; for that destroys only the child, this, its mother besides![19]

> Did that angel babe which died in your arms go to heaven? Then that unborn infant you destroyed has gone there likewise. Do you expect to meet the former at that "great judgment day"? Expect also that one whose life you took before it breathed to "rise up in judgment" against you when and where you would not be thus publicly accused and condemned.[20]

Fowler indicted the clergy for failing to deal with their errant parishioners:

> Ministers of the Gospel know that this sin is often perpetrated by "mothers in Israel," even by some of their own flock at that, without one shadow of excuse but "total depravity," "yet open not their mouths!" If they do not know of this sin, they are certainly too ignorant

and verdant to preach well. What are they if they do? If they knew a
murderer heard them every Sunday would they feel justified in omitting
all allusion to his crime? Nothing can justify this significant clerical
silence. It gives consent.[21]

Fowler was aware of Archbishop Spalding's recent efforts and, as noted
earlier, apparently believed that Spalding "and some others" had influence the
Pope's 1869 Bull, given the following that also demanded additional efforts by the
clergy and others:

> The Catholic Bishop of Baltimore, and some others, have
> anathematized it, and turned St. Peter's keys against its perpetrators.
>
> The Old School Presbyterian Church, thank God, has also
> condemned it! New School, Baptist, Methodist, Swedenborgian,
> Episcopalian, Universalist, Unitarian, Trinitarian, Arian, Spiritualists,
> and all others, follow suit. The tocsin now just sounded gives hope.
> Clergymen to the breach!
>
> "Young Men's Christian Association," put that plank into your
> platform. Teachers, teach that. Lecturers, lecture against that. Editors,
> edit that. Lawyers indict, judges condemn, and sheriffs punish that.
> Awake all to its extermination![22]

Fowler quoted "A Western Physician" who discussed physicians' duty:

> "I am often solicited by married ladies who, or whose husbands, want
> no more 'family,' and piteously implored by unfortunate unmarried
> 'ton,' and by parents to hide the disgrace of an aristocratic family, and
> sometimes by church members, by producing abortion; shall I offici-
> ate or decline? And why? Let *science*, not prejudice, say what I shall
> do."

The physician continued his conversation with Fowler:

> "Do? Do nothing. … In *principle*, wherein differs it from murder, but
> in being the worst form? Death pains are trifles, in either case, com-
> pared with life. Are you willing to do, and thus oblige yourself to re-
> member, *that* deed forever? Besides,
>
> "You break the august laws of the land; become a culprit and a
> felon; indictable and punishable any subsequent hour, by the friends
> or foes of either party. And all for what? Money cannot pay you. No."
>
> It finally came home to his daughter. But he shook his head,
> "Never;" he, she, and family less disgraced than by adding infanti-
> cide.[23]

It is not clear whether the daughter's illegitimate pregnancy was a hypothetical one raised in the conversation or a real one that actually produced disgrace for the physician and his family.

Another very popular book, *The Physical Life of Woman: Advice to the Maiden, Wife and Mother,* first published in 1869 by the physician, George Henry Napheys, also included a strong condemnation of abortion.[24] The short-lived Napheys was esteemed for both his medical and popular contributions. A sketch of Napheys claimed the Gynaecological Society of Boston elected him as a Corresponding Member "shortly after the first publication of the *Physical Life of Woman,* ... as a direct tribute of respect to him as the author of that work, thus obtaining for it the testimony of the highest body in that specialty then existing in our land."[25] The sketch probably was written by Daniel Garrison Brinton, co-author with Napheys on another popular book, and holder of the copyright for the 1890 edition of *The Physical Life of Woman* where this sketch appeared.

Napheys' chapter on criminal abortion included:

> *From the moment of conception* a new life commences; a new individual exists; another child is added to the family. The mother who deliberately sets about to destroy this life, either by want of care, or by taking drugs, or using instruments, commits as great a crime, is just as guilty, as if she strangled her new-born infant, or as if she snatched from her own breast her six-months' darling, and dashed out its brains against the wall. Its blood is upon her head, and, as sure as there is a God and a judgment, that blood will be required of her. The crime she commits is *murder, child-murder,*—the slaughter of a speechless, helpless being, whom it is her duty, beyond all things else, to cherish and preserve. ...
>
> We appeal to all such with earnest and with threatening words. If they have no feeling for the fruit of their womb, if maternal sentiment is so callous in their breasts, let them know that such produced abortions are the constant cause of violent and dangerous womb diseases, and frequently of early death; that they bring on mental weakness, and often insanity; that they are the most certain means to destroy domestic happiness which can be adopted. Better, far better, to bear a child every year for twenty years than to resort to such a wicked and injurious step; better to die, if needs be, in the pangs of childbirth, than to live with such a weight of sin on the conscience.[26]

Napheys' book was frequently reprinted, including an edition in German. An earlier sketch of Napheys, written a year after Napheys' suicide in 1877, claimed that a quarter of a million copies of *The Physical Life of Woman* had been sold.[27] One reason that Napheys book may have been so popular was that Napheys recommended contraception and, to a limited and erroneous extent, advised how to achieve it. He told the woman to exploit the periods of infertility "between her monthly illnesses" and while she was nursing.[28]

The Professor of Theory and Practice at Chicago's Hahnemann Medical College, Nicholas Francis Cooke, quoted much of the condemnation of unnecessary abortion from Napheys' *Physical Life of Women* in his own book, *Satan in Society: By a Physician*, and followed them with: "This has the ring of true metal. We like and indorse every word of it."[29] However, Cooke found fault with other sections of Napheys' book, particularly Napheys' advice to women on family limitation. Cooke's chapter on abortion, "The Sacred Rights of Offspring," began with a brief discussion of abortion among Roman women and then discussed how "[t]his monstrous heresy against religion, science, and common sense is not without its imitators in our own time."[30] Cooke then described a clergyman who wrote Cooke about his concern that his wife might be pregnant. His letter included:

> If Mrs._____ is in such a condition, it would be entirely proper now, before life or animation has commenced, that something be done to bring on the regular periods. We are both very anxious it *should* be done, and in her present condition there would be nothing at all wrong. But knowing her, and also our general circumstances, as I do, it seems to me a Christian duty. Had life commenced the case would be different.[31]

Cooke responded "immediately." He discussed the probable pregnancy of the clergyman's wife and the danger of interfering, particularly if she were not pregnant. He pointed out that both science and religion "declare positively that the child in the womb, from the very moment of conception, has being and soul, and consequently 'life or animation.'" Cooke guessed the clergyman meant by before life or animation, before the time "when it could maintain existence independently of the mother." "Why not, then," Cooke continued, "decide that it might be a 'Christian duty' to murder the infant six months or a year after birth, or, for that matter, at any time before it is old enough to defend itself?" This killing of the born child would be simpler and "and no danger to life or health would attach to the mother." He continued:

> Come, Reverend sir, I will as soon help you do the one as the other— suppose we try it? Certainly you can as well persuade me of my 'Christian duty' in the one case as in the other. It does not alter the case that physicians can be found ready to undertake your 'little affair.' Any physician who would undertake it is a monster and a scoundrel, and would murder you and your entire family as readily, 'for a consideration,' provided the chances of detection were equal. By the Almighty God who rules in Heaven, I conjure you do not this thing! nay, do not even contemplate it![32]

Cooke concluded his response by discussing the numerous consequences for the minister's wife if she were to have an induced abortion. These were hemorrhage, inflammations, insanity, barrenness, and "female weaknesses." "The long train of sad and tedious phenomena indicated by this popular term, is absolutely multifarious," Cooke continued, "congestions, ulceration, and prolapsus uteri, diseases of the bladder, urethra, and rectum, incontinence of urine, spinal irritation, sciatica, and other things, of which the greatest misfortune is that they do not kill, but simply render life insupportable." Cooke continued:

> It is due to these parties to mention that the arguments set forth in our response, had the full effect intended, and that they now rejoice in the possession of the mature product of that pregnancy—a living refutation of the assertion that man can ever usurp the functions of Divine Providence. The health of the mother has been fully restored through the very process which, in the fallible judgment of man, appeared most calculated to destroy it. Were this the place, or did space permit, we could adduce many remarkable facts within our own observation illustrative of this truth. A few must suffice:[33]

Cooke then described five more cases where women wished their pregnancies to be terminated, were talked out of it, and where each set of parents was delighted with their new child. "Numberless similar instances are within the knowledge of physicians," he continued, "and every practitioner of experience could add some dozens to the list." Even if Cooke is exaggerating to some extent, it is probable that the "[n]umberless similar instances" amounted to thousands of children, probably hundreds of thousands of children each year. Perhaps it is not necessary to again point out that they became the ancestors of millions.

Cooke next took on Edwin Moses Hale:

> A medical writer of some note, ... published, in 1861, a pamphlet, in which he declared himself the hero of three hundred abortions. In speaking of a certain instrument well adapted to the infamous purpose, he claims to have used it "several times since this little work was commenced, and always with success." In a subsequent work the same writer admits that he only found abortion necessary to save the life of the mother in four instances, thus publicly confessing that in an immense number of cases he has performed the operation on other grounds; and yet, in the face of all this self-accusation, several attempts at his expulsion from his county medical society have been defeated, and he is accounted "a brother in good standing" of several learned bodies, and holds an enviable position in a fashionable Church and fashionable society.[34]

Hale's 1860 pamphlet, "On the homoeopathic treatment of abortion," included phrases nearly identical to those Cooke quoted and certainly was the pamphlet that Cooke discussed as "published in 1861." Hale's "subsequent work," *The Great Crime of the Nineteenth Century*, included: "I have been obliged to cause the destruction of the foetus but *four* times, and in each instance it was done *to save the life of the mother.*" This was hardly "publicly confessing" that he had frequently "performed the operation on other grounds," but Cooke apparently assumed Hale's previous discussions about numerous inductions of abortion constituted such a confession. Cooke may have been incorrectly blaming Hale for being lax about the crime. However, in 1888 Hale agreed to perform an abortion on a "Girl Reporter" of the *Chicago Times* who feigned an illegitimate pregnancy (See Chapter 22). Nathan Smith Davis provided a letter to the *Chicago Times* during their expose calling for Hale's arrest as an abortionist. Another Chicago physician made the flat claim that Hale "has been in the business for twenty-five years and made his money principally in this nefarious pursuit."

Cooke's *Satan in Society* was tremendously successful and there were editions every year from 1869 through 1884 and the book was still published as late as 1895. Numerous editions exist in libraries and are currently available for sale by many dealers in old books.

The Ohio physician, Franklin Wayne Intrikin, published a book in 1871 called the *Woman's Monitor*.[35] Intrikin's last chapter dealt with and condemned unnecessary abortion. The author frequently quoted from Storer's *Why Not* and Cooke's *Satan in Society*. Unlike the widely distributed books discussed earlier, the *Woman's Monitor* probably was not a major factor in the physicians' crusade. It is mentioned because Intrikin provided the unique claim that some physicians had provided abortions in the past as a result of the "urgent demand of a wealthy friend or an influential patron," but "having since looked carefully into the nature of intra-uterine life," now could not be induced to perform such abortions "for all the wealth of California."[36]

CHAPTER 18
PHYSICIAN ABORTIONISTS

In April 1870, the *Boston Medical and Surgical Journal* published a paper that Obed Chester Turner had recently read to the Bristol North District Medical Society.[1] Turner graduated from Tufts College in 1859 and obtained his M.D. from the Medical School at Georgetown in the District of Columbia in 1864. He served as Assistant Surgeon on a ship in the Potomac Flotilla in 1865 and, after the war, returned to his hometown of Attleborough, Massachusetts where he was practicing in 1870.[2]

Turner claimed that there were regular physicians who performed unnecessary abortions and other regular physicians who may not have performed abortions but defended the practice. He began by outlining the problem:

> Mr. President and Gentlemen,—There is a subject which deserves the gravest consideration of medical men, and which pertains to the most vital interests of society, but which is, or appears to be, unthought of, or at least untalked of, in our meetings. There is an ever-deepening shadow creeping over the face of the land, like a destroying plague. There is a soul-staining crime which is corrupting the community, a flood undermining the very foundations of our civilization, and which demands our united efforts to resist and sweep back. Physicians, whose efforts should be put forth to save and prolong life, connive and assist in destroying it. Parents, whose natural and Heaven-given instincts should lead them to cherish their offspring and multiply their species, debase themselves far below the level of the brute creation, and for their temporary convenience stain their hands with blood and their souls with sin. Where the Asiatic cholera or any other dreaded pestilence takes one this takes ten, and for every hundred that consumption, that scourge of our race, demands, this Moloch receives a sacrifice of thousands. Legislators overlook it, or at least make no efficient attempt to stay its progress; the press and the pulpit are almost silent in regard to it, and so the carnival of death goes on unchecked. Gentlemen, you know to what I refer, the slaughter which out herods Herod, *Criminal Abortion.*[3]

Turner's belief that the subject of criminal abortion was "unthought of, or at least untalked of, in our meetings" may seem incorrect, given the large number of society presentations and articles already discussed in this book. The same point had been made by the Pennsylvania physician, H.A. Spencer, and other physicians would comment about the lack of professional attention to the subject. One explanation, and one implied by Turner, is a contrast effect where other life-threatening diseases and accidents were frequently addressed despite a much lower death rate than that occurring for the aborted unborn children and even despite fewer deaths than occurred to women as a result of criminal abortion.

There was no question that Turner viewed criminal abortion as murder unlike a "defender" of abortion who told Turner: "There is no life in the foetus until respiration is established after birth." Turner responded:

> With respiration? That is only one added function. There was circulation previously, and the power of nervous action and motion. Why is not a foetus alive when it is diving and plunging in its mother's womb? Simply because its lungs are not inflated? Out on such nonsense! One might as well say that a child born blind was not alive because it did not use its eyes.[4]

Turner continued by indicating that only pelvic deformities that prevented live births justified abortion. He indicated the "girls who have 'got into a scrape'" should not be saved by the physician "from a just measure of disgrace." However, he indicated that it was married women who obtained the bulk of the abortions.

Turner then turned to the physicians who provided them and their motivations:

> "But," says the professional murderer, "if I don't do this some one else will; and I may as well have the money as these quacks." Here is the prime reason of his strong desire to save people from disgrace. A member of the medical profession, in good standing apparently, and not unknown to all of us, told me that not a day passed that he did not procure an abortion for somebody, and perhaps more than one.* He used the above argument in justification, but what weight has it? None at all.[5]

Edwin Moses Hale had hinted that abortionists took sexual advantage of their clients. Turner was more explicit:

> They are in our very midst; we all know what they are. Unscrupulous, lecherous, adulterous perhaps (for we know that under certain circumstances, having a woman's secret at his disposal, the abortionist can make demands of her which she dare not refuse), ready to commit crime for a few dollars—why may we not suppose that he would be willing, for a small fee, to remove an aged parent from the path of an anxious heir, or perform any other crime which could be done easily and secretly?[6]

Turner concluded:

> The remedy rests with ourselves. Let us refuse, under any and all
> circumstances, to be accessory to the crime of which we have spoken.
> Let us discountenance any practitioner who persists in performing it.
> He is not worthy of recognition, either as a physician or a man. His
> manhood is blotted out since he has prostituted his medical
> knowledge to the service of crime.[7]

Turner moved from Attleborough to Vermont and then to Cambridge,
Massachusetts where he became the Assistant City Physician. He died there on
October 31, 1882 from typhus contracted while treating a family of recently
arrived immigrants. His obituary honored his death in "active service,"
comparing it to the death of a surgeon serving on the Gettysburg or Wilderness
battlefields.[8]

Addison Niles, a leading physician of Quincy, Illinois, presented a paper
"Criminal Abortion" to the Illinois State Medical Society on May 16, 1871. He
indicated that during his "third of a century" of medical practice he had
witnessed increasing demand for criminal abortion. His sources were
confidential communications from "the practitioners themselves" and from their
patients, "many of whom were in high standing in the communities in which
they lived."[9]

Of particular interest was Niles' discussion of medical society members
who were abortionists:

> Physicians undoubtedly have a duty to perform, and if every regular
> practitioner were true to himself and his profession, much could be
> effected. But it is useless to deny that regular physicians in good
> standing in the profession are deeply implicated in the crime. The
> question, in many places, is not who are abortionist[s]? but who, if
> any, has kept his skirts free from "blood guiltiness" in this matter?
> Members known to be abortionists should be expelled from medical
> societies, and in counties where they control them, the honest portion
> should withdraw and organize themselves.[10]

By indicating abortionist *control* of some societies, Niles showed that physician
abortionists were not the small minority, or at least were no longer the small
minority, that most physicians had earlier claimed. Their larger incomes may
have made them the prominent members and even controllers of their local
medical societies.

More accusations that regular physicians were abortionists were made at
the 1870 Meeting of the American Medical Association in Washington, D.C.
The Ireland-born, Jefferson-Medical-College-educated Maryland physician,
Dominick A. O'Donnell, proposed the following Resolutions and they were
accepted unanimously by the attending members:

> *Resolved*, That a committee of three be appointed whose duty it shall
> be to represent the evil of criminal abortion in its proper light, and to

take into consideration the best course to be pursued by the profession in arresting its progress, and in forcing from our ranks all who now, or may hereafter, pursue this iniquitous course. And that the said Committee shall report at the next annual meeting of this Association.

   Resolved, That the members of this Association, in expressing their unqualified denunciation of such persons, are acting in accordance with the high trust reposed in them, and paying a just tribute to their individual characters, and to a noble and honorable profession.[11]

The Committee on Criminal Abortion that was appointed consisted of O'Donnell, Washington L. Atlee, of Pennsylvania, and Henry F. Askew, of Delaware.[12] Nathan Allen also was present at the 1870 meeting and presented a paper, "On the Physiological Laws of Human Increase." In the published version, Allen only briefly discussed criminal abortion as a factor accounting for differences in the number of births for "Irish, English, Scotch, and American women." "A partial explanation was soon discovered," Allen wrote, "viz, that some portion of the latter used various means to prevent conception, and in case of pregnancy to procure abortion."[13]

Allen may have expanded on this in his spoken presentation and this may have caused the new Committee to cite Allen as the authority on criminal abortion in their Report on Criminal Abortion presented a year later at the Annual Meeting in San Francisco.[14] Their Report made no mention of Horatio Storer, the preceding 1859 Association Report on Criminal Abortion, or the Association's appeals to state legislatures and state medical societies that had caused and probably were still causing major revisions in the abortion laws. This probably reflected the animosity between Washington L. Atlee and Storer who were competing ovariotomists. Atlee's antipathy toward Horatio was shown at the 1871 AMA meeting in a debate on recognition of women physicians (Storer opposed and Atlee supported this).[15] O'Donnell himself may have developed a dislike of Horatio at the 1870 AMA Convention where Storer was a principal in at least three controversial issues.[16]

Although Nathan Allen had made only a brief reference to abortion in his 1870 AMA paper, he expanded his discussion of criminal abortion in other articles and one of these longer paragraphs was quoted in the 1871 Report. It read:

"The only remaining cause [of the reduced birth rate], 'prudential considerations,' cannot be passed over so lightly. These have had their influences in a great variety of ways; in postponing marriage till a later age in life; in regarding the care and expense of children as a burden, as well as in preferring pleasure and fashion to domestic duties and responsibilities. To such an extent has this 'prudence' been carried, that a great variety of means have been adopted to prevent conception, and in case of pregnancy to produce abortion."[17]

The quote continued with Allen's theory that a "radical change in the organization of women" accounted for women's loss of "natural instincts," their low estimate of "the value of human life," and their willingness "to defeat one of the most important objects of the marriage institution."

The 1870 Resolutions expressed "unqualified denunciation" of those who pursued the "iniquitous course" of criminal abortion. The 1871 Report expanded on this:

> These modern Herods, like their prototype, have a summary mode of dealing with their victims. They perform the triple office of Legislative, Judiciary, and Executive, and, to crown the tragedy, they become the executioners. They seem impatient for the sacrifice; the "fiat" goes forth, and those innocent and helpless victims are not permitted ever to breathe that vital air which God in His providence has destined for their use in common with the rest of the human family. Their resting-place is rudely invaded, and that which would grow and ripen into manhood is cut off from existence by the hand of an educated assassin. Mark the monster as he approaches his work! With a countenance which generally characterizes the movements of the interior—which serves as an index to a corrupt heart, he stands by the bedside of his victim, with poisoned cup or instrument in hand, ready to proceed to the work of destruction. Does any compunction assail his corrupt soul, as he gazes on the field of his labors? Does he measure the extent of the foul deed he is about to commit? Or does he not fear that the uplifted hand of all avenging God will suddenly fall on his guilty head? No; Judas-like, he solaces himself with the prospect of thirty pieces of silver, and this forms the climax of his aspirations![18]

The women who sought abortion also came in for rough treatment:

> And woman, whose high destiny was to be instrumental in propagating the human family; who ought to be the appropriate representative of a refined age, a model of purity, the centre of honor and affection—she descends from her high position, associates with these degraded characters, and becomes a participant in the destruction of her own offspring. She becomes unmindful of the course marked out for her by Providence, she overlooks the duties imposed on her by the marriage contract. She yields to the pleasures but shrinks from the pains and responsibilities of maternity; and, destitute of all delicacy and refinement, resigns herself body and soul, into the hands of these unscrupulous and wicked men. Let not the husband of such a wife flatter himself that he possesses her affection. Nor can she in turn ever merit even the respect of a virtuous husband. She sinks into old age like a withered tree, stripped of its foliage; with the stain of blood upon her soul, she dies without the hand of affection to smooth her

pillow.[19]

The Report included much discussion about when life began. For example:

> By some it is supposed that at a certain period after conception, at a
> certain stage of development of the human embryo, a second concep-
> tion takes place, or, in other words, that God, as in the case Adam,
> breathes into it a living soul, and that from that period the presence of
> that soul, or life, becomes manifest. The other and the more rational
> view is, that God by His eternal "fiat," at the moment of conception,
> creates and breathes into the product of that conception a living soul,
> and that that soul under the same general law and guidance inhabits
> its frail tenement, until by its appropriate nourishment that tenement
> has assumed definite proportions to enable it (the new being) to move
> and give other evidences of life. … It matters little, however, what
> view may be taken of this subject, or what stage of development the
> embryo may have reached, it is to be the man of other days, and is
> more entitled to life than he who meditates its destruction.[20]

Although increased penalties for inducing abortion were mentioned, reform of statutes was not the major recommendation for eliminating criminal
abortion, as was the case in Storer's 1859 Report. Foremost, was getting rid of
the abortionists, and regular physicians were viewed by the author or authors as
a major problem. The following final paragraphs reiterated this and clearly show
that the overarching concern of the authors was the loss of human lives:

> It is time that the seal of reprobation were placed on these characters
> by all honest men; it is time that respectable men should cease to con-
> sult with them, should cease to speak to them, should cease to notice
> them except with contempt; and we are inclined to think, if such a
> course be pursued towards them, they will soon be induced to seek
> another locality, where they will find it to their advantage to pursue a
> more honorable course.
> If in the foregoing report our language has appeared to some
> strong and severe, or even intemperate, let the gentlemen pause for a
> moment and reflect on the importance and gravity of our subject, and
> believe that to do justice to the undertaking, free from all improper
> feeling or selfish considerations, was the end and aim of our efforts.
> We had to deal with human life. In a matter of less importance we
> could entertain no compromise. An honest judge on the bench would
> call things by their proper names. We could do no less.[21]

The new AMA Report called on physicians to visit members of the clergy
and influence them to publicly condemn abortion. This tactic was included in
the following Resolutions proposed by O'Donnell and Atlee that were adopted
by the membership:

Resolved, That we repudiate and denounce the conduct of abortionists, and that we will hold no intercourse with them either professionally or otherwise, and that we will, whenever an opportunity presents, guard and protect the public against the machinations of these characters by pointing out the physical and moral ruin which follows in their wake.

Resolved, That in the opinion of this Convention, it will be unlawful and unprofessional for any physician to induce abortion or premature labor, without the concurrent opinion of at least one respectable consulting physician, and then always with a view to the safety of the child—if that be possible.

Resolved, That we respectfully and earnestly suggest to private teachers and professors in public institutions the propriety of adopting, according to their judgment, the means best suited for preserving their pupils, and those who may hereafter come under their care, from the degrading crime of abortion.

Resolved, That we respectfully call the attention of the clergy of all denominations to the perverted views of morality entertained by a large class of females—aye, and men also—on this important question, and the ruin which has resulted and continues to result daily to the human family from such views.

Resolved, That we respectfully solicit the different medical societies, both State and local, to send delegates to the clergymen in their respective districts to request their aid in so important an undertaking.

Resolved, That it becomes the duty of every physician in the United States, of fair standing in his profession, to resort to every honorable and legal means in his power to crush out from among us this pest of society; and, in doing so, he but elevates himself and his profession to that eminence and moral standard for which God has designed it, and which an honorable and high-toned public sentiment must expect at the hands of its members.[22]

This 1871 Report with its six Resolutions appears to have produced little action by the membership of the American Medical Association. Viewing this 1871 effort, Horatio Storer may have recalled his words in the 1859 Report: "Mere resolutions and nothing more, are therefore useless, evasive, cruel." However, it clearly shows that the primary concern of its physician author or authors was the "execution" of the unborn child. What is more, there was no mention of the need to reduce competition from irregular practitioners and there was little discussion of protecting women from dangerous operations or preventing "foreigners" from becoming dominant over "Americans."

In August 1871, Butler's and Brinton's *Medical and Surgical Reporter* provided a long editorial, "Killing no Murder,"[23] that dealt with "destroying a fetus in order to save the life of the mother." Brinton discussed his early study of medicine in Europe and he contrasted the unwillingness of "timid old fogies" of the Academy of Medicine of Brussels to even discuss the question of abortion with what he heard "the venerable Velpeau" say: "the fetus has no independent life and no claims upon our consideration on any such account—that it is, in short, nothing more than a vegetable."[24] Brinton did not agree with Velpeau, but he did criticize a case where premature labor was not induced and "a woman was left to die, and did die." Brinton claimed that "an unusual timidity about what people might say, prevented the physician from doing his obvious duty, and destroying the foetus." The editorial concluded:

> We are second to none in opposing *criminal* abortion; every physician should condemn it with his utmost strength, but the hue and cry against it must not prevent him from doing his duty, and his full duty to defend his patient. It is the lawyer's duty to defend his client by every legal means; and, far more so is the physician called upon to save the life of his patient by every resource of ingenuity and art.[25]

Although certainly not the intended result, Brinton's strong defense of therapeutic abortion may have emboldened some physicians to help women end pregnancies that were far from life threatening.

CHAPTER 19

NEWSPAPERS BRIEFLY JOIN THE CRUSADE

At the May 18, 1871 meeting of the New York Academy of Medicine, resolutions were adopted commending Judge Gunning S. Bedford for the way he conducted the trials of two "notorious abortionists and enemies of mankind," Dr. Michael A.A. Wolff and Thomas Lookup Evans. Judge Bedford was the son of Dr. Gunning S. Bedford who died on September 5, 1870. The resolutions were reported in the *New York Times* on May 23, 1871 and were reprinted in the June 15, 1871 issue of George F. Shrady's *Medical Record*.[1]

Wolff was charged with manslaughter in the death of a woman on whom he had performed an abortion. At his January 1871 trial, Wolff's lawyer asked Judge Bedford to "direct a verdict of acquittal on the ground that the medical experts in the case were unable to tell the cause of the abortion." Bedford refused. Wolff's lawyer then indicated that the defense would produce no witnesses, and that the prisoner would not testify, as professional obligations sealed his lips."[2] The jury found Wolff guilty of manslaughter and Judge Bedford delivered his sentence with the following:

> Wolff, you are a well-known abortionist. But a few days ago, Judge Dowling inaugurated throughout this City an admirable system for the suppression of this rapidly-increasing crime. That system is now being faithfully carried out with telling effect by Superintendent Kelso. ... In one word the authorities have declared war to the bitter end against the fraternity which you, today, so guiltily represent. Let every professional abortionist—male and female, rich or poor, in this City—take warning, for on conviction their fate shall be the same as yours, namely, confinement in the State Prison for the period of seven years, the longest term allowed under the statute.[3]

The other abortionist, Thomas Lookup Evans, was indicted for manslaughter for procuring an abortion in August 1870 and his trial began May 13, 1871. This time the mother survived and was the "complainant." The news article continued: "The details of her description of the operations that he performed, and the death of her twin children subsequently, are of a revolting character, and totally unfit for publication."[4]

A later article indicated that Lookup Evans was convicted of second-degree manslaughter. The judge sentenced him to three years and six months in the State Prison. As with Wolff, Judge Bedford warned other professional abortionists: "He wished all persons engaged in the same business to distinctly understand that they would receive the merited punishment when justly convicted, and that no mercy should be extended to them."[5]

This strong support of these judicial efforts against abortion by the *Times* and other New York newspapers reflected a recent change in newspapers' relationship to criminal abortion. Prior to 1870, newspapers generally provided indirect support via their more-or-less veiled advertisements for abortionist services and for drugs that were claimed to produce miscarriage. In 1869, the *New York Times* ceased printing such advertisements and became strongly involved in antiabortion efforts. The editor was Louis Jennings who not only reported on abortion trials and wrote antiabortion editorials, but actually created news by having undercover reporters visit abortionists.[6]

One of Jenning's reporters, Augustus St. Claire, visited the major abortionists of New York with a female friend and pretended to seek an abortion for the woman. While at the offices of "Dr." Jacob Rosenzweig in the summer of 1871, St. Claire and his friend observed a beautiful blonde woman who apparently was waiting for an abortion. A few weeks later, she was found dead crammed inside a small trunk in a railroad baggage room. Many sensational stories for the *Times*, *New York Tribune*, and for other newspapers resulted about Alice Mowlsby, the poor "orphan" girl from New Jersey who died as a result of the abortion; about Rosenzweig who was arrested and convicted; and about Walter Conklin, the man who seduced her, arranged the abortion, and after confessing this, committed suicide.[7]

Judge Bedford's charge to the grand jury in the Rosenzweig case began by discussing the "murder most cruel in its nature" of the young woman who "in a moment of utter hopelessness and frantic despair, she gave herself up, and was robbed of her existence by the murderous hand of the abortionist." He then asked: "can crime so fearful and atrocious be perpetrated in the very midst of a Christian community, embracing within its jurisdiction more than a million of souls, and where the religion of heaven is preached and its holy mandates observed?" He concluded:

> Let the warning word this day go forth, and may it be scattered broad-cast through the land, that from this hour the authorities, one and all, shall put forth every effort and shall strain every nerve until these professional abortionists, these traffickers in human life, shall be exterminated and driven from existence, and the majesty of the law be fully vindicated in all cases of this fiendish character. And now, gentlemen, to conclusion, let me express the earnest hope (shared in, as I feel confident it will be, by you and all other right-minded citizens) that the Legislature, at its next session, will so amend the Statute Book so that ... the crime of abortion, shall be declared to be murder in the first degree, and punishable as such with death, instead of, as now, but manslaughter in the second degree punishable by imprisonment not exceeding seven years.

At the conclusion of this address there was loud applause in Court.[8]

George F. Shrady commented about the trunk murder in his *Medical Record* of September 15, 1871. He discussed the probable good result of all the sensational publicity. On the one hand, it would, "temporarily at least," halt the operations of most of the abortionists. On the other, it "cannot fail to awaken the public, not only to a positive knowledge of the enormity and growth of the crime, but the better to prepare it for solving the important question of prevention." Shrady noted that the "persistent efforts of the medical profession" to present the subject in its proper light had overcome "a false prudishness" and the newspapers now were willing to state the facts in abortion cases. He also noted that the public was becoming aware of the enormity of the crime and was applauding the actions of judges against abortionists and supporting the clergy in their denunciations.

Most noteworthy was Shrady's claim that the public was associating the crime with certain death for the woman. He saw this as a good thing that the medical profession should not contradict, but encourage:

> If the prospective victims of the abortionists could be made to understand and to believe this, a more efficient means of prevention could be adopted than any appeal on behalf of humanity to the unborn could effect. To many the contemplation of the crime of consenting to the death of the offspring is nothing compared with a reasonable certainty that death to the mother may be more than probable.[9]

Shrady then quoted the six Resolutions from the 1871 AMA Report and recommended them as guides for physicians in their efforts to combat criminal abortion. He also complimented Judge Bedford for his recommendation that the crime be made one of first-degree manslaughter.[10]

When the Gynaecological Society of Boston met on September 26, 1871, Dr. George H. Bixby, the Co-Editor of the Society's *Journal*, read much of Gunning Bedford's charge to the grand jury and Bedford's words were later published in the "Proceedings" of the Society. Bixby then asked for and received support for the following Resolution:

> "*Resolved*, That the Gynaecological Society of Boston has received, with unqualified approval, the charge to the Grand Jury of the Court of General Sessions, by Judge Bedford, of New York, upon the crime of abortion; and as in this great missionary work, to which it has pledged its aid, it believes in recognizing, fostering, and encouraging every effort in the right direction, from whatsoever source it may come; that it recognizes in this address the advice of a wise counselor, the opinion of an eminent jurist, and the sentiments of a good citizen and a Christian gentleman, and would, therefore, tender to Judge Bedford its sincere thanks."[11]

The New York Academy of Medicine also praised Judge Bedford with a preamble and series of Resolutions. The preamble quoted much of Bedford's charge to the jury with additional emphasis of Bedford's "shall be deemed guilty of murder in the first degree." Their Resolutions read:

> *Resolved*, That, in the opinion of the New York Academy of Medicine, the author of that language has, by so public a declaration of his sentiments, his intentions and his hopes, gives us reason for renewed expression of highest commendation, has vindicated the already widely-expressed support from the medical profession of the country, of the course he has hitherto pursued, and has, we trust, greatly strengthened the esteem and confidence in which he is held by the public.
>
> *Resolved*, That this Academy, in the discharge of the duty its professed objects commend—to promote public health and public morals—pledges all its influence and efforts, in support of any legislative or other measures which our law-officers may propose, as offering a reasonable promise of mitigating, if not removing, the pestilence of criminal abortion which is upon our country.
>
> *Resolved*, That to remove all doubt from the public mind, in regard to the position of the New York Academy of Medicine in this important matter, to secure the influence upon the State authorities desired by this expression, and to stimulate the medical profession generally to similar acts, a copy of this preamble and these resolutions be forwarded to Judge Bedford, to District-Attorney Garvin, and to the New York Bar Association; and the leading daily papers of this city, and its medical journals, be furnished with the same; and that the secular and medical papers and journals throughout the country be requested to copy.[12]

The "journals throughout the country" obliged. Shrady included the preamble and Resolutions in the October 16, 1871 *Medical Record*. The preamble and resolutions appeared in the *Boston Medical and Surgical Journal* on November 16, 1871. Their source was the *New York Medical Journal* who had copied it from the *Proceedings of the New York Academy of Medicine* for September 21, 1871. No doubt other medical journals also followed suit.

The New York newspapers were not alone in covering the "trunk murder." Marvin Olasky in *The Press and Abortion* mentioned newspapers in four other states that covered it and implied that many other newspapers covered it as well.[13] One Missouri newspaper's coverage of the murder led to a rare physician objection to the typical physician claim that criminal abortion was highly prevalent. J.P. Chesney, of St. Joseph, Missouri, published a letter in the *Medical and Surgical Reporter* that began:

> The literature of our profession has, within the last few years, contained many, very many articles, paragraphs and *assertions* in regard to "criminal abortion," particularly as to its existence and rapid increase in the United States. Now, I have never been a believer in the

prevalence of this abuse to the extent that the medical periodicals of the day would have us think, and for this reason: I have been an active practitioner of medicine for thirteen years past, and I can solemnly affirm that I have never been applied to but *one* time to relieve a female of her unwelcome encumbrance, nor have I known but a single instance where such an act has been performed by any of my professional acquaintances, and they are many.[14]

Chesney then discussed the recent newspaper interest in abortion, including the "late Conkling-Bowlsby tragedy in New York." Their investigations had led to

some of the "dailies" finding out since then that one woman in the highly moral city of Boston had in the last 17 years produced 20,000 abortions, as could be verified from "verbal and ledger testimony." That statement I have no doubt is as worthy of credence as many we see stated in our own professional literature, and yet does any one believe that a woman in Boston or anywhere else has procured *three and one-fifth abortions every day* for the past seventeen years? It is simply an absurdity.[15]

"Before there is much more said upon this subject," Chesney concluded, "let us have reliable facts and figures upon which to base our statements, and not swallow bare assertions and get alarmed over them."

It may be that Missouri women were less inclined to seek abortions than their counterparts in the eastern states. However, Montrose Pallen had not believed this to be the case for St. Louis and another Missouri physician, John W. Trader, would shortly describe the frequent requests for abortions in his area (See Chapter 20). What is more, three or more abortions per day may not have been such an "absurdity." The June 6, 1868 letter in the *Medical and Surgical Reporter* discussed earlier reported that a Philadelphia woman seeking an abortion from a female abortionist "found quite a number waiting for the same purpose."

No response supportive or critical of Dr. Chesney was located in subsequent numbers of the *Reporter*, although an Albany, New York physician, Thomas Davison Crothers, provided an article in that journal two weeks later dealing with a young woman who died in Albany following a criminal abortion by "Doctress" Emma Burleigh.[16] Crothers described the denial by a pair of physicians that the death had been a result of an abortion, an unusual delay on their part to examine the uterus for evidence of the cause of death, and their denial that the girl had recently been pregnant, despite testimony to the contrary. "These and many other obscure facts," Crothers concluded, "throw an unpleasant suspicion over the medical history of this case, as determined by the jury at the inquest."[17]

This case prompted a *Medical and Surgical Reporter* editorial which used satire, on the one hand, to discuss the high profitability of the popular "specialty" of abortion, and, on the other, to discuss the unwillingness of many newspapers to tackle these abortionists who provided them so much advertising revenue. Although the *New York Times* had dropped the advertisements for abortion, many other newspapers continued to take them. The Editors claimed this totaled $150,000 per year in New York City. In the following excerpt, "Margaret Campbell" was the 22-year-old woman who died in Albany at the hands of "Doctress Burleigh." Alice Bowlsby was the New York trunk murder victim.

> Naturally enough, editors and proprietors of newspapers, a class who always know which side of their bread is buttered, cannot but grieve to see such a handsome addition to their incomes dwindle away through an illiberal public opinion.
>
> We are not surprised, therefore, when a *contretemps* of the Alice Bowlsby kind occurs in the respectable City of Albany, in the hands of Doctress Burleigh, who has long been a liberal patron of their advertising columns, the large dailies, with one exception, have nothing to say about it.
>
> Whether bribed to silence, or ashamed to speak (the latter is hard to believe), it is true, so a correspondent in that city writes us, that *The Evening Times* is the only daily which has dared boldly to stigmatize in proper terms the authors and abettors of Margaret Campbell.
>
> This unfortunate young woman's history, is the same old story, seduction, pregnancy, attempted abortion at the hands of the doctress mentioned, death. But, position, money and influence are interested to keep back the truth about her fate. The Coroner's jury returned an evasive verdict, which does not touch the point at issue, the daily papers with the honorable exception of the *Evening Times* were prevailed to keep silence by such means as are usually efficacious, no doubt, and the *two medical men*, regular practitioners in reputed good standing, who apparently aimed to shield the criminal and avert justice, were not mentioned in the papers. They made the *post mortem*, and it looks as if they connived to defeat the laws.
>
> What else can we expect when papers of the widest circulation admit advertisements which invite to abortion? Are not such papers accessory before the fact?[18]

Horatio Storer persisted in San Francisco long after the meeting of the American Medical Association and contributed to the October 1871 "Editorial Notes" of the *Journal of the Gynaecological Society of Boston* from there.[19] He discussed the prevalence of malaria in the West and its contribution to uterine disease. He also discussed the proposals for sanitation in San Francisco that would make the city "the healthiest city of its size upon the continent." George H. Bixby concluded the "Notes" with a discussion of a recent Boston newspaper editorial condemning criminal abortion. "We heartily commend it," Bixby wrote, "for its truthfulness, boldness, and for the clear and comprehensive manner in which the editor has treated the subject." Bixby noted that the newspaper editor had claimed "'much can be done by the Press.'" Bixby agreed, and continued:

> A free discussion of this subject by every respectable journal in the land, would, we believe, carry conviction into many, many hearts, and save to the world innumerable precious lives, and untold moral and physical pangs. But what would be the use of free discussion, and such united action as that suggested in the noble sentiment of the editorial in question, when over against it in the same issue, or perhaps in a more conspicuous column, there appear the flaming announcements of notorious quacks and abortionists, or long lists of lauded nostrums, with their insidious cautions to women, in italics, against "their use by ladies in an interesting condition"?
>
> Is the press intended for the public weal or public woe? According to our observation in nine-tenths of the cases of criminal abortion, so often resulting in the death of both mother and child, the poor victim has found her information in the columns of some respectable newspaper.
>
> When we consider the extent of this crying evil, the very thought is appalling. We cannot serve God and mammon. We doubt the efficacy of the prayer of "Good God and Good Devil." No, gentlemen of the press, either lend us your powerful influence, undivided and unalloyed, in this humane, ennobling, Christianizing work,—an object worthy of the highest aspiration of the human soul,—or forever hold your peace.—G. H. B.[20]

The Special Committee on Criminal Abortions of The East River Medical Association of New York provided a Report that was approved by the members on December 5, 1871.[21] The authors began by noting the high prevalence of criminal abortion in New York City and claimed that one factor contributing to this was the sale of "nameless and numerous nostrums so extensively advertised and sold as powerful remedies for the removal of all female obstructions." They indicated that the advertisements for these drugs, "in language too plain to be misunderstood," often provided the "first impulse to abandon the path of virtue."[22]

Another problem was the unwillingness of physicians to report professional abortionists to the authorities. They denied "that any member, in good standing, can be justly charged with being engaged in or with countenancing this abominable practice."[23] However, they claimed that by refusing to implicate the patients who required their services after consulting abortionists and thus protecting the abortionists as well, criminal abortion continued virtually unchecked.

However, of most current interest was their claim of the large role of unregulated physicians in the problem and their proposal to use the sharp increase in public concern about abortion as a means to achieve needed regulation of the medical profession. They wrote:

The recent developments of the horrid practices of professional abortionists has dispelled the hitherto prevailing apathy of the people and authorities, and has aroused a justly indignant public to demand the adoption of measures for the suppression of the unrestrained practice of medicine. Much credit is due to the public press for the severity with which it has denounced this evil; and too much can not be said in praise of the judiciary for the noble sentiments it has uttered on this subject, as also for its prompt and vigorous action toward criminals of this class, as was made evident by the results of the recent trials. *Your committee deem the unrestrained practice of medicine as the main cause for the existence of professional abortionists, and the want of proper laws to regulate the practice of medicine as encouraging knaves to assume and practice under titles which institutions duly chartered by the State alone have the right to confer.* Our laws know no distinction between the duly authorized physician and the imposter. They grant no privileges to the one which are not equally enjoyed by the other.[24]

The Committee then discussed ways to get "a justly indignant public to demand the adoption of measures for the suppression of the unrestrained practice of medicine." They wrote:

We call upon our chartered colleges, and upon the entire medical faculty of this State, not to allow the present opportunity to pass by without making one united and earnest effort to induce our next legislature to pass laws which, while they would tend to protect the morals and the health of the community, would at the same time afford that protection and encouragement to a profession honored and fostered by every civilized government except this.[25]

In support of this, the Report included a draft of "AN ACT TO SUPPRESS CRIMINAL ABORTIONS, AND TO REGULATE THE PRACTICE OF MEDICINE AND SURGERY IN THE STATE OF NEW YORK." The first section laid out the penalties for inducing abortion. The second did this for the administration and advertising of drugs for this purpose. The next three sections, respectively, prohibited unauthorized persons from practicing medicine, prohibited practice under a fictitious or fraudulent diploma, and established a register of physicians judged certified to practice.[26]

Mohr in *Abortion in America* made the valid claim that this Report was evidence that opposition to criminal abortion was being used by regular physicians as a means to legally control medicine.[27] However, it was the new *public* opposition to criminal abortion that they wished to exploit for this purpose. The long-standing *physician* opposition to criminal abortion had led to few earlier calls for regulation of medicine. The 1859 and 1871 American Medical Association Reports on Criminal Abortion did not call for such government regulation of medicine as a means to curtail the crime, nor did a score or more of antiabortion papers and editorials by physician communicating their intense opposition to criminal abortion. As we have repeatedly shown, the most common solutions to the problem of criminal abortion offered in these documents were improving legislation specifically directed at the crime and changing minds about the desirability of ending unwanted pregnancies. The same was true of reports and articles *following* this East River Medical Association Report. Rarely, if ever, did these repeat the East River proposal to use public opposition to abortion as a tool for achieving medical regulation. This may have been because public opposition to criminal abortion returned to former low levels after the intense newspaper and judicial opposition to the practice of the early 1870s. Opposition to criminal abortion again became the province of the regular physicians, or at least the large majority of regular physicians who were not part of the problem.

It was inappropriate for Mohr to claim that physicians were opposing criminal abortion as a means to regulate the medical profession and that the special abortion committee of "the East River Medical Association Report expressed this concern of American regulars unambiguously."[28] He was extrapolating from this single Report that would exploit the brief period of strong *public* opposition to criminal abortion as a way to obtain legislation regulating medicine and from its and the many other physician calls for elimination of irregular abortionists. Unfortunately, this false claim that physicians opposed criminal abortion as a means to regulate the medical profession would be repeated by dozens of writers after Mohr (See Foreword). And many people today no doubt believe that the early physician opponents of abortion opposed it for such "professional" reasons and were not particularly concerned about its unborn victims.

Government regulation of medicine in the United States did become a fact later in the nineteenth century. Mohr claimed that criminal abortion decreased by the end of the century, at least among married women.[29] This in part was because he, like the authors of the 1871 East River Report, believed that regulation would reduce criminal abortion.[30] However, there is no evidence that criminal abortion decreased among the married by the end of the century. Almost all physicians writing about the subject at that time claimed that such abortions were prevalent and increasing (See Chapter 24).

In November 1871, the Syracuse physician, Ely Van de Warker, republished articles he had placed in the *Journal of the Gynaecological Society of Boston*. Van de Warker's monograph included this dedication:

> Inscribed to
> Horatio R. Storer, M.D., LL.B.
> As an humble evidence of admiration for his genius; as a slight return
> for his brave words to the men and women of his country upon this
> crime of the period, and as a grateful consideration for his cordial
> recognition of the labors of the author.[31]

Horatio's belief that his words were actually having an effect "upon this crime of the period" was illustrated at the meeting of the Gynaecological Society on February 6, 1872. The "Proceedings" included a discussion of the imprisonment of a notorious abortionist in the Nebraska Territory. Following this: "Dr. Storer commented upon the growing sentiment of the community that this crime must be suppressed. It was evident that efforts that a few earnest men had made in the face of doubt and ridicule were now producing their perfect work throughout the country."[32]

At the next meeting of the Society, Storer was present, although shortly thereafter he would be stricken with near-fatal blood-poisoning from a surgical wound. It is possible that the wound occurred just prior to the meeting when he removed a chestnut-sized cervical polypus that was exhibited at the same meeting.[33] Horatio read the suppressed portion of his father's Introductory Lecture of November 1855. Horatio also discussed the reasons for the suppression of this section of his father's Introductory Lecture and the failure of some recent authorities to give his father proper credit for bringing the moral and medical problem of criminal abortion to the attention of the profession. The "Proceedings" indicated:

> Dr. H. R. Storer stated the circumstances under which his father's paper had been written (in 1855,) and those under which its publication had been suppressed. He himself had always regretted that the "injudicious" counsel had been followed. So far from the publication having been likely to have injured the interest of the Harvard Medical School, it was well known that the school had been very nearly ruined by just such a timid, vacillating no-policy, of whose fear of taking a manly stand, even upon purely scientific matters, the present was one among many proofs.[34]

Horatio then discussed the history of local efforts to improve the laws against abortion and proposed the Society take further action on this. The "Proceedings" indicated that Horatio reminded the members of the failure of the Massachusetts Medical Society to recommend to the legislature changes of its abortion laws and of his protest of Jacob Bigelow's action in his 1858 absence. The "Proceedings" also recorded that:

> Dr. Storer thought that the time had at last come, so great a revolution was occurring in public sentiment, when steps for a betterment of the statutes might be taken with success. The New York Medico-Legal Society for instance, had lately been acting with vigor and success. He would therefore move the appointment of a committee to consider the propriety of a memorial from the Society to the Legislature. He himself should decline serving upon it, as he feared he was considered by his friends a fanatic upon this subject, but he would aid the committee by every means in his power.
>
> The motion was seconded by Dr. Hazelton, and Drs. Greeley, Hazelton and Bixby were appointed.[35]

Like the East River Medical Association Committee, Horatio saw the heightened public objections to abortion as a means to effect legislation. For Horatio it was "betterment of the [abortion] statutes," not new statutes to regulate the medical profession.

George F. Shrady was an active member of the New York Medico-Legal Society that Horatio praised. Shrady discussed the advantages societies made up of doctors *and* lawyers had for making laws in the area of medicine and described the Society's proposals for revision of the New York statutes:

> Heretofore one of the main troubles has been that medical societies proper, from the want of an intelligent examination of existing statutes, have not proved themselves capable, in their efforts to procure laws, of disposing, in a practical manner, of the technical objections to the enforcement of just penalties. This difficulty, we believe, has been overcome by a union of the two professions of law and medicine in the committees. The Society has given its attention, through such committees, to two very important subjects, not the least of which is one referring to a law for the proper punishment of abortionists. The committee having this matter specially in charge have examined the whole subject in a very thorough manner from a legal as well as medical standpoint, and have culminated their labors by recommending the following act, which has been endorsed unanimously by the Society:—[36]

The section of the draft law that followed stated that any one "who shall administer to any woman with child, or prescribe for any such woman, or advise or procure her to take any medicine, drug, substance, or thing whatever, or shall use or employ, or advise or procure her to submit to the use or employment of any instrument or other means whatsoever, with intent thereby to produce the miscarriage of any such woman, unless the same shall have been necessary to preserver her life or that of such child, shall, in case the death of such child or of such woman be thereby produced, be deemed guilty of a felony, and upon conviction shall be punished by imprisonment in a State prison for a term not less than four years."[37]

Shrady wrote that every precaution had been taken in drafting this law to cover both direct offenders and accessories before the fact. He noted that punishment could be as large as life imprisonment. He accurately predicted that it would soon become law. The new legislation made the abortion-related death of the fetus or the woman a felony and also made the woman guilty of a felony if she submitted to an abortion or performed an abortion on herself.[38] However, in 1968, this successful effort of the Medico-Legal Society to protect the unborn child with legislation would be dismissed as the pronouncements of an aberrant group of "Nineteenth Century fanatics" by the lawyer, Cyril Means, when he presented his case that New York's law was not constitutional.[39]

Storer was confined to his bed early in April and the May 1872 "Editorial Notes" probably were written earlier when the suppressed portion of his father's Introductory Lecture of 1855 was published in March 1872. They were largely a restatement of the circumstances leading to suppression of that portion of the Lecture. Novel in this rendition, however, was attribution of the opposition in 1855 that caused the suppression to Dr. Henry J. Bigelow and apparently to him alone.[40]

It is tempting to speculate that Bigelow, the established Professor of Surgery, had something to hide when it came to forced abortion and that this motivated his successful suppression in 1855 of the antiabortion section of Horatio's father's Introductory Lecture. Bigelow had spent years in France where he had been a student of the French surgeon, Velpeau. We earlier presented Brinton's Velpeau quote: "the fetus has no independent life and no claims upon our consideration on any such account—that it is, in short, nothing more than a vegetable." Brinton disagreed, but Henry J. Bigelow may have taken this to heart and operated accordingly.

Horatio Storer remained critically ill for a number of months and underwent surgery to remove infection from his left knee on more than one occasion. By October, he had recovered sufficiently to travel with his family to Europe where he hoped to achieve recovery of the function of his knee. He returned to the United States in August 1877 and settled in Newport, Rhode Island. His diseased knee would not bend and Horatio spent the rest of his long life on crutches or with a cane. He made brief returns to medical practice and was an important medical and surgical consultant in Newport. He also made important contributions to Newport's sanitation, government, history, civil rights, and natural science.[41] He briefly returned to active opposition to criminal abortion in 1897 and this is discussed in Chapter 24.

CHAPTER 20

PHYSICIANS OF BOTH SEXES JOIN THE CRUSADE

Scores of physicians continued the physicians' crusade against abortion that Horatio Storer began in 1857. One was J.C. Stone whose "Report on the Subject of Criminal Abortion" was published in the 1871 *Transactions of the Iowa State Medical Society*. Stone provided long passages from Hodge's Introductory Lecture and quoted Storer's statistics to show the high rate of criminal abortion. He added: "Iowa fills her quota of crime as surely as she filled the broken ranks of her regiments during the late war."[1]

Stone discussed how "individuals claiming to be *medical men*" procured abortions for "those who insist that this abominable work of abortion shall be done at any cost, even at the risk of their own lives." He mentioned the frequent claim of these requestors "that prior to quickening, the embryo is a mass of inanimate matter, not yet endowed with vitality!" He noted that even some physicians "urged" this argument.[2]

Stone then indicated the public's perception of abortion had to be changed:

> Even if legislation were practicable in any case, it can do little until this custom is branded *as* a crime; until the unwarranted discrimination between the murder of a child in one condition of its being, and that in another, is broken down, and a social judgment shall condemn each equally as a violation of human and natural law, and until the opinion everywhere prevails that the due course of maternity is not a disease to be treated, but a course of nature which cannot be interrupted without calamitous results.[3]

Another physician sustaining the crusade was P.S. Haskell from Stockton Maine.[4] Haskell began by "reminding" his Maine Medical Association audience of the alarming increase of criminal abortion in Maine, "the apathy which exists, both in the profession and out of it, as to the results of the same," and the dangers of criminal abortion to the life and health of the woman. He continued with a counter example to the usual claim that the maternal instinct increased as pregnancy advanced:

> You have seen, too, the demoralizing effect upon the wife, leading the woman who, at first, could not feel it right to destroy a foetus after *motion* was experienced, to come to be willing to be delivered of her burden at most any period; and hearing a feeble wail from her child, just born, instead of being moved by a mother's feelings of sympathy and affection to beg of you to save her child, the rather to cry out to

you who have been called to finish the dirty job another had begun, "Don't let it live"! "don't let it live"! or again, to strangle it with her own hands, or smother it between her beds.[5]

Haskell claimed Maine was not as "cursed" by abortionists as some States, but "the midnight bell, at the close of every year in the State of Maine, is a funeral dirge to not less than *two thousand* helpless victims to the abortionists!" He argued that criminal abortion was dulling the moral sensibilities of all concerned and this "cheapening of human life" was one reason that criminal abortion was not "condemned, often and earnestly, from the press, the pulpit and the forum." He noted that "women's rights lecturers and women preachers" were not making any "earnest, continued effort" against criminal abortion, but instead were devoting all of their efforts to obtaining the vote.[6]

Haskell then provided some unique observations about the favorable view of abortionists held by the "masses" and the plight of "the honest physician."

> But strange as these things may seem, it appears to me that the course of the honest physician is stranger still, for he, of all men, is suffering, being disgraced in the minds of a part of mankind because he associates with the abortionist as an equal, and degraded in the minds of the rest by comparison with the abortionist, for I verily believe that the masses think that the "common kind" of a doctor, as they call him, has not the knowledge how to produce an abortion, nor the courage to do it if he knew, and that there is more knowledge and skill in the little finger of one of these destroyers than could be packed into the craniums of a car-load of M.D.'s of the honorable stamp.[7]

James S. Whitmire, a surgeon during the Civil War with the 56th Illinois Infantry, presented a paper, "Criminal Abortion," on October 21, 1873 to the Woodford County Illinois Medical Society.[8] Whitmire indicated that criminal abortion occurred frequently "for the sole purpose of getting rid of responsibilities that may come to disturb their secular pleasures or to increase the family expenses." This was true among women in all classes and conditions including "those who possess a respectable standing in the church, and are apparently, from all outward appearances, patrons of morality." He noted that the presence of the crime among such "patrons" "would startle the well-meaning, but innocent and uninitiated, and cause them to lose faith in their kind, but it cannot be avoided; it is nevertheless true, whitewash it as you will."[9]

He noted that "professional abortionists" were "generally known by the lewd of both sexes for miles around," and that they also were "known to one another in the different cities, so that if a case is likely to be too close at home for complete safety to all parties, the victim is sent to the next bloody station where the operation is performed." He continued:

> Persons who engage in this crime, whether they are professional or self-abortionists, have lost all the natural instincts of humanity; they have

neither principle nor good morals, and are, hence, an eyesore to society, a plague-spot upon communities where they exist—lepers, whose infectious breath undermines the very foundation of the morals of the people, and should not be tolerated for a single day, when and where they are known.[10]

Whitmire also characterized the woman who habitually resorted to abortion:

You see her tottering, not walking—pale, discouraged, sallow and languid—along your streets; she has prolapsus uteri, probably displacement of the os uteri; her sexual organs are in a flaccid condition; she has profuse leucorrhoea; is afflicted with menorrhagia at her menstrual periods; in short, her health is virtually gone, broken down by those violent means used either by herself or others for the purpose of producing abortion.[11]

Whitmire concluded:

Certainly the whole of the evil we cannot avert, but we may add our mite and put forth our hand to stay this monster iniquity. This is not the work of the medical profession alone, but the church, the bar, our law-makers, and all good men and women, should engage in it for the benefit of public morals, for the preservation of our national characteristics, and the general well-being of our people. It is a labor of love that we owe to ourselves, to society, and more especially to the opposite sex; and no less to the health and general well-being of mankind.[12]

An editorial two months later in the same journal mentioned that a notorious Chicago abortionist, "'Dr.' Earll," was convicted in Cook County of the murder of a woman by abortion and was sentenced by the jury to one year in the penitentiary.[13] The editors, J. Adams Allen and Walter Hay, made the points that the sentence was far too light for the offence and that the "murder of the unborn child was entirely overlooked." The editors indicated that this failure of justice was the result of "false teaching to which society has been subjected, both in physiology and morality—false teachings which have become a part of the moral character of the greater portion of society, under the sanction of mischievous laws, their inevitable outgrowth." The editors described a future appreciation of unborn children by society that would lead to appropriate justice for abortionists. They concluded with the following initial strategy for achieving this:

Let physicians cease to throw the mantle of professional confidence around applications for the production of abortions. Let these be regarded, as they undoubtedly are, as suggestions to the commission of felony, and let them be treated as would be a suggestion to commit robbery, forgery, or perjury. Let information, under oath, be laid before the proper authorities that the crime of abortion is meditated, and we will see it rapidly diminish, and perhaps cease altogether.[14]

This proposal to report requests for abortion to authorities was novel and, if carried out, might well have caused criminal abortion to at least "rapidly diminish." As will be seen, the proposal would be made again in 1887 by a physician writing to the *Journal of the American Medical Association* and by the Editor of the *Canada Lancet* in 1889.

In October 1874, the Missouri physician, John W. Trader, read a paper on criminal abortion before the Central Missouri District Medical Association.[15] He claimed its "revolting features silence the tongue of the general teacher of morality." "From this fact alone," he continued, "it becomes the duty of this assembly and of medical men everywhere, to give forth no uncertain sound in regard to this matter, and to resolve to bear the shame in silence no longer."[16]

Trader followed with a long history of abortion, noting its rarity among the Jews, but its common occurrence in Greece, Rome, and ancient Germany. He indicated that, bad as the old days were, "the evidence will bear out the assertion, that *in no age of the world* has there been a more reckless disregard for the lives of unborn human beings than this present age, and among the civilized and professedly christianized nations of the earth."[17] Trader provided personal evidence of this, describing how women sought abortions from local physicians with the claim that they would "do any thing in the world—even suffer death—before they will bear another child." He indicated that "if it was thought their pleas would be heard or requests granted," the physician would be faced with "daily" requests for abortion.[18] Unstated was the probable fact that physicians and others who provided abortions did have such daily business.

Canada also was plagued with criminal abortion. The Windsor, Ontario physician, Alfred A. Andrews, began his paper, "On Abortion," by discussing two cases in his own practice "about thirty years ago."[19] He noted that he had procured abortion for a woman with "extreme pelvic deformity" rather than put her through the craniotomy violence that she had thrice undergone and that had resulted in vesico-vaginal fistula. He indicated that faced with a similar situation today, he would recommend the Caesarean section.[20]

He described his second case where his diagnosis of pregnancy caused the couple to believe the wife's death was inevitable since her previous physician had claimed she would not survive another pregnancy.

> [The husband] called himself her murderer, entreated her pardon, and seemed beside himself. She strove to soothe and console him, and finally brought matters to the climax, by conjuring him, "After I am gone, don't allow any woman (she was too kind to say stepmother) to ill use my darlings—our darlings; promise, for my sake, Charles." ...
> I saw and verified a letter from her former attendant, in which he urged that abortion was the sole means of averting otherwise inevitable death. ... I was not satisfied of the absolute necessity of the act, and yet I assumed the responsibility—undertook and effected

abortion. *"Mea culpa!"* I was wrong, very wrong; responsibility cannot be delegated. Upon a subsequent occasion, when I came to know the lady better, I cheered her spirits, raised her hopes, and safely delivered her at term of a living child, with much less difficulty, danger or suffering than I have encountered in scores of cases.[21]

Andrews described a successful case of early delivery that enabled a woman to finally have a living child. Her previous pregnancies had ended when the unborn child died in the womb in the last trimester of pregnancy. Andrews called this professional abortion. He then moved to "Felonious Abortion," and indicated he had had scores of applications "for this murderous act." He indicated the applications from young unmarried women that were hard to resist, given the "terrible penalties inflicted by society on the female sex for incontinence." He described the case of a young woman who indicated that if not "relieved," she would avert exposure by suicide, rather than "disgrace her recently-married sister and kill her mother." "Thank God, I have no confession to make in this case;" Andrews said, "I did not yield, but my heart bled when I refused her." He noted that she traveled to a distant "watering-place" for "her poor health" and "returned cured." "Believe me, gentlemen, you may be subjected to severe temptation, but being forewarned, you must be forearmed."[22]

Andrews then moved to applications for abortion from married women and indicated that he had "hundreds." Andrews noted that the "fearfully prevalent" crime was more damaging to the community "than Typhus or Small-pox" and that it could not be addressed in the public press or the pulpit. He provided this *medical* prescription for restraining it:

I had for many years noted and wondered at the fact, that of the married women who sought my co-operation, nearly all were Protestants. Being myself a Protestant of the broadest Orange stripe, and not ready to acknowledge any marked moral inferiority in my co-religionists, I was for a long season puzzled, but I think the solution is this. The Pulpit is debarred, but the Roman Catholic Priesthood, have in their confessional an opportunity of instructing and warning their flock. Protestant women do not go there, but we, and we only, have the private confidential ear of the whole sex, and it is, I conceive our duty, to lose no opportunity of diffusing the information we possess in this regard. Let us purify the moral atmosphere. Let us make the whole sex know that it is murder, when the embryo is but four weeks old, as completely as if the nine months of foetal life had been reached or passed. We have a duty to perform, and we have countless opportunities of doing it.[23]

In 1876, Homer O. Hitchcock, President of the Michigan State Board of Health, provided a "Report on Criminal Abortion."[24] The Kalamazoo physician claimed "people, otherwise of good intelligence appear to be entirely ignorant of the first principles of embryonic life, or else smothering their consciences for the time by the vapors of an intense selfishness, make themselves believe a lie." He indicated that there also were physicians "who really believe this old error, or at least do nothing towards removing it from the minds of their patrons, and in many instances, it is to be feared, too easily excuse themselves for being *particeps criminis* in this work of real child-murder." He made a strong case for changing the Michigan abortion statute that made inducing abortion a lesser crime before quickening.[25]

A more extensive discussion of criminal abortion was provided a year later by Edward Cox, the President of the Michigan State Medical Society. The Battle Creek physician claimed that when he began medical practice in 1839 only "the unfortunate maiden or brazen courtezan [sic] were guilty of the crime." He cited Storer, Gardner, and Blatchford as concurring that criminal abortion among the married was "scarcely known" 40 years earlier, but now "has become frequent and bold."[26] "Every city, village and hamlet has its *specialist*, plying this homicidal vocation," Cox continued, "who has sufficient patrons and friends, equally guilty with himself, and too often among the officers of the law, to hide his crime from publicity, and, in case of prosecution, to shield him from conviction."[27] He discussed one of "these modern Neros" from Detroit who confessed to 2,500 abortions on his deathbed.[28]

Cox estimated that there were 100,000 criminal abortions in the United States each year and 6,000 associated maternal deaths. His statistics would be widely quoted by other physicians over the years as evidence of the high frequency of criminal abortions.[29] However, as has been and will be shown, several other physician estimates of the number of criminal abortions were higher. Cox went on to discuss the many injuries to health for women who survived the criminal abortion and made reference to claims that "these lesions produce reflex irritation of the brain, and directly and indirectly are often the cause of insanity." He also claimed that "subsequent children" of these mothers "are feeble in body and mind." Cox continued:

> A combination of circumstances has produced a depraved and debauched public sentiment that not only winks at but condones, palliates, and defends the crime. It goes further in many instances: it recognizes the abortionist as a useful member of society, and even extols him as a benefactor. It will take line upon line, and precept upon precept, facts, figures, and eloquence to overcome this false and pernicious sentiment.[30]

Included in Cox's "combination of circumstances" was the common belief that there was no life in the embryo until the fourth month of pregnancy and state laws that reflected this belief. He cited the various inappropriate reasons married women gave to justify such abortions and particularly condemned "she whose god is Fashion."[31] He also mentioned the press that published advertisements of abortionists and nostrum manufacturers and the druggists who sold the supposed abortifacients. "Very few of these are efficient," Cox wrote, "but the mind becomes poisoned thereby, the individual becomes desperate, and perseveres until she succeeds in her undertaking."[32]

Given all of the factors leading to "the toleration, perpetration, and defense of criminal abortion," Cox saw reform as "almost a hopeless undertaking." He continued:

> But when we contemplate that annually in this country foeticide is perpetrated 60,000 to 100,000 times, that 6,000 or more women in consequence lose their lives, the misery that results from so many families bereaved of wife and mother, the thousands of sickly women transmitting disease of body and mind to tens of thousands of children, the increase of licentiousness and various forms of vice, the direct consequences of this practice, our minds are filled with horror at the atrocity of the crime, and we believe that all philanthropists should join in an intelligent, persistent and united effort for reform."[33]

Cox then named the "philanthropists" that needed to join the effort. He called on the Governor to make recommendations and the Legislature to pass laws based on "the rational views of our profession—that 'to extinguish the first spark of life is a crime of the same nature, both against our Maker and society, as to destroy an infant, a child, or a man.'" Judges needed to charge prosecutors and grand juries "to inquire into and present all such cases. This will tend to prevent crime, by enlightening the bar, the jurors, and through them the people."[34]

"Educationists" needed to make girls more aware of "the laws that govern their physical as well as moral and mental organizations and also the danger of violating the same." Social scientists needed to add criminal abortion to the evils they were successfully attacking. "Boards of health and sanitarians" should make people aware of the dangers to health, including death, and Cox indicated this "will do more to stop the practice than any argument that can be offered." Political economists needed to point out "the great loss to the State." The press needed to use its talents to fight criminal abortion and thereby redeem itself from its alliance with "abortionists and vendors of abortive drugs." By following this new course, the press "will be hailed as one of the greatest benefactions of mankind."[35]

The "Church" received special attention and Cox indicated it could do more "to abate this vice" than any other organization. He then discussed ministerial responsibilities:

> The physician must not leave his post in time of pestilence, the surgeon in time of battle, nor can the sentinel be caught sleeping at his post, without incurring the penalty of death. Neither should ministers of the Gospel be deterred by "sensitive minds," wealthy, influential and guilty parishioners, fear of censure, loss of popularity, place or position, from presenting this subject in an intelligent, forcible manner to "the congregations committed to their charge," and he that

has a knowledge of this crime and cowardly neglects his duty, should be censured, like the sentinel caught sleeping at his post, or the surgeon who neglects to apply the ligature to the severed artery.[36]

Cox gave credit to Bishop Coxe and Rev. John Todd for their strong opposition to criminal abortion. However, he claimed Protestant efforts in general were meager. He contrasted them with the lead taken by Roman Catholics whose "ministers work systematically, hold special services, give special instructions on this as on other social evils." Cox indicated that in his 40 years of practice attending the mothers of "nearly 3,000 children, we have never known the crime perpetrated by a married Catholic woman."

He let a member of the clergy, almost certainly Henry Ward Beecher, help make his point about deficient Protestantism:

A popular Brooklyn clergyman said, in the course of a late sermon, "Why send missionaries to India when child-murder is of daily, almost of hourly, occurrence? Aye, when the hand that puts money in the contribution-box to-day, yesterday, or a month ago, to-morrow will murder her own unborn offspring. The Hindoo mother when she abandons her baby upon the sacred Ganges, is, contrary to her heart, obeying a supposed religious law; and you desire to convert her to your own worship of fashion and laziness, and love of greed. Out upon such hypocrisy!"[37]

Cox then lifted much of what Gardner had said about modest clergy and immodest abortion seekers:

I see no resort left, no staying this tide of sin, unless it be in the power of the church. There should be no queasy sensibilities, no mawkish delicacy; the sin should be grappled with and crushed out. The pulpit of every denomination should make common cause and fulminate its anathemas against every abettor of this enormity. I know not why such tenderness of speech on the part of the clergy, for there is no such modesty on the part of the actors concerned. Arrayed in gorgeous silks, covered with gems, they enter the physician's office and ask him to perpetrate the crime as coolly as they would order a steak for dinner.[38]

Remiss as the Protestant clergy was, Cox indicated that the medical profession was worse. The prevalence of criminal abortion and the associated public tolerance of criminal abortion were described as failures of the profession in its duties "to give counsel to the people on subjects of medical police, hygiene, and legal medicine," and "to enlighten the public on all matters of public health, physical, moral and mental." Physicians had "year after year, witnessed the rapid increase of the crime" and could not plead ignorance. They had frequently become "accessory to the crime" by failing to inform applicants for abortion, their husbands, advisors, and friends about "the great moral and physical wrong she is about to perpetrate upon herself, her family and society."[39]

Cox also criticized physicians for inappropriately keeping secrets of the applicants when these "violate the moral laws, our own consciences, and the ethics of our profession." He noted that various medical associations had passed resolutions condemning criminal abortion and mentioned "the valuable works of Dr. Storer" that he incorrectly claimed resulted when the American Medical Association "offered a prize."[40] He indicated that physicians were the best informed and thus best qualified to provide the needed instruction to the groups who could contribute to reducing criminal abortion. He proposed sending delegations from medical societies to instruct legislators, educators, boards of health, sanitarians, social scientists, members of the press, "and last, though not least, the various theological bodies, where, we doubt not, they will be received as the representatives of an honorable profession, and will obtain their cooperation."[41]

Cox then described how to deal with the woman requesting abortion:

> The wiles, artifices and strategems [sic] which women use when be-sieging their physician for the commission of this unnatural practice should not only be met with firmness and decision, but with such teachings and instruction relative to the nature, consequences and criminality of the practice, as is due them from the guardian of their physical condition. Treat the abortionist as a wretch dangerous to so-ciety, ostracise him socially and professionally, teach the people to avoid him as the plague or pestilence; and if, with brazen impudence or serpent-like cunning, he intrudes upon your friends, warn them that he "is unclean," advise them "to pass out of his way and make room for the leper." Room! Room![42]

Cox concluded by asking his audience to take active measures against criminal abortion, even if they were not the ones he had suggested. This was to be done

> so that before the heads of our young members become "silvered o'er with age," they may have the happiness of knowing, that this most cowardly crime is made odious, and is no longer perpetrated with impunity; that the depraved public sentiment which tolerates and causes it no longer exists, and the satisfaction of having done their part in rescuing the people occupying the land recently wrested from Indian paganism from a condition leading to a *half-civilized heathenism.*[43]

Cox's Battle Creek colleague and the inventor of Corn Flakes, John Harvey Kellogg, provided an immensely successful book, *Plain Facts For Old and Young*, in 1879 that included a strong condemnation of unnecessary abortion. Kellogg included extensive quotes of Storer, Gardner, and other physicians. However, the following account of a dialog with a married patient who requested an abortion was his own:

> A number of years ago, a woman called on the writer, stating that she had become pregnant much against her wishes, and earnestly desired that an abortion should be produced. The following conversation ensued:—
>
> "Why do you desire the destruction of your unborn infant?"
>
> "Because I already have three children, which are as many as I can properly care for; besides, my health is poor, and I do not feel that I can do justice to what children I now have."
>
> "Your chief reason, then, is that you do not wish more children?"
>
> "Yes."
>
> "On this account you are willing to take the life of this unborn babe?"
>
> "I must get rid of it."
>
> "I understand that you have already borne three children, and that you do not think you are able to care for more. Four children are, you think, one too many, and so you are willing to destroy one. Why not destroy one of those already born?"
>
> "Oh, that would be murder!"
>
> "It certainly would, but no more murder than it would be to kill this unborn infant. Indeed, the little one you are carrying in your womb, has greater claims upon you than the little ones at home, by virtue of its entire dependence and helplessness. It is just as much your child as those whose faces are familiar to you, and whom you love.[44]

Kellogg followed with a discussion of how the woman "continued to bemoan her condition, and allowed her heart to be filled with enmity against the innocent being that was in no way responsible for her afflictions." He was fairly certain that no attempt at abortion was tried. She gave birth to "a puny infant, which barely survived the perils of parturition, and came into the world the most wretched of all human beings, 'an unwelcome child.'" Kellogg indicated the puny infant caused untold suffering to the mother before its death several months later. "Vain is her effort to undo the wrong she had done her little one;" Kellogg concluded, "but let us hope that by genuine repentance and the many months of faithful and patient watching, she has made a full atonement for her sin."[45]

Many women readers probably were influenced not to abort by this dialog demonstrating the moral and physical problems associated with abortion. On the other hand, Kellogg's doubtful conclusion about the bad effect of not wanting a child on the child's intrauterine development could actually have been used by some women with an unwelcome pregnancy as a justification for abortion. Readers also would have been aware of another Kellogg claim that a woman who attempts abortion, but is unsuccessful, would undoubtedly stamp her "murderous intent" upon the character of her unwelcome child, "giving it a natural propensity for the commission of murderous deeds."[46] If this were accepted as a fact, the woman seeking abortion would make sure her attempt was successful.

Kellogg claimed in a preface to the second edition of *Plain Facts* that nearly 100,000 copies had been distributed. Other evidence of the book's large circulation is the fact that libraries in the United States have editions of the book with publication dates ranging from 1879 to 1917 and only the year 1885 is missing between 1879 and 1895. Other extremely popular books by Kellogg, such as *The Home Hand-Book of Domestic Hygiene and Rational Medicine*, first published in 1880, also strongly condemned abortion and contributed to Kellogg's antiabortion crusade.[47]

In February 1878, Anthony Comstock, the Federal Government's special agent for the enforcement of his own 1873 "Act for the Suppression of Trade in and Circulation of, Obscene Literature and Articles of Immoral Use," tricked Madame Restell into disclosing her abortionist occupation by pretending to need an abortion for his girlfriend. Searches of her mansion followed and confirmed the existence of instruments for procuring abortion. She was briefly jailed, out on bond, and her case was scheduled for trial on April 1, 1878. However, she slashed her throat with a butcher knife the night before the trial and died in her bathtub.[48]

Satan in Society author, Nicholas Francis Cooke, addressed the Homoeopathic College of Physicians and Surgeons of Michigan in 1879. The thrust of his paper, "Licensed Foeticide," was that induced abortion was almost never justified.[49] Cooke described how he sent a long extract from Edwin Moses Hale's 1860 *On the Homoeopathic Treatment of Abortion* for comment to various eminent homeopathic physicians. Some of Cooke's respondents discussed the adequacy of homeopathic methods for dealing with the "diseases and complications of the state of pregnancy" that Hale had claimed were indications for abortion and Cooke summarized these by stating: "baby killing should be left entirely out of the question so far as these diseases are concerned." Cooke continued:

> But the open and earnest advocates of the art of baby killing, are your semi-respectable practitioners, who owe what they possess of detestable popularity and financial prosperity to their known willingness to undertake "the little affair for a consideration." Sharp, shrewd and cunning are they—these hyenas of the medical profession! They *force* themselves on the faculties of medical colleges—they write pamphlets and magazine articles (and always find publishers!) to show how often and skillfully they have murdered babies, and whine and whine when lashed for their beastly work— making each new castigation the occasion for further advertisement! They clothe themselves with fashionable church memberships—they ape respectability—they adopt the nasal twang and show much

sclerotic expansion—and wear always an air of injured innocence, as who should say: "Behold me, virtuous, yet calumniated!"[50]

This diatribe probably was aimed at Hale who wrote pamphlets and whom the Chicago Homeopathic Medical College included on their faculty, whether they had been forced to or not. Hale also had responded to an attack from Dr. Gaylord Beebe, a former faculty colleague, with something describable as "Behold me, virtuous, yet calumniated!"[51]

Cooke concluded by preparing his audience for "the most vital" battle against abortion.

> For, if our mission be to save life and health, how can we more surely fulfil [sic] it than to interpose first, the fiat of science, and afterward, and as a necessary sequence, the strong decree of the criminal law, in arrest of the slaughter of the innocents, thereby saving hundreds upon hundreds of thousands of maternal and foetal lives? What, in comparison, are our grave discussions of prophylaxes against "plague, pestilence and famine," our learned discussions of the therapeia of this, or that, or the other, stalking shadow of what we call death? What, indeed? They number at most but a few thousands of victims, while this vast MOLOCH of destruction gathers in his burning bosom I think it safe to say, *one half the annual increase of humanity in our "glorious republic!"*[52]

The American Medical Association remained involved in the fight against criminal abortion. Edward Hazen Parker, provided a paper, "The Relation of the Medical and Legal Professions to Criminal Abortion" to the Section on State Medicine at the Annual Meeting of the Association in New York in 1880.[53] This was the same Dr. Parker who strongly supported Horatio's Suffolk District Medical Society efforts as editor of the *New-Hampshire Journal of Medicine* in 1857. Parker began by discussing three cases of criminal abortion that went to court. In the first, the lawyer for the abortionist "was allowed to bully and coax" the girl into changing her testimony which had been made when she was near death as a result of the abortion. As a result, the charge of abortion was dropped. In the second, the girl died. A witness who saw a sharp instrument passed under the bedclothes and saw it withdrawn covered with blood was late at the trial of the operator. The judge decided the case was not important enough to wait for the witness and discharged the prisoner. In "Case III," the abortionist actually was convicted of the crime, but the judge requested the governor of the state to pardon him and he served but half of his sentence.[54]

Parker used these examples to point out the large differences in perception of criminal abortion between the medical profession and the legal profession and this may have been the first published physician claim that some in the legal profession were lagging in their opposition to the crime. According to Parker, physicians were aware that killing the unborn child at any stage of its prenatal existence was an immense crime, while lawyers saw the crime as against the mother and gave little regard to fetal life, at least prior to quickening.[55] Parker provided examples showing that the community shared the lawyer's position on criminal abortion:

> Married as well as unmarried women apply to medical men to have an abortion produced with as much if not more readiness that they do to have a cancerous breast removed. Mothers will say that they prefer the life of the daughter shall be imperilled [sic] rather than have disgrace fall upon her. I have been told when refusing to do the operation on a married woman that I was too squeamish. A professional friend refusing to operate for a fee of five hundred dollars was told that it was a great loss to the community when Madam Restell died.[56]

Parker called for a "determined effort on the part of the courts to enforce the laws—which are, I am told, quite sufficient—and a rigid holding of the criminal to the full amount of his sentence." He concluded by describing the need for physicians to carry out

> a decided and continued effort to enlighten the community in general, and the legal profession especially, upon the enormity of the crime of foeticide. The peril to the woman great as it is, is safely escaped by very many—exactly what proportion it is impossible to say—but an abortion is of necessity fatal to the child, and the number of human lives thus destroyed is enormous. I therefore respectfully present the following propositions, urging their adoption by this Section and, if possible, by the whole Association:—
> 1. Abortion should never be brought on by the use of medicinal or instrumental means unless necessary to the safety of the mother in consequence of pathological complications.
> 2. The destruction of the foetus in utero for any other reason, properly ranks with other forms of murder.
> 3. Abortion produced artificially always places the mother's life in jeopardy and thus becomes a double crime.
> 4. The severe punishment of the operator when possible, without any probability of executive clemency, is due in justice to the honorable members of the medical profession, and yet more to the community at large."[57]

When the members of the Section on State Medicine discussed these Resolutions, there was an initial motion to accept the paper and refer it to the Association for publication. Three members indicated that there was no need for the Section to adopt the Resolutions, since the laws of the states already were "sufficiently explicit" and made criminal abortion a felony. Parker countered that he offered the Resolutions as a source of "moral force" to strengthen "weak-kneed" physicians. The motion to accept the paper and refer it to the Association for publication was carried. Another motion to table the Resolutions "was carried by a rising vote."[58] Although not adopted by the Section or the full membership as Parker hoped, his Resolutions at least accompanied his paper into the *Transactions* and may have actually helped some "weak-kneed" physician refuse a patient's request for abortion.

The March 1881 meeting of Boston's Suffolk District Medical Society included a long discussion of the failure to convict an abortionist in a case where the woman obtaining the abortion died. The failure to convict was largely because of the testimony of medical experts regarding the cause of death. This was cited as an example showing how Boston abortionists had developed a fairly effective network of lawyers and medical experts to protect their business.[59] However, this failure to convict was only one such instance in four trials of abortionists in Massachusetts that occurred following replacement of the coroners with medical examiners four years earlier. The advantages of the medical examiner system over the coroner system were discussed a few months later.[60] The article described the successful conviction of "an individual of fifty or more, styling himself a homeopathic physician and prefixing 'doctor' to his name." His attempt at abortion caused the death of the young unmarried woman. The editor, George B. Shattuck, discussed the salutary effect of the conviction: "When such individuals are made to feel that five, ten, or twenty years' imprisonment is the certain result of attempting to procure a criminal abortion, then, and not till then, will the business which has reached such proportions in Boston begin to diminish."[61]

Shattuck then described the problems that such a trial could create when "counsel question the experts, and compel them to disclose to an audience composed of any and all who choose to come, the exact methods by which abortion can be procured, the best instruments to use, and the time in pregnancy at which the operation can be done with the greatest safety to the mother." He was concerned that almost anyone could set up an abortion business with this information since "students in a medical school rarely get better instruction in this branch than can be obtained at a trial like this."[62]

A Special Committee on Criminal Abortion was appointed at the 1881 Michigan State Board of Health Convention. It provided its report a few days later and it consisted of an abstract of Edward Cox's 1877 address discussed above.[63] The "new" Report called for physicians to "agitate" the subject "upon all occasions likely to educate the people." The "press and pulpit" were seen as "the greatest in-struments to instruct the people in the needed reformation." The Committee noted that Catholic women were rarely obtaining abortions and "believes that if the Prot-estant clergy would properly present the subject to their congregations with the assistance of the press and other auxiliaries, the crime would soon become as rare among the Protestant as the Catholic women."[64]

The Report concluded with the committee recommending that the Board of Health pass the following resolution:

Resolved, That the State Board of Health be requested by this convention to correspond with municipal boards of health, physicians,

civil authorities and such others as it may deem proper, for the
purpose of obtaining information relative to criminal abortion, to
publish in documents and newspapers all things relative thereto
proper to be published, and that physicians, sanitarians, educationists,
social scientists, civil authorities and others be requested to
communicate to the Board all information in their possession relative
to the same, and that the clergy and press be earnestly solicited to
acquaint themselves with the subject and to educate their hearers and
readers as to the causes, prevalence, consequences and moral
depravity of this the great curse [sic] of the nineteenth century.[65]

An Episcopal clergyman, J. Morgan Smith, indicated that it was
inappropriate to call criminal abortion "the great crime of the nineteenth
century." "Somebody gets up the next minute and says intemperance is the
greatest crime," he continued, "and so we have a half-dozen of the greatest
crimes of the nineteenth century." He called for a change in the language of the
report or resolution since it "seems to imply that the whole clergymen of this
country are derelict in the matter." Smith also indicated that there were "obvious
reasons why the pulpit should not be always used to denounce crimes of this
nature. To do it continually would be to turn the pulpit and church into a place
that many people would not like to visit."[66]

Dr. Cox responded: "The committee believes every word of it." He
reiterated his statements that he had never known a Catholic woman to have an
induced abortion and mentioned a Dr. Klein of Detroit who claimed the crime
was "very rarely" perpetrated by Catholics. The implication was that, relative to
the Catholic clergy, the Protestant clergy were indeed "derelict in the matter."[67]

Two other ministers, Rev. D.C. Jacokes and Rev. Mr. Barnes, agreed with
Rev. Smith that the Protestant clergy was not derelict on the matter of criminal
abortion. Jacokes then contradictorily indicated that the clergy were ignorant of
the problem. Barnes denied this, indicating that ministers were in contact with
physicians, buried the dead, and were not ignorant. For Barnes the question was
whether the subject was to be presented "in the promiscuous audience" or "more
privately."[68] Implicit in this was a shared concern with Rev. Smith about the
"pulpit and church" becoming an unpleasant place that would not be visited.

Dr. Cox called on a Battle Creek Judge, R.F. Graves, for his views and the
Judge "fully agreed" with the committee's report. He saw the problem rising
from the ignorance of people regarding the criminality and immorality of
abortion. Laws would have no effect on reducing the crime until the people were
enlightened to the fact that "it is murder and nothing else." Following the
Judge's comments: "The resolution was then adopted."[69]

The parade of physicians addressing their medical societies about the problem of criminal abortion continued. Jno. S. Pearson, of Louisiana, Missouri, read
a paper, "Criminal Abortion," before the Linton District Medical Society in
Mexico, Missouri on November 8, 1881. Pearson began by noting that criminal
abortions were induced both by non-physicians and by "those who call them-

selves physicians, with diplomas, and [who are] licensed by reputable medical colleges." He was ashamed to admit that the latter "lend themselves to this great crime in total perversion of their true mission."[70]

Pearson indicated that the taking of life *"at any time"* after conception was "the foulest and grossest of murders, on whomsoever practiced or by whomsoever done."[71] His next comments echoed Storer's 1857 proposal to increase the legal penalty for criminal abortion when induced by a physician:

> But if the production of abortion is wrong and criminal by the subjects themselves, and those without the profession, it is doubly vicious in the physician. Why? Let us consider the sphere of the physician— his scope. What is his mission to others in life? What to himself as a reasonable and reflective being? Obligations arise, exist and assert themselves in all the varied relations of life, and are peculiar to each calling therein. The higher, the more responsible and sacred the calling in life, the greater and more sacred the duties and obligations.[72]

J. Miller, M.D., Professor of Orthopedic Surgery in the Medical Department of the University of Kansas City, published an article, "Criminal Abortion," in the initial number of the *Kansas City Medical Record*. Miller began by discussing various organizations such as temperance organizations "whose object is protection of some kind to some thing." He continued:

> It is claimed by temperance advocates and lecturers that a large per cent of the crimes that are perpetrated are due to alcohol. This I will not undertake to deny, but desire to call attention to one class of beings upon whom there is being a terrible crime perpetrated, and for which alcohol is not to blame. A class of being who have no organization for their protection, no adequate law by which they may seek redress, and no earthly tribunal before which they can lay their grievances and sue for justice; I refer to the malicious and criminal destruction of unborn children.[73]

Miller provided estimates of the number of abortions based on a formula that criminal abortions were 7.5 percent of the total number of births. For the year 1880 he came up with "121,002 antenatal murders" and "12,100 women sacrificing their lives."[74] He discussed as causes women's unwillingness to raise children, training of girls on anatomy and physiology that gave them knowledge for self-abortion, and laws that did not recognize that the embryo had life during the first half of the pregnancy. He also included the advertisements of "villainous pills and compounds" by the press and by druggists. He quoted Michigan's Dr. Cox on causes including Cox's note that the public "recognizes the abortionist as a useful member of society, and extols him as a benefactor."[75] Also following Cox, he criticized the clergy for failing to address the issue and claimed that they had to be aware "that this is the greatest crime known to God's law."[76]

Miller included a letter "from a leading physician," from whom he had requested information on abortion cases "that would be interesting to the profession." The physician indicated "the one of most importance" was a married woman whom he attended who was "flowing freely" and from whom he extracted a fetus of two months. The woman indicated her miscarriage resulted from a fall. He was skeptical and she admitted that she had used a flexible male catheter to induce this and "four or five" previous abortions. She had induced at least 12 abortions altogether in ten years with the earlier ones induced with a crochet hook. She indicated that she had been able to recognize the fetus in every case. She bragged to the Kansas City physician that she was "still quite a healthy woman."

Miller commented on the case:

What a regret to some and what a relief to others that our eminent ministers have in the last few years abolished hell? If this woman had died before hell was abolished, and presented herself for admission at the golden gate, there would have been *twelve little angels* crying out: "Don't let her in; she was our mother on earth, and she murdered us."[77]

Although the term "woman physician" meant "abortionist" in some circles, there were women physicians who shared the regular physicians' typical abhorrence of criminal abortion, including the most famous early woman physician in America, Elizabeth Blackwell. Her biographer claimed that she wrote in her diary: "The gross perversion and destruction of motherhood by the abortionist filled me with indignation, and awakened active antagonism. That the honorable term 'female physician' should be exclusively applied to those women who carried on this shocking trade seemed to me a horror. It was an utter degradation of what might and should become a noble position for women."[78] Blackwell was intent on showing that the true woman physician strongly opposed the practice. Repeatedly in her letters she condemned unnecessary abortion and Madame Restell was a major object of her condemnation when she practiced medicine in New York City from 1853 to 1869.[79]

James Mohr made reference to Anne Densmore, a physician who provided a series of lectures in 1868 where she stated that abortion was murder. A teacher who attended the lecture wrote that "'several' of the women in the audience who had practiced abortion fainted at the thought of having committed murder."[80] Anita Tyng was a Massachusetts physician and surgeon who served as Horatio Storer's assistant in the mid 1860s. Dr. Tyng's friend, Caroline Dall, wrote in her diary, that Dr. Tyng was frequently approached to provide abortion, but refused to comply with such requests.[81]

Dr. Charlotte Lozier was noted for her antiabortion efforts. The New York City physician made the newspapers in November 1869 when she turned over to the police a man who approached her seeking an abortion for his girlfriend. The feminist magazine, *The Revolution*, praised Dr. Lozier for her actions and reproduced portions of a pair of newspaper articles expressing their pleasure that a physician would take action against those seeking illegal abortions, despite criticism from other physicians for violating privacy. The editors of the *Springfield*

[Massachusetts] *Republican* reported their belief that an increase in women physicians would help to eliminate a crime that they implied men physicians were not sufficiently concerned about. Dr. Lozier died during childbirth a few weeks after this episode.[82]

A number of strongly antiabortion women physicians were identified in an 1888 expose of abortionists in Chicago by the *Chicago Times*. These included Jennie E. Hayner, Julia Holmes Smith, Catherine J. Wells, Odelia Blinn, and Sarah Hackett Stevenson (See Chapter 22). Although many midwives and several male physicians were willing to induce abortion, only one woman physician, Emilie Siegmund, agreed to perform the operation and it is doubtful that she was a *bona fide* physician.

Women physicians also contributed to popular antiabortion literature. In 1883, Alice Bunker Stockham, M.D., published *Tokology: A Book for Every Woman*.[83] It was written to help women avoid the pains of childbirth and she quoted Horatio Storer's: "There is probably no suffering ever experienced which will compare, in proportion to its extent in time with the throes of parturition." In her chapter on abortion she initially discussed miscarriage and its prevention, but concluded with a discussion of "*produced* abortion." Stockham noted that many women believed the child was not alive until quickening and she quoted John Brodhead Beck to show the fallacy of this. She continued:

> When the female germ and male sperm unite, then is the inception of a new life; all that goes to make up a human being—body, mind and spirit, must be contained in embryo within this minute organism. *Life must be present from the very moment of conception.* If there was not life there could be no conception. At what other period of a human being's existence, either pre-natal or post-natal, could the union of soul and body take place? Is it not plain that the violent or forcible deprivation of existence of this embryo, the removal of it from the citadel of life, is its premature death, and hence the act can be denominated by no more mild term than murder, and whoever performs the act, or is accessory to it, in the sight of God and human law, is guilty of the crime of all crimes?
>
> By what false reasoning does she who feels that the life of the babe who draws its sustenance from the snow white fountain, is more precious than all else to her, whose heart is thrilled with a pang of agony at thought of least danger to its life, convince herself that another life equally dependent upon her for its existence, with equal rights and possibilities, has no claim from her for protection? More than this, she deliberately strikes the red hand of murder and terminates its existence with no thought of wrong, with no consciousness of the violation of law.
>
> The woman who produces abortion, or allows it to be produced, risks her own health and life in the act and commits the highest crime in the criminal calendar, for she takes the life of her own child.[84]

Unlike most physicians, Stockham had no qualms about "preventing conception of a life, but once conceived it should not be deprived of its existence." She next provided a list of "incentives to produce abortion." The unmarried desired "to shield her good name." Some married women simply were unwilling to have a child that would "interfere with their pleasures." "Others," she continued, "who are poor or are burdened with care or grief, or have licentious or drunken husbands, shrink from adding to an already overburdened existence." The unmarried and "overburdened" married had Stockham's sympathy, but not a married woman who requested abortion so that she could travel to Europe:

> She returned the second and third time even, armed with a lawyer's sophistry to endeavor to persuade me to be accessory to the diabolical deed. No doubt one cause of her persistency was fear of trusting her secret to me unless she could persuade me to be an accomplice.
>
> She probably found some one to assist her out of the "trouble" for she took the proposed trip, but I was not astonished to know in three or four years from that time she was lying at death's door with consumption. How many times she produced abortion I know not, but I was told for months she suffered from uterine hemorrhages and in the weakened state of her system a violent cold settled upon her lungs which soon terminated her life. This was the physical result of the crime she had committed.[85]

Numerous editions of Dr. Stockham's book were published during her long life. The author's copy is the twenty-third edition and it was published in 1885 only two years after the first. This strongly suggests a major early effect of the book on attitudes about forced abortion. It is probable that *Tokology: A Book for Every Woman* was as influential in decreasing abortion for its two generations of readers as Horatio's *Why Not? A Book for Every Woman* was for a prior generation.

Women physicians also contributed to the medical antiabortion literature. The New York surgeon, Mary Amanda Dixon Jones, wrote a long article for the *Medical Record* in 1894 discussing ways that physicians could reduce abortion and describing her own successful persuasion of a dozen women seeking abortion to have their children instead. A Denver physician, Minnie C.T. Love, condemned women seeking abortions and the people who provided them in a 1903 paper. So did Inez C. Philbrick, a Lincoln, Nebraska physician and women suffragist from in 1905. Their efforts are described Chapters 25 and 26.

CHAPTER 21
A PROPOSAL TO CONTROL JUSTIFIABLE ABORTION

Perhaps the most insightful paper of the latter half of the century dealing with the problems of criminal and therapeutic abortion was presented to the Gynaecological Society of Boston in 1886. The paper, "The Ethics of Abortion, as a Method of Treatment in Legitimate Practice," was given by James E. Kelly.[1] Dr. Kelly had recently arrived in Boston from Ireland via New York. An earlier paper by Kelly listed his affiliations as "Member of the Royal Irish Academy; Fellow of the Royal College of Surgeons, etc."[2]

In an introductory paragraph, Kelly referred to "many able writers" who had dealt with criminal abortion, but he failed to mention the Gynaecological Society's founder. This may have reflected ignorance associated with his previous Ireland residence. The paragraph concluded:

> I write this paper for the purpose of inducing the thoughtful physician to reconsider his duty and responsibilities, as well as to investigate the basis of the popular idea, that owing to the adoption of the most humane calling, a physician should be expected to produce abortion at the behest or for the benefit of any individual. I have appended a few suggestions indicating a possible method of relieving the profession from this unjust and odious responsibility, while extending to the parent and the foetus the fullest measure of human justice.[3]

Kelly discussed the beginning of life at conception and the very early appearance of all major functioning organs other than those associated with respiration. He indicated the perception of pain by the fetus was probably possible in the fourth month following development of "the sensory zone of the cerebrum." This may have been the first physician reference to the pain experienced by the fetus during abortion. Kelly continued:

> The conclusion at which we must arrive, a conclusion corroborated by the teachings of religion, is that from the instant at which impregnation occurs and the ovum receives life, the foetus is human, and at all periods differs in degree and not in kind from the infant and the adult. Therefore, we must regard it as a "human being" with an inalienable right to life, and that its destruction is homicide.[4]

Kelly indicated the various circumstances such as war or self-defense that could justify homicide and showed that induced abortion did not fit any of these categories. He also indicated that the premeditated aspect of the act made it "nothing less than willful murder." He continued:

> But is it not still a greater crime? Crimes are divided into natural and unnatural, the latter consisting of all those acts which are contrary to the great fundamental and natural instincts of self-preservation and reproduction of species. Abortion is an act which is directly antagonistic to reproduction, and as such, like suicide and other crimes which are unnamable, it is unnatural. Consequently it is a greater crime even than willful murder; a "Murder most foul and most unnatural."[5]

Kelly continued:

> It is often contended that the undeveloped condition of the foetus and its dependent and defenceless state detract from its claim to existence, but if we exclude the element of birth, this is an argument which with equal propriety may be advanced against the rights of many adults, most children, and all infants. ... Another defence of abortion is based upon the futile and deceptive comparison of the relative value of the lives of the mother and foetus. This is but an effort to contrast the known with the unknown, for the natural development of this unborn being may possibly result in a career greater than any with which the old world or the new has ever yet been blessed, greater even than that of a Caesar or a Socrates, an Aquinas or a Washington.[6]

Kelly followed with this plea:

> The prevalence of abortion as an established procedure in modern medicine, the freedom with which it is practised and the enthusiasm with which it is advocated by gentlemen of great professional influence in this city, some of whom I heard in public indignantly denounce other individuals, medical, lay, and clerical, because they conscientiously refused to assist or sanction the destruction of the embryo, are the circumstances which convince me that no existing enactment, either human or divine, can prevent many physicians from practising abortion in good faith, and consequently that some "new laws" are needed which shall tend to limit its application to the minimum, and to alleviate, in the juridical sense at least, the repugnant act of abortion into "justifiable foeticide."[7]

No names of these influential Boston physicians who enthusiastically advocated abortion were given, but during the discussion of Kelly's paper, W. Symington Brown claimed that Kelly's "whole plea was based on the authority of the Church," presumably the Catholic Church, and "could not hold water." Brown claimed that abortion was justifiable in some circumstances where "the welfare of the patient demands it."[8]

Kelly's proposed method to limit abortion to the minimum and insure that it was "justifiable foeticide" was to have authorities establish "a tribunal for the purpose of restraining those practitioners who are not deterred by ethical considerations or religious scruples." He continued:

> According to precedent it might consist of the presiding officer or judge, a physician of the highest professional probity and juridical reputation; an able practitioner as the counselor defendant of the foetus, the parent being represented by her personal medical attendant, and the fourth member of the court would be the executive officer. That such an officer as a State abortionist should be appointed is apparent, owing to the many instances in which no power could compel the attending physician to perform so repugnant an operation, while even if he were willing to undertake it, his opportunities might not afford him the essential skill and experience. It would hardly be in keeping with that rigid impartiality so desirable in a presiding officer if, as the executioner of his own mandate, he were to perform an operation for which he would necessarily be remunerated; neither would it be in keeping with the function of the physician to whom we have alluded as the representative or defender of the foetus, to destroy the life of his client. With such a tribunal the operation would be shorn of some of its most objectionable features.[9]

Kelly's "tribunal" appears to have been the first proposal for a committee to evaluate the appropriateness of requests for therapeutic abortion. It apparently never got beyond the proposal stage. Such committees would become commonplace six decades later, although they may not have safeguarded the fetus as well as Kelly's would have.

A few months later, the *Journal of the American Medical Association* included the following suggestion of "a correspondent" for reducing criminal abortion:

> "When we shall have passed a law binding all physicians, upon their honor, to make public the desire of any person who may ask the performance of an abortion, we can then hope to check, in a measure, the wholesale murder of the unborn. Secrecy in regard to patients who come to us for advice should be sacredly observed, but the audacious insult of requesting an honorable physician to procure an abortion should be publicly resented by openly reporting the party."[10]

However, the editors disagreed. They claimed it was rare for women to make such direct requests for abortion. Patients instead pleaded for something to restore their blocked menses. They indicated that most of these women immediately abandoned any efforts to have an abortion following positive assurance that they were pregnant and a description of the physical and moral dangers of abortion. They also said that publicly identifying the few who would continue requests for abortion would simply send patients directly to known abortionists. The editors also noted that the patient reported to authorities might sue the physician for libel and it would be rare for any witness to be available to support the physician. "We fear such a law would prove more dangerous to the honorable physician," the editors concluded, "than helpful to the cause of public morals and humanity."[11]

In 1857, the Nashville physician, James W. Hoyte, wrote Horatio Storer that there were no criminal abortions in Tennessee.[12] Three decades later, another Nashville physician, John Bryan Ward Nowlin, read a paper to the Tennessee State Medical Society that indicated things had greatly changed.[13] Nowlin began by questioning whether the medical profession itself was not "criminally responsible," since "thousands of abortions are annually produced, which might by judicious management have been prevented, and living children preserved to the world." He indicated that there were contingencies requiring therapeutic abortion, but he saw them as "very rare," and he had never found it necessary to produce abortion during his 31 years of practice. He noted that the frequent use of abortion in instances where there was no absolute necessity, led the public to regard abortion as a matter of little legal or moral concern. Nowlin claimed the prevalent "evil of committing promiscuous and unwarranted abortion" pervaded all social classes but found "its most congenial soil" "among the rich, refined and educated."[14]

Nowlin claimed women frequently attempted to trick doctors into introducing the uterine sound to correct a feigned problem with the uterus, knowing that it would produce the desired abortion. Women also made use of professional abortionists and "[e]very neighborhood and town has its old hag who is ready, for a consideration, to lend her assistance in the nefarious scheme."

Nowlin continued:

> It has been urged in extenuation of this practice that the child has no individuality as such, until the period of quickening occurs. That the profession is, to a considerable extent, responsible for this popular error is unquestionably true. The great Velpeau says: "For my part, I confess I can not balance the life of a foetus of three, four, five, or six months, a being which so far scarcely differs from a plant, and is bound by no tie to the external world, against that of a woman whom a thousand social ties engage us to save."[15]

Nowlin's Velpeau quote actually shows somewhat more consideration of fetal rights than the one provided by Brinton: "The fetus has no independent life and no claims upon our consideration on any such account—that it is, in short, nothing more than a vegetable." But Nowlin obviously viewed Velpeau as part of the problem, despite referring to him as "the great Velpeau."

Nowlin again implicated the "legitimate profession" in criminal abortion:

> Unfortunately, some members of our profession are not perfect, and in the face of temptation and fear of the lash have not the courage to assert their manhood and maintain the true dignity of the profession, yet it is exceedingly hard to catch them in *res delictu*. Like the fox in the snow,

they wipe out their tracks with their tails. Madam _____, a rich client, calls upon him with a plethoric purse. Tells him that she has unfortunately become *enciente*; that such a condition is utterly incompatible with her health and the demands which society makes upon her; that something must be done. ... To refuse, he knows that he will not only lose the practice in her family, but also provoke her hostility among a large circle of influential families.[16]

Nowlin proposed the following remedies:

What hoe can be used to dig up these thistles in the fallow fields of society? What means can be resorted to, to purify our moral atmosphere? What disinfectant to heal this great, foul cancer upon the body politic? I answer, in the first place, by the profession teaching the public the facts of embryology, in so far as they relate to the enormity of this crime. Let us all repudiate any assistance in this matter of abortion, save in our own ranks, based upon well-assured facts demanding its performance. And should any member be so lost to a sense of his high professional dignity, cut him off root and branch, and let him no longer cumber the ground and hold association in an honorable profession.

    The Society should speak with no uncertain sound in this matter. The American Medical Association should take up the cudgel. Thoroughly instruct our law-makers, so that laws may be formulated which will let no guilty one escape. You owe it to the dignity of the profession, you owe it to the conservation of public morals. Then let this Society at this meeting express itself by resolution in this matter, and request the American Medical Association to take a similar step.[17]

    The American Medical Association did appoint a special committee in 1887 "to report at its next meeting, upon the *criminality of foeticide* and such measures as may be commended for legislative action for its prevention and punishment." This, however, was at the request of the New Jersey physician, Isaac N. Quimby, who delivered an address, "Introduction to Medical Jurisprudence," at the Annual Meeting in Chicago.[18] One of the first problems Quimby addressed was foeticide that he described as "alarmingly prevalent." He decried the meager misdemeanor crime that was associated with unnecessary abortion and the fact that the quickening concept still mediated punishment of the crime. He called for physicians to counter the common belief that there was no life until quickening by pointing out that it was murder to destroy the fetus at any period of gestation. He lamented the fact that there were some "who call themselves physicians" who willingly responded to the numerous entreaties from women to end their pregnancies.

    Quimby continued:

The physician's responsibility in this matter is very grave, and they should do all in their power to discourage this prevailing tendency of the times to foeticide, and teach that life commences with conception.

God forbid that anyone calling himself a physician should be tempted by any appeal however pressing and piteous, or by any fee however large, to become the assassin of the unborn, in any stage of its development. I suggest that a special committee be appointed by the Association to report at its next meeting, upon the *criminality of foeticide* and such measures as may be commended for legislative action for its prevention and punishment.[19]

A footnote indicated that a committee was appointed consisting of Quimby, W.B. Atkinson, of Pennsylvania, and William Heath Byford, of Illinois. However, the next year after Quimby read the report of the Committee on Foeticide, "the whole subject was laid upon the table."[20] Unlike for some other addresses, there was no motion to publish. Shortly thereafter, however, the proceedings of the Annual Meeting indicated this initial tabling of the subject was overturned: "After much discussion, on motion of Nathan Smith Davis, the report by Dr. Quimby on *Foeticide*, was taken from the table and referred to the Section on State Medicine."[21] The next year there was no discussion of the subject in the Proceedings of the main meeting, the minutes of the Section on State Medicine, or the Address on State Medicine by W.H. Welch, of Maryland. Apparently the motion was effectively tabled in 1888, despite not being tabled formally.

The *Journal of the American Medical Association* published the proceedings of the October 1, 1887 meeting of the Medico-Legal Society of Chicago that included a paper, "The Medico-Legal Aspect of Criminal Abortion," by Dr. A.K. Steele and a discussion of its legal aspects by Judge O.M. Horton.[22] Steele admitted that his paper represented nothing new, but, despite this, it was worthwhile to provide a retelling of "old truths" and to expose "old errors and present crimes." He described the existence of "vitality" from conception and indicated it was homicide to destroy this being with its "inalienable right to life." He stressed the need for more than one physician to agree that an unborn child was a sufficient threat to the life of the mother to justify its destruction. He called on additional education of the public and, particularly, of the profession related to the moral aspects of the crime. He also claimed "conviction of a few of the principals with their accessories would go far towards correcting this terrible evil."[23] A more detailed version of Steele's paper published in the December 17, 1888 *Chicago Times* included Steele's claim that abortionists were "in our medical societies—some of them perchance, even in this society."[24] The *Journal of the American Medical Association* perhaps did not want to broadcast this claim that medical societies harbored abortionists.

For his part, Judge Horton talked about the necessity of lawyers and physicians working together to get rid "of the quacks and shysters—the leprous excrescences that fasten themselves upon both professions."[25] He described the Illinois abortion laws that made it a criminal offense to destroy the fetus at any stage of development and contrasted them with earlier laws that made it a crime only after quickening. He then made a plug for a 20-year-old book:

Allow me here to commend to your consideration a small volume, of about 200 pages, upon "Criminal Abortion, its Nature, its Evidence and its Law," by Dr. Horatio R. Storer. The collection of evidence and statistics showing the prevalence of this crime would astonish those who have not given especial attention to the matter, even members of the medical profession. I am indebted to this writer for some of the conclusions here presented.[26]

Horton continued with discussion of the frequent failures to bring violators to justice. Reasons cited included the "general absence of all fear of detection, the prevailing of a feeling of 'false modesty,' the number of persons practicing as physicians who will commit the crime or contribute towards its commission, and the sacredness of the professional confidence of the regular physicians." He called on "honorable practitioners" to "drive from the public mind the too prevalent opinion that *money* will induce almost any physician to perpetrate a crime against the laws of God and man." The judge then quoted, Storer's "Of the mother, ..." sentence, presumably to emphasize the depravity of requestors and providers of the "crime against the laws of God and man."[27]

The report of these Chicago proceedings concluded with the claim by one physician discussant, "Dr. Sawyer," that abortion was not as frequent as Steele had claimed and the contrasting claim of the Chicago physician, Fernand Henrotin, that the crime "was a very common one." Henrotin described how in "former years" he had had many opportunities to investigate criminal abortion and "had the pleasure of bringing several of these criminals to justice."[28] As will be seen, the *Chicago Times* investigation one year later would also show that a large number of Chicago's physicians were willing to provide abortions and numerous letters from physicians to the newspaper during their expose claimed that unnecessary abortion was highly prevalent.

The Belmont, Texas physician, Henry Clay Ghent, addressed the Texas State Medical Association in its 20th Annual Session in Galveston in April 1888.[29] Ghent began by citing the abortion prohibition of the Hippocratic Oath and followed this with the first 1859 American Medical Association Resolution on Criminal Abortion to illustrate "that the standard of our profession has not been lowered." Ghent continued:

> We know of no subject within the entire domain, or field of medicine, of more importance in its relations to woman, to the family, to society, to government, to humanity, to the race, to morals, to the medical profession, than that of foeticide, or criminal abortion. On the other hand, we know of no subject, within the same field, that has received as little attention at the hands of our profession, in proportion to its magnitude in the relations alluded to, as the one we are about to discuss.[30]

Ghent made a tribute to Horatio Robinson Storer, although two of his dates were incorrect:

In 1865, the A. M. A. offered a gold medal for an essay upon "The, Physical Evils of Forced Abortion." This medal was awarded Dr. H. R. Storer, of Boston, Mass., and his essay was published in the Transactions of the Association for that year. At the meeting of the Association next year, 1866, it was voted to reprint the above for general circulation. This was done under the title, "Why Not? A Book for every Woman." This work has been very highly eulogized by the medical press and medical profession.[31]

In a section describing "the awful conspiracy, to forcibly enter the portals of life for the purpose of destroying a living, human being," Ghent reproduced Storer's "Of the mother, ..." sentence. He no doubt judged this appropriate, given its discussion of mother, father, and abortionist conspiring to destroy the unborn child. Ghent next provided a long quote from Storer's *Is It I?*, which emphasized the conspiratorial contributions "by us men."[32]

Ghent also discussed the "duty of the medical profession." This was to teach the rest of humanity that life began at conception and that it was an enormous crime to end it in the womb. The dangers to women's health and life also needed to be taught. He saw no other group as capable of providing the education needed to change the pathological state of the public. He concluded by discussing his own successes in preventing abortion and may have been the first physician to describe the resulting children:

> We are satisfied we have been able to convince many fathers and mothers of their erroneous notions and criminal intent, and to-day could point to scores of bright, beautiful, living monuments of different ages and of both sexes, as so many attestations of the truth of the statement. Who, then, can do most to stay the dark tide of this fearful crime in its onward course to disease and death? We take the liberty and assume the responsibility of saying, the honest and upright physician, the family doctor, who is ever the true, tried and trusty friend in all the troubles and trials and sorrows, the result of sickness and pain and anguish, physical and mental. He is the one, above all others, in whose bosom are all the secrets of the family entrusted.[33]

CHAPTER 22

MARKHAM'S TREATISE AND THE
CHICAGO TIMES EXPOSE

Two years after publishing James Kelly's paper, the *Journal of the American Medical Association* published another insightful article on abortion.[1] The Independence, Iowa physician and former Civil War surgeon, Henry C. Markham, read the paper to the Section on Medical Jurisprudence at the May 1888 Annual Meeting of the American Medical Association. Markham began:

> In approaching the consideration of the subject of foeticide we are at the outset confronted by two facts, both of which possess an important significance. We first note that the highest crime—from some standpoints at least—of which criminal humanity is capable, and whose prevalence doubtless exceeds the highest estimate, is of no more judicial importance, in either treatise or statute, than when the evil was scarcely known, and motherhood was everywhere the crowning glory of woman. The second fact is little less an anomaly: that in the presence and despite the elevation, culture, refinement and more than all else, the religious training and influences operating upon and in modern social life, that in the class of society making in all these respects the highest claims, this vice has developed, the enormity and extent of which is but feebly recognized outside the medical profession.[2]

Markham claimed that criminal abortion did not receive proper attention because there had been no agreement on whether it was the province of "the law, the church, or medicine." He continued:

> To the moralist and jurist it presents a barrier of delicacy whose sacred realm they instinctively shrink from invading. The resistless power, also, of social pride and ambition would seem to leave little hope of reform through moral agencies. The highest level of ethical profession, in the geography of the modern social world, is honeycombed by this lurking and hideous evil. The conditions insuring perfect concealment and the absolute certainty of the ignorance of the public as to its commission impart characteristics both unique and formidable to the crime. Foeticide is also the one great crime in which the chief victim, or sufferer, is wholly defenseless and without hope of an advocate.[3]

He continued:

The champions of the temperance cause, in order to enforce and prove their claims, have only to point to the living victims of dissipation. Those espousing the cause of social purity easily refer to living illustrations of the evils they seek to remove. Statistics are the weapons most feared by the foes of public good. But foeticide enjoys immunity from all these methods of attack. As this important subject is, for inherent reasons, unsuited for judicial investigation, and successfully opposes religious influences, the obligation necessarily rests upon the medical profession to propose a method for checking the fearful progress of the evil.[4]

Markham briefly touched on the "diabolical attributes and features of the crime from a moral standpoint" and on its medical results, "both pathological and physiological." He regretted that time did not permit discussion of these important subjects. He described instead the need for physicians to report criminal abortion to the authorities when they became aware of it, since this, like smallpox, was a danger to the public that circumvented traditional physician unwillingness to disclose their patients' secrets and confidences. Patients believed that physicians would not only keep an attempt at abortion secret, but would save them from the danger that might ensue.

"Probably no fact is indirectly more promotive of foeticide than the absence of laws regulating medical practice;" Markham wrote, "thereby enabling abortionists, disguised as members of an honorable profession, to pursue their nefarious avocation with comparative impunity."[5] However, this single sentence reference to regulation of medicine hardly makes a case that regulation of medicine was the *reason* that Markham was expressing his opposition to criminal abortion before the Section on Medical Jurisprudence.

Markham mentioned the "wrong inflicted upon the husband who suffers willful betrayal of his hopes and expectations of offspring." "Medical men will verify this as being no fancy or rare event," he continued, "as too frequently, when called to rescue the victim from her self-induced peril, has it been a duty to impart to the anxious husband the cause of the danger and the first knowledge of his already severe loss."[6]

Markham concluded by discussing the "facilities" that were "disseminating criminal knowledge of the practice." This no doubt was a reference to the newspaper advertisements of abortionists and abortion-drug sellers. He called for them to instead provide "a popular presentation of the evil as such."[7] It may not be a coincidence that six months later the *Chicago Times* provided its "popular presentation of the evil as such," i.e., their expose of criminal abortion. Much of Markham's paper was reprinted in the *Times* in a subsequent "Remedy" segment.[8] Markham also published two letters in the newspaper, one during and one following the expose.[9] If Markham himself were not an instigator of the *Times* expose, the Chicago-based editor of the *Journal of the American Medical Association*, Nathan Smith Davis, may have adopted Markham's suggestion and caused the *Times* to undertake the effort.

The editor of the *Chicago Times* was James J. West who had only recently taken the position. During November 1888, West sent a male and a female reporter to the offices of scores of midwives and physicians and they were able to persuade dozens to agree to perform an abortion on the "Girl Reporter" who feigned an illegitimate pregnancy. The young woman claimed that she was from Memphis and the other reporter claimed at times to be the father of the child, a friend of the girl, or her brother. Some of the interviews with potential abortionists were conducted by the girl alone, a few by the "brother" alone, but for the most part, both reporters visited physicians. The interviews were published in the *Times* from December 13 to December 25, 1888.

Editor West never identified the physician or physicians who stimulated his crusade. One Chicago physician, Isaac Prince, included in a letter "indorsing" the crusade: "If I had not believed in the need of reform in the medical profession, I should not have asked you to seek to unearth and break up the satanic and murderous practices you are making public."[10] This may indicate that Prince was an instigator. There was strong editorial emphasis on Nathan Smith Davis, "founder of the American Medical Association."[11] Early in the series of published interviews, Davis made a comment at a meeting of the Chicago Medical Society that "other [Society] members might be written up."[12] These factors suggest that Davis may have had some role in the etiology of the expose.

Another possible instigator of the expose may have been the Chicago physician, John Floyd Banton. The "Infanticide" section for December 16 began with additional editorializing about the problem, including a long quote from Banton who discussed the barbarous nature of "infanticide in utero." Banton also wrote: "America stands today without a parallel among the nations of the world for the wholesale murder of human souls." These quotes were from Banton's 1885 pamphlet, *Revolution in the Practice of Medicine*.[13] It included some of the harshest words uttered by a physician against women who sought abortions:

> "The Hindoo women did cast their offspring into the waters of the Ganges, but this was the result of ignorance and superstition: their babes were offered as a sacrifice to the gods of their worship. But the women of our country murder their little ones purely from their vile concupiscence, and this terrible crime is inflicted on the victims while yet imprisoned within the womb of one perverted and changed from a human being to a fiend. Let me say to all men that the woman who can thus destroy the life of one nourished by her own blood and protected by the wall of her own womb in a manner marvelous and beyond the comprehension of man, such a creature, though fair to look upon and charming with entertainments, would much more easily take your life; did circumstances arise giving birth to the idea in the brain[,] the hand would not be constrained."[14]

Other published quotes of Banton repeated the notion that the woman who desired to abort but failed, created a child that had the same murderous intent "and it is from this source that our prisons are filled." There also was the claim that criminal abortion "gives full control of our government and country to the foreigner in less than a score of years." The editor followed the Banton passages with: "Such is the language of one who has given his life's labor to the elevation of man and woman kind, not above the degradation of barbarism, but above that deeper and more damnable degradation which results from the interference of scientific knowledge with the handiwork of nature and the laws of God."[15]

Still another possible instigator was Edmund J. Doering, President of the Chicago Medico-Legal Society. "Infanticide" for Monday December 17 began with his letter to the editor:

> DEAR SIR: I desire to thank you for your investigation of the crime of "infanticide" as committed in this city. On behalf of the Medico-Legal Society of Chicago—composed of representative physicians and lawyers—I can promise you moral and financial support to bring these abortionists to justice, as one of the objects of this society is the punishment of criminal practices of the medical profession. The most infamous, the foulest of all crimes, is the murder of the unborn, and its punishment should be *death*, nothing less, as it *is* murder in the first degree. Hoping that public sentiment will be aroused and opportunity given to rid this city of these human monsters whose very existence is a plague and a public calamity, I am very respectfully, Edmund J. Doering, M.D.[16]

The next day, Doering's letter was reprinted in a cartoon and reprinted again on the editorial page. Long excerpts from Dr. A.K. Steele's October 1, 1887 paper to Doering's Chicago Medico-Legal Society also appeared in the *Times* on December 17. Doering may have included Steele's original paper as an enclosure to his letter to the editor.

The newspaper provided names and addresses of physicians who were interviewed and classified them on their willingness to perform abortion, their refusal to do this, or their willingness to refer the woman to some abortionist, although unwilling to perform the abortion themselves. Many totally refused to perform abortion, but a score or more were willing to do so. One physician who agreed to perform the abortion was Edwin Moses Hale.

The Girl Reporter discussed the interview with Hale:

> By the time we had reached the door of Dr. E. M. Hale, 159 Twenty-second street, my attendant had himself metamorphosed into my brother, and I became a girl of wealth but no discretion. An interview between the brother and doctor took place, in which the former related the conditions and the latter at first demurred from assuming connection with it. It was then found advisable for the brother to instance a case or two in which the doctor had prominently officiated. This mode of procedure brought down the persimmon handsomely. No further demur was made, the doctor remarking that he would have nothing to do with cases of this complexion excepting in families of the most unquestioned

standing and aristocracy. I was then politely shown out of the private room, during an interview I was not to hear, between the two. My "brother" informed me, when we had taken our departure, that the conversation related to arrangements for my accommodation.[17]

Hale's plan was for the girl to check into a hospital where unmarried women stayed until delivering their babies. The physician who ran the hospital did not allow abortions. However, the girl was to pretend she took pills (that Hale actually provided) before arriving and this would force Hale to "complete" an abortion, although he really would be inducing one. An Editorial on December 18 hypothesized about the interaction that would have occurred:

> This Dr. Hale was quite shrewd—quite shrewd. He managed his part of the case, or thought he did, with consummate skill, but the best laid plans, as you have heard before, gang aft aglee. He would call upon the unfortunate girl and say: "Ah hem, let me see." Then to the nurse in attendance he would say: "Ah, hem, has this young woman taken any medicine?" The nurse would reply: "Yes, doctor. She tells me that somebody gave her pills. Here are some of them; I wouldn't let her take them." The doctor in an agitated tone would say: "What? You have taken them! Why, my dear young woman you have put yourself beyond my power, I am afraid. But I will do what I can for you. Nurse, go down and get me— —," And while the nurse was gone he would do what he could for her.
>
> Is this a diagnosis of the doctor's case? THE TIMES thinks it is, and a good one.[18]

Hale would claim in a letter to the paper that he had been misunderstood.[19] However, the paper held fast in its claims and provided additional details in subsequent editions.[20]

Several physicians wrote claiming that Hale was an abortionist. "For twenty years," Dr. S.V. Clevinger wrote, "some of these wealthy scoundrels have been protected by church and social influence while enjoying open reputations as abortionists."[21] This almost certainly was a reference to Hale, given the similar criticism that Cooke had made about Hale's "enviable position in a fashionable Church and fashionable society." "Medical Student" wrote that Hale "has been in the business for twenty-five years and made his money principally in this nefarious pursuit."[22] "It is a crime for a physician to have in his possession any instruments or medicines for the purpose of committing abortions," Nathan Smith Davis claimed, "and there is no reason why Dr. Hale should not be convicted."[23] Some accused physicians brought suit against the newspaper for being identified as willing to produce abortion. Hale, however, was not mentioned as doing this, despite having the harshest treatment of any.

The President of the Chicago Medical Society, J.H. Etheridge, referred the reporters to "the northeast corner of Wabash avenue and Harmon court [where] I think you will find a man who would get the lady out of trouble."[24] Etheridge was briefly included on the list of physicians who would refer the patient to an abortionist. However, the newspaper then went to great lengths to remove Etheridge from the awkward position into which they had placed him. A few days later a reporter interviewing Etheridge suggested that Etheridge's referral of the girl was just a trap whereby the abortionist at Wabash and Harmon would be apprehended. Etheridge actually denied that that was the case, but did indicate that if anything had happened to the girl, he would "get a hold on" the abortionist.[25] The *Times* was unrelenting in its attacks on Edwin Moses Hale, but surprisingly kind to Etheridge.

One physician willing to perform the requested abortion was the Police Department Surgeon, Dr. C.C.P. Silva.[26] He was fired by the mayor, John A. Roche, two days after his interview was published. Another physician who agreed to perform the abortion, Dr. E.H. Thurston, was expelled from the Chicago Medical Society.[27] The city physician, Dr. Andrew J. Coey, agreed to perform abortion, but was able to extricate himself from firing or Society expulsion by showing that he was working to investigate the girl who he believed was faking pregnancy. He had a plain-clothes police officer present the next day when there was to have been another appointment with the girl.[28]

A cartoon in the December 20 *Times* showed "Hercules," depicted as a tall ancient Greek with a belt labeled "THE TIMES," patting Mayor Roche on the back and saying: "Bravo again, John A. As a headsman you are a bright and shining example to the fathers and husbands of Chicago. The police abortionist has gone. Will the family abortionist go also I wonder?" The Hercules cartoon for December 19 showed Hercules observing King Herod who was sitting on an outside throne supervising the slaughter of infants whose corpses littered the courtyard around him. The title read: "IT OUT-HERODS THE DAYS OF HEROD." The caption read:

> Hercules—It is a second massacre of the innocents, more damnable in its extent; and in its atrocity than the first. Let us continue to murder the children of American mothers during the next twenty-five years at the same ratio of increase as during the past, and where, I wonder, will the American men and women of the future come from? Is the Anglo-Saxon-American race to be driven out by the healthy sons and daughters, morally and physically, of Celtic, Teutonic, and Latin origin? Americans, patriots, think of this seriously, and answer me: Will you stop this annihilation of American children?

It is intriguing to speculate where Editor West came up with the verb "Out-Herod." Storer had talked of "wretches who out-Herod Burke and Hare." Storer also expressed concern about the drop in American births and warned that the lands that were opening up to the west would be populated by immigrants. Storer's name did not come up in the *Times'* articles, letters, or editorials, but Judge Horton's reference to *Criminal Abortion: its Nature, its Evidence and its Law* was part of the discussion of Steele's paper to the Chicago Medico-Legal Society. The *Times* reprinted Steele's paper, but not the portion of Horton's discussion that referred to Storer. However, Editor West would have been aware of Storer's book from the full version of Steele's paper and it seems highly likely that he obtained and read it.

Many physicians totally refused to perform the requested abortion. These typically were praised by the editor and the Girl Reporter. Four of these, H.M. Hobart, W.T. Belfield, Evan E. Guinne, and J.E. Gilman, were professors at Chicago medical schools and they were cheered and presented with floral tributes by their students after their refusals were made public.[29]

Three women physicians were particularly singled out for their response to the abortion request. The Girl Reporter visited Dr. Sarah Hackett Stevenson alone, "to test if womanly sympathy could be led to override principle." Dr. Stevenson was quoted as saying:

"My dear, you have broken one commandment; for that, suffering must come. But, is it any reason why you should break two? Think of the gravity of taking a life. You have no more right to make yourself the judge of whether it should live or not after life has once begun than you have to decide that any person you know is injurious to society, and for that reason it is your privilege to put him out of the way. Only one thing is before you, which will in any way atone to the child for the wrong you have done it. Legitimatize it by marriage, even if the latter be but a step toward divorce. If utterly uncongenial to you, you do not need to live together, but have that care for the child. No one but a quack or charlatan would commit the deed you ask me to do. If you can not marry, God help you, my child. I can not. But do not place another sin upon your conscience, for your mother's sake, or that of the unborn."[30]

Dr. Stevenson elicited much praise from the Girl Reporter that ended:

Mrs. Stevenson, God bless her, spoke many kindly words that I have not reported here, and she sent me away feeling that bad as the world may be it is not all bad. There was no compromise in her. She did not respond to my appeal with a "You know it is a dangerous thing," or "It is an illegal thing." No; she stood upon higher ground than that. She would not touch the case because her honor, her conscience, and her womanhood protested against it.[31]

The Girl Reporter had similar praise for the similar reaction of two other women physicians who were visited, Julia Holmes Smith and Catherine J. Wells.[32] The responses of these women would be cited by Junius Hoag, Professor of Obstetrics at the Post-Graduate Medical School of Chicago, when he countered a claim that "educated and refined married women" believed that abortion should be a woman's right (See Chapter 23). Hoag himself provided a letter to the *Times* during its expose calling for a lying-in hospital as part of "The Remedy" to Chicago's abortion problem.[33]

Over a hundred physicians wrote letters in support of the *Times*' effort with over 60 published in one Sunday edition (December 23). Most were responses to a "postal" that the newspaper sent out to a substantial number of Chicago physicians. The response from Arthur Hinde shows the content of the postal:

> To your queries "Do you believe in reform in the medical profession?" "Are you willing to aid in crushing out malpractice?" there can be only one answer. Yes! I am with you tooth and nail, root and branch. Foulness must needs be so long as sewer-holes exist and are untouched, and bad odors will continue to offend the nostrils of the pure and impure alike.[34]

Although the physicians were faced with the request for abortion from what was claimed to be an unmarried woman seeking abortion, it quickly became evident in the letters from physicians that married women were much more likely than the unmarried to seek abortions in Chicago. There also were claims that it was the higher class of women and the members of Christian churches who were guilty.

Several editorials in the *Times* called for ministers to take up the cudgel against these women seeking abortions. A pair of sermons resulted, but the editor claimed on December 25 that both sermons neglected the heart of the problem, their own parishioners.

> They deplored infanticide as something wicked, horrible, godless, practiced here in a Christian community, but not tolerated or tolerable among church members. Bishop Fallows thinks the church may lend a hand for the relief and reformation of outsiders; he never dreams, apparently, that the reformation is needed within the churches. ... And Dr. Fawcett, like Bishop Fallows, all unconscious that the worst offenders, the people who make society, the worshipers of Christ, whose mother carried him into Egypt to escape the murderous designs of a king, the occupants of fashionable pews, the rich, the well-to-do, the respectable, the intelligent, the progressive, and all that, are the very worst offenders. ...
>
> Until the Nathans of the pulpit speak to the Davids of the pew saying, "Thou art the man," we may not hope for much change of heart or conduct among the adults of the childless churches.[35]

One interesting facet of the expose was the repeated claim that women seeking abortion were exploited sexually by some abortionists. For the unmarried, this apparently often started or reinforced a path to prostitution. On December 27, the Girl Reporter expressed her views on the subject:

> A strong impression I dared not state at the time, gathered from various interviews in my pilgrimage of disgrace, was that some of these ready to use the steel or drug were held in abeyance from unprofessional fa-

miliarity only by the character of my personality. Worse than vampires, ready to bleed the helpless victim not only of every dollar of earning but of the honor, without which a woman is better dead.

I pictured to myself unfortunates placing themselves in the hand of these, only to discover later they had crossed the dead-line and there was no return to virtue.

One of the most pathetic recitals I have recently read is a letter I possess, through THE TIMES, from an abandoned woman, who from the bitter depths of her blightedness begs that the scoundrels may be driven from the face of the land so far as possible. She states in a way to be believed that her fall was due to the degradation imposed upon her by one of the class now awaiting public sentence.

Such statements, sent for no selfish purpose, carry strong truth with them. The balance of judgment is certainly in favor of a place where unfortunates will be safe from doctors.[36]

The Girl Reporter obviously believed that abortionists were not only taking the money of the unmarried woman but were having sexual intercourse with them. The "place where unfortunates will be safe from doctors" was a lying-in hospital that the newspaper and many of the physicians were proposing for Chicago.

Married women also were not immune. "Do husbands stop to think when they allow their wives to start on an expedition of this kind for relief," wrote S.L. Rea, M.D., "that the nature of their errand is such that any one immoral enough to commit that crime would not hesitate to demand, as part of his consideration, something he (the husband) would be very slow to concede?"[37] One physician abortionist by the name of Higgins was apparently notorious for taking sexual liberties with his patients. Irate husbands and boyfriends threatened the doctor for his behavior and at least once shots were fired at him. Another man divorced his wife because she repeatedly returned to Dr. Higgins to be insulted.[38]

The stated goals of the newspaper's expose were to strengthen legislation and the power of the state board of health as means to curtail the abortionists, to open a lying-in hospital where unfortunates could have their babies, and to change public opinion about abortion, many people not seeing it as criminal. A Dr. D.R. Brower was interviewed and was pessimistic. He viewed existing laws as inadequate, but saw no possibility of passage of better legislation. He saw the *Times'* agitation as doing good:

> "We may be able by the agitation to form public opinion so as to induce the legislation needed; it will certainly do much toward bringing many doctors who will commit the crime to abandon it, and it will, I believe, start such a reflection on the subject by the women as will deter many from seeking to have it done. Certainly it is in this line that a great revolution is needed. But you have started them to talking about it. A woman was in to see me the other day and said that as far as she was concerned she and her husband would not have any more children if they did not want them, it mattered not what was said and

written on the subject. Of course a case like this tells its own story. It was a woman of wealth and prominence."[39]

The last sentence indicates that public opinion about criminal abortion may not have been greatly changed by the expose. As will be seen, criminal abortion continued to be a large problem in Chicago. A lying-in hospital was started a few years later, but this apparently was not due to this 1888 newspaper expose.

About a dozen newspapers around the nation commented on the expose and their comments were republished in the *Times*.[40] For the most part, these were highly supportive of the effort. An editorial, "Professional Abortionists," dealing with the newspaper's effort was published by the *Journal of the American Medical Association*. Davis' editorial included: "Men that will commit abortion are unfit for citizenship in any civilized state, are too far lost to moral responsibility for the profession of medicine, and to degraded to be associates of honest men."[41]

Management of the victim of the criminal abortionist would come to dominate much medical writing on criminal abortion late in the nineteenth century. T. Gaillard Thomas published a series of six lectures on abortion that he gave at the 1889-1890 session at the College of Physicians and Surgeons in New York. The book, *Abortion and Its Treatment, From the Stand-Point of Practical Experience*, went into at least seven editions from 1890 through 1899.[42] The bulk of the lectures dealt with treatment of abortions arising spontaneously and from other sources, including those induced criminally. However, the book's popularity may have reflected Thomas' fairly liberal indications for therapeutic abortion. For example, he called for an early induced abortion instead of the later caesarian section in cases where the pelvis was too small to allow a natural birth.[43] The book's large readership also may have reflected his explicit presentation of techniques for inducing these therapeutic abortions.[44] The same techniques were useful for the professional abortionist and the physician who only occasionally and reluctantly induced an unnecessary abortion.

Denslow Lewis, Professor of Gynecology at the Chicago Policlinic, delivered a lecture, "Criminal Abortion and the Traumatisms Incident to Its Performance," at the Cook County Hospital in Chicago which was published in the Fall of 1895. Lewis first noted that such traumatisms were prevalent at the Cook County Hospital that was devoted to the care of "the pauper, the friendless, and the unfortunate." He also noted that less unfortunate unmarried women and even married women also resorted to abortion and experienced similar traumatisms.[45]

However, Lewis went beyond description and treatment of these abortion-related problems. He described women who pretended not to be pregnant and requested dilation of the cervix because of dysmenorrhoea, a suspected polypus, or fibroid. "[T]hey will come to you with their lessons well learned,' he claimed, "they will surreptiously [sic] endeavor to induce you to make use of a uterine sound or dilator, in fact they will try most cunningly to persuade you to undertake some form of intra-uterine examination, well knowing that the outcome of your manipulation will be the accomplishment of the result they so earnestly desire."[46]

Others came right out and asked for abortion:

> They apparently expect you to produce an abortion very much as they
> would ask you to lance a boil. Then the reasons they give, how ludi-
> crous they would often seem were there not always a life at stake. The
> women want to go on a summer trip, they expect visitors whom they
> must entertain, or very often they will state that they cannot afford any
> more children. Others will relate the difficulties of their last labor or
> explain how debilitated they became, in consequence of persistent vom-
> iting or some other unpleasant concomitant of a former pregnancy. Still
> others will expatiate on family troubles; they will tell a tale, only too of-
> ten true, of marital infelicity.[47]

According to Lewis, knowledge that the fetus was alive did not deter such
women:

> It is of no use speaking of wrong and of sin. These women will admit
> the truth of all you may say on that score when applied to others; they
> fail to see its applicability in their own individual cases. It is astonishing
> to observe religious women, even the daughters of clergymen, ac-
> knowledge cheerfully the justice of your remarks in one breath, and in
> the next still persist in their efforts to convince you why you should
> make an exception with them.[48]

Lewis instead would tell the requesting woman "that in her case the danger
of abortion is infinitely greater than that of labor." He was contrasting the septic
environment of the abortionist with "labor occurring under aseptic conditions."
Lewis then admitted he would prevaricate to some extent:

> I acknowledge that under certain conditions physicians, after due con-
> sultation, are sometimes compelled to interrupt a pregnancy in order to
> save the mother's life. I am forced to admit that under these conditions
> the operation is usually devoid of danger, and then I often make another
> statement, which, I regret to say, is not in strict accord with my knowl-
> edge of the facts. I add that no decent medical man can be induced to
> undertake this operation except in the most serious cases. I explain that
> if the patient succeeds in finding any one to do as she wishes, it will be
> a disreputable person, probably unskillful, and most certainly ignorant
> of proper aseptic measures.
>   An argument of this kind is apt to succeed. The woman will not
> fear sin, for through some process of reasoning she will find a way to
> absolve herself, but she does fear death.[49]

An 1889 *Canada Lancet* editorial echoed Iowa physician, H.C. Markham's
call for physicians to report their knowledge of criminal abortion, but also identified reasons why they often did not.[50] The Editor was John L. Davison, Professor

of Materia Medica and Therapeutics in Toronto's Trinity Medical College. He noted the prevalence of abortionists in "cities and towns, not to say villages," and that "these criminals practise their nefarious trade among us with comparative impunity." Only rarely, after the "dangerous illness or death of these unnatural mothers," was an abortionist convicted and penalized. The reasons were that the public and even some physicians concealed the activities of abortionists "in order to avoid an exposure of the fair sinner, and prevent her family from suffering the scandal necessarily consequent."[51]

Davison then discussed the dangers faced by physicians as a result of their refusal to comply with the "many applications, often accompanied by a consider-able bribe." He complimented physicians for resisting temptation in most cases, particularly new young physicians with few patients and few fees. However, these turndowns produced enmity in the applicants and it was not uncommon for the very physician who refused to provide the abortion to be charged with it.

> Numerous instances could be mentioned where false charges of this na-ture have been made, possibly to screen the actual criminals, or to grat-ify the resentment of those on whom exposure has fallen through the abortionist's mismanagement and the subsequent illness or death of his victim, on whom the medical man had declined to operate. Indeed, more than one instance could be quoted where innocent physicians have committed suicide from the mental worry and distress caused by false charges of this character.[52]

Davison then claimed this threat to innocent physicians was a major reason that physicians should notify the authorities whenever they received an application for a criminal abortion. When the public became aware that they would be re-ported to authorities for such applications, this would end the applications "and the temptation and danger incurred to medical men [would be] obviated." Davison believed this incrimination of abortion applicants would also lead the public to regard "the detestable practice" "with greater abhorrence." This, in turn, would make it easier to obtain sufficient evidence to convict abortionists. He also antici-pated that the increased abhorrence of criminal abortion would increase young ladies' motivation "to resist the wiles of the libertine."[53]

Davison's call for physicians to report requests for abortion to authorities followed the similar 1874 and 1887 proposals from American physicians already described. Davison apparently was unaware of the arguments against such report-ing given by the editors of the *Journal of the American Medical Association* in March 1887. No report has been located that indicated the results of actually giv-ing authorities such information.

CHAPTER 23
A CALL FOR ABOLISHMENT OF LAWS AGAINST ABORTION

The string of condemnations of unnecessary abortion in medical journals was broken by a paper calling for abolishment of laws against abortion that appeared in the New-York-based *Medico-Legal Journal* in 1889.[1] The anonymous author, "a Member of the Medico-Legal Society," read the paper before the International Medico-Legal Congress in New York on June 7, 1889 and again before the New York Medico-Legal Society in September. The author discussed "our wives" and almost certainly was male. He was assumed to be a lawyer by Junius C. Hoag, who quickly challenged his call for legalization of abortion (See below).

The writer discussed the history of laws against abortion, noting that, although the earliest written records in English-speaking countries made it a crime, it "has been substantially a dead letter upon the statute books, and rarely enforced." He continued:

> This has been due, doubtless, to the fact (unpleasant and unpalatable as it may sound, to state it) that it was against the common and almost universal sentiment of womankind; she who was the greatest sufferer and victim of the social conditions, under which its practice became necessary and inevitable; she who dreaded more the consequences as affecting her social condition than she feared legal penalties, never in her heart respected the law nor held it binding on her conscience.[2]

The writer then asked if a woman had the right to determine whether or not "she will take upon herself the pangs and responsibilities and duties of maternity?" He gave this answer:

> It does not need any argument to establish a fact well known to every careful student of political economy, to every medical man, in general practice, that the educated, refined, cultured women of this country, in married life, have, by a very large majority, decided these questions in their own favor, and have set at nought and at defiance the statute laws upon this subject, as binding on neither their consciences nor their actions.[3]

"The laws are in violation of the universal sentiment of woman," he continued, "though no one has, apparently, dared to say so, and all that is said has been said by man in support of existing statutes; and so far as action has been taken, it is all in the line of increasing the severity of the laws, and adding to the penalties, without the slightest perceptible or probable effect upon women, either in preventing the practice, or diminishing its frequency in the slightest degree."[4]

He continued:

> Writers, of which Dr. Storer, in his work, is an example, have very generally denounced the practice as a horrible and detestable crime. The medical professions, as such, in all public or private utterances, with singular unanimity, condemn it, and none more loudly than those who, as family physicians, have been many times compelled, by the exigencies of their own practice, to aid the unfortunate mothers, who have attempted it, or had partially succeeded in doing so, before their family physician was called in.
>
> The question is worthy the consideration of the body I address.
>
> 1. What are woman's rights in this matter?
>
> 2. Why keep laws on our statute books which are against the public sense of womankind, and
>
> 3. Why not have the courage to meet the issue fairly, and abolish all our laws upon the subject, as did the laws of Moses.[sic] and leave the question to the moral sense and training of our women, as the Jews were left, remembering that where there was no law, there was no transgression.[5]

The writer noted that there was no evidence that any married women obtaining criminal abortions had ever been convicted under the laws. As for the unmarried, he asked whether any "lawyer with human blood in his veins" "would condemn the fair young daughter of his best friend" for saving her honor by having a criminal abortion. He asked the same question of a father if his own daughter did the same and asked whether any man would behave differently if in the unmarried woman's place.[6] He suggested that many women for reasons of "modesty and shame" ended their own lives instead of "seeking that aid from medical men, which the law now makes it a crime in them to grant."[7]

After discussing how "Hindoos do not hesitate to kill children who come too rapidly," and citing another way the population was reduced when Chinese sailors were forbidden to rescue their mates who fall overboard, he surprisingly brought up issues of when life began.

> There can be little doubt, that in the present state of our knowledge as to the embryo, that life in the human being commences at a very early date indeed, and that the arrest of foetal development involves much the same ethical questions at two weeks as it does later, so far as the suppression or extinction of a human organization is concerned.
>
> What is called quickening in the law is simply such a state of foetal growth or life as is capable of a given muscular phenomena at that period.
>
> The human entity is there before as certainly as after quickening, this being only a manifestation of a certain period of foetal activity.[8]

However, these facts were not raised to condemn the killing of the unborn, as they had been raised for that purpose by scores of physicians. Apparently he was showing that one could prevent overpopulation by killing the "human entity" early as well as late.

"Let us take our choice as free untrammeled men of science without fear of popular clamor," the author concluded, "and let our only fear be that of violence to truth, to right, and to conscience."[9]

The Chicago Professor of Obstetrics, Junius C. Hoag, provided an article with the objective "to direct your attention to a recent apology for abortion, and to make a few comments upon the statements therein contained."[10] Hoag took it as a given that his physician audience considered unnecessary abortion "to be sinful as well as criminal." He did not "care to consider" questions about the fate of the soul of the unborn child who died in abortion, but did make the following request, apparently in all seriousness: "I hope that if there be abortionists who hold with certain religious creeds that the souls of the unbaptized are lost, they will not forget this rite in the midst of their employment."[11]

Hoag then discussed the large effect existing laws had on the frequency of abortion.

> We well know with how few children the instincts of maternity can be satisfied when only motives of purely personal convenience are considered; and when once these instincts were satisfied what a slaughter there would be of the undesired offspring! The abortion specialist, grown skilful from much practice, would soon be able to assure his patients of the complete safety of his methods. A few such specialists could pretty nearly depopulate the largest city and they would certainly have such opportunity afforded them and could old Malthus revisit the scenes of his former labors, he would have a much more difficult problem to solve than that of proportioning human reproduction to the means of human sustenance.[12]

Hoag belittled the anonymous writer's "arguments" for ending these important laws, claiming they were not arguments, "not even sophisms," which require "subtlety and acumen." He indicated that the writer's "vapid utterances," could only influence the "unthinking—the class of people to whom I alluded at the outset." "But as this is, perhaps, a somewhat numerous class," Hoag continued, "I have thought it proper to make some answer to an essay which can do no good and may possibly do some harm."[13]

Hoag indicated that the writer's claim that abortion was not contrary to divine law "was sufficiently covered by the sixth commandment of Moses." He next responded to the writer's claim that "educated and refined married women" believed they had the right to terminate unwanted pregnancies:

> If the writer is, as I apprehend, a lawyer, he probably knows less about the sentiments of refined women in this regard than does the average physician. As bearing upon the subject, however, I would like to have

our anonymous writer read what some of the educated and refined women of this city have said. I quote from interviews held by an attractive appearing young woman reporter, who, under pretense of being pregnant, sought and importuned various physicians for assistance in her supposed extremity, among whom there were several women physicians. One of these said: "You have broken one commandment, but is it any reason why you should break two? Think of the gravity of taking a life. You have as much right to make yourself the judge of whether it should live or not after life as once begun, as you have to decide that any person you know is injurious to society and for that reason it is your privilege to put him out of the way. Two wrongs cannot make one right." Another said: "I do not kill, I try to preserve life. Have you forgotten your womanhood? I am not one of those who think in such a case the woman is more sinned against than sinning; you share the guilt and are going through the fire for it. Let the fire purify you. Don't add to your load, for I believe forgiveness would be doubtful with the guilt of two such crimes combined." A third said: "I could not commit any such wrong; it would be wronging you as well as another creature."[14]

"One such expression is more weighty than a hundred idle utterances emanating from women who have given the subject but a passing consideration," Hoag continued, "or whose opinions have been biased by the force of personal and selfish motives."[15]

As to the practices of the ancients, "Mohammedans," "Hindoos," and Chinese, Hoag wrote: "We know that human life among them was and is very cheap; but the fact that they habitually commit the crime of abortion does not justify us in following their example; neither does the custom of the Feejee Islanders of consuming their fellows as food warrant us in adopting a revolting practice."[16]

Hoag concluded with further discussion of the value of the statutes the writer wanted abolished.

I cannot at all agree with him in this; if they do nothing else these laws certainly enable us now and then to rid the community of an infamous physician, who would otherwise have continued his abominable practices to the end of the chapter. Who shall say how much good is done, both directly and indirectly in putting a stop to the crimes of one such an individual? A woman bent upon ridding herself of an encumbering, unborn child, is often deterred from her purpose by the words of advice and warning that come to her from well-meaning physicians. Many a woman starts out upon her quest for such aid with little idea of the full meaning of her plans; if she does not upon the very threshold of her inquiry meet a human vampire, the chances are that her better nature will respond to the words of wisdom from conscientious advisers.

In the laws concerning abortion we find an outspoken expression of the best sentiments of society. The law is a constant monitor; the clergy and all other educators may fail in their duty to properly instruct the people, but we still have left instruction in the law. The man who would remove this barrier to crime, lays the axe at the very root of civilization, society, home. Why one should wish to do so, I cannot comprehend. Our anonymous writer appeals in feeble language to our sentiments of compassion, but he offers not one sound argument in favor of his dangerous plan.[17]

Although not another call for abolishment of laws against abortion, an article published two years later caused a similar controversy because of the author's defense of abortion in a multitude of instances.[18] The author, Charles H. Harris, of Cedartown, Georgia, was born in 1835 and after studying with a Tuskegee physician, obtained his M.D. in April 1857 from "the University of New York state," probably the Medical Institute of New York. He served as an assistant surgeon to a North Carolina unit in the Civil War and later moved to Georgia where he began practice in December 1866. According to his son, "a year had not past before he had acquired a large practice, which he held for thirty years." Harris and his wife raised ten children.[19] Ironically, in 1934, another of Harris' sons, the eminent Alabama physician, Seale Harris, would provide one of the strongest twentieth-century condemnations of avoidable abortions like those recommended by his father.[20]

Harris began by admitting that his thesis would not be well received in some quarters:

"Dr. Jones, Specialist in Abortion."—How would that look in a medical journal. [sic] Who would have the temerity, the hardihood, who would dare to place such an advertisement before the profession. [sic] Of course it would not do for the newspapers, nor yet for an office window. It would be something like "Sansom the Executioner" and the dear doctor would be besieged by an array of beauty never yet lavished on canvas. An [sic] yet "The Specialist in Abortion" exists. He is no ideal drawn from the mystic realm of fiction, but an actuality, a real live man and a good one. He is the guardian of virtue and womanhood and above reproach.[21]

Harris continued:

The profession in its dread of crime and interest in the embryo have monopolized all guardianship in posterity, and have become its blind partisans. The poor women are to suffer and sacrifice everything at the shrine of maternity as if it was for this alone they were made. Here is a chapter in the warfare of science well worth our study.[22]

Harris then called for quickly emptying the uterus in every instance where there was the slightest threat of an abortion. He indicated that it also did not make sense to continue pregnancies in women with diabetes, albuminuria, excessive nausea, "the slightest dilatation of the cervix," blood spots from the womb, or any disease that would be endangered by labor. He continued: "The older doctors will frown at this rule and stand ready to make the fur fly. The young man in the profession who is the coming doctor and whom the people always welcome 'can see a thing or two' and 'knows a good thing when he sees it.'"[23]

At 57, Harris arguably was among the "older doctors," but he appeared to share the "good" perspective of the "young man in the profession who is the coming doctor." He described the "surest and quickest way of treating abortion," and it no doubt also was his idea of the "surest and quickest way of" *performing* abortion. This involved "curetting and snaring with instruments that are adjustable in utero." He described the two "snares" and their use and claimed the "operation" "may be safely brought to a finish in a few minutes[,] frequently within an hour and very rarely in two sittings." Dilatation of the cervix was not required for Snare No. 1 and it could be used to dislodge and break up "the products of conception" in cases "where pregnancy interferes with treatment." In these instances where "there is suspicion of pregnancy," the dislodged and broken up result of the snaring usually would be discharged by "the unaided powers of the uterus." However, he noted that the patient should be carefully monitored since dilatation and curetting with Snare No. 2 might be required.[24]

Harris concluded:

> Snares are troublesome and should be carefully kept. The spring-steel wires and watch spring are prone to rust and should not remain in the staff but [be] thoroughly wiped and dried and wrapped in close paper. They are, however, well worth the trouble and yield to the earnest doctor handsome returns—returns in the shape of reputation and prestige and fat fees for special services—returns in good conscience and duty performed—more than all[,] returns in the satisfaction of adding to human life and lessening suffering.[25]

Harris no doubt saw this as "adding to" the quality rather than the quantity of "human life."

A Brooklyn surgeon, Mary Amanda Dixon Jones, and a Boston physician, Ernest Watson Cushing, would single Harris out for criticism. Dixon Jones did this in an article, "Criminal Abortion, Its Evils and Its Sad Consequences," that may have been the most passionate condemnation of criminal abortion in the last decade of the century.[26] She wrote:

> Abortion, induced at any time, or for any purpose except for the mother's welfare, or for the preservation of the life of the foetus, is a crime and a murder. This foul taking off has been the cause of the destruction of an uncounted number of children; and has, in unnumbered instances, resulted in the death or ill health of the mother.[27]

Dixon Jones discussed the not infrequent maternal deaths consequent to induced abortion and the diseases resulting from interruption of the normal pregnancy process and from the septic, unskilled, and brutal techniques of the abortionist and self-abortionist. She then moved to discussion of the "holocaust—a great army of little children" destroyed as a result of the very frequent resort to criminal abortion. She continued:

> But, if possible, there is yet a greater evil. The woman who entertains such thoughts, who has such intentions, the other who thus seeks the destruction of her own child, thereby perjures and blackens her own soul, and demoralizes her whole moral being. It is a prostitution of all her higher nature. To think of a mother contemplating the murder of her own child! Studying to destroy the being that rests nearest to her own life, and bound to her by every tie of kindred, love, and interest. What a soul-staining! Could anything be more debasing and blunting of all the finer feelings and affections?[28]

Dixon Jones followed with a brief discussion and rebuttal of several excuses married women gave for seeking abortion. She then criticized the lack of instruction of women "as to the wonders of their own being, or even of the simplest laws of life and health." These included the beginning of life at conception and she maintained that destruction of the embryo "in the earlier periods of existence, is as much murder as it would be in the latter months of pregnancy, or in the earlier periods of infancy." She then addressed quickening:

> Some have asserted there is no life till it moves, or what is understood as the "period of quickening." At the first moment there is motion, every moment of its existence. The new being unceasingly moves, and the powers, processes, and changes, even at this early period, are marvelous. It is then a human being. To destroy it is worse than vandalism. To attack it thus, in the dark borders of its existence, in the vestibule of its being, when it is so helpless and defenceless, is a most cruel warfare, a most unfair battle, more cowardly than the midnight assassin, or he who puts the dagger in the heart of the unsuspecting. ... What if the mother of Washington, of Shakespeare, of Lincoln, or of Milton had so acted? In eternal light there will be just as sad reckoning, in every case. A sin so terrible brings its full and increasing evil, with arithmetical progression. The responsibility is not all in the simple act, it carries a weight beyond. Are those who help women to do this deed any less to blame? Is not their work the blackness of darkness, by whomsoever performed?[29]

Dixon Jones described 21 requests for abortion she had received from women dating from 1866. Dixon Jones did not know the outcome in 4 cases. In 12 cases her admonitions and explanations had the desired effect and the women bore their children. In 5 cases, the woman ignored her pleas and found some means of having the abortion. One of these, an unmarried woman, was seen a few years later. She was an invalid and although she had married she had not been able to bear children.

"Many are now walking the streets that I have saved—," she wrote, "have prevented their mothers from destroying them."[30] Probably there were more children saved than the 12 she described in her article, but if it were 12, one would predict 20 or more offspring being born to these 12 "beautiful little children," 40 or more grandchildren of these 12, and over one hundred descendants of these 12 in our current generation.

Dixon Jones then rebutted claims that the medical profession itself was responsible for many criminal abortions. She took particular issue with the 1892 Harris article and with an editorial in the same journal. The editorial had claimed "foeticide, in the early months of gestation, is constantly performed with the flimsiest excuses, by prominent reputable men and women too, in every community." She wrote:

> I absolutely deny the assertions, though, four times lately, I have heard physicians say, "All do it;" and a member, at the annual meeting of the Tennessee State Medical Society, asserted, "I fear that the profession frequently takes a hand in the nefarious business." This also is untrue. It is not the profession. It is a few unworthy ones in it. In no profession are there men of more exalted morality, nobler aims, and purer integrity than the medical profession.[31]

To make this point, Dixon Jones referred to numerous objections to abortion by physicians, including Hippocrates, Hodge's Introductory Lecture, Storer's 1859 Committee on Criminal Abortion Report, the *Boston Medical and Surgical Journal* editorial praising Storer's 1860 book and condemning abortion, and the New York Academy of Medicine's September 1871 Resolutions.[32] Her review of literature was certainly the best of any physician writing on the subject of abortion at that time or later.

Dixon Jones then attacked Charles Harris:

> The writer ... remarks: "Poor women are to suffer and to sacrifice everything at the shrine of maternity, as if it were for this alone they were made." I reply, maternity is woman's highest mission, and should be her greatest pride. While a woman may possibly accomplish, in other directions, all that is high, noble, and good, yet everything should bow to maternity. This is the shrine to which she brings her noblest offerings. Is she educated, has she physical health, and physical perfection? Are her mind, heart, and soul cultured and highly endowed? It is that she may give birth to more perfect and beautiful children. This is the end, and should be her highest aim. ...
>
> The writer ... continues: "What sense is there in allowing a woman with diabetes, albuminuria, and the grave forms of disease, to run the gauntlet of pregnancy and labor? At once empty the uterus." This, when life is endangered, may be judicious; but, in general, if one's individual judgment may decide whether it is best for a child in utero to live, may not the same individual judgment decide whether it is

expedient for a boy or girl of five or ten years of age to live. ... A physician has no more right to destroy a human foetus, because he imagines it, in future years, may be sickly, than he has a right to destroy the delicate baby, because it possibly may have before it years of invalidism.

The writer of the same article next gives explicit directions as to how abortion shall be produced. ... "Snare No. 1 is passed into the uterus; sweep the staff around the globe of the ovum. Pull gently with the forceps, until the mass is extracted entire or cut in twain. In the latter event, repeat the procedure until it" (the baby!) "is chopped into fragments of easy extraction!" Hail horrors! lay on, Macduff. One almost shivers in reading these descriptions, and for this horrible work the writer holds out the inducement of "handsome returns and fat fees for special services."

I maintain that all this work is murderous, unprofessional, and degrading to the high office of a physician. A physician stands as a preserver of life, and should be the embodiment of honor and high morality.[33]

Dixon Jones herself had earlier been the subject of charges that she performed unnecessary abortions. These first arose in 1883 and resurfaced when she was sued for malpractice in 1889 and a Brooklyn newspaper joined the plaintiff in attacking her. On the other hand, her biographer doubted that she had performed unnecessary abortions. "Clearly she was not an abortionist," Regina Morantz-Sanchez wrote, "though one can imagine a variety of reasons why she might have been willing to go through with the procedure for selected patients whose health was threatened by pregnancy."[34]

Charles Harris was not the only physician in the early 1890s advocating liberal indications for inducing abortion. A 36-year-old Cortland, New York physician, Francis W. Higgins, published an article, "Abortion and Manslaughter," that made reference to a single article "daring to raise a voice in the question of the law on the subject."[35] Higgins indicated it was authored anonymously and he almost certainly was referring to the *Medico-Legal Journal* article criticized by Hoag.

Higgins' major theme was that the fetus at early stages of development was still just an animal. He cited the prevalent but false belief that the embryo went through various animal configurations as it developed. He first mentioned "fish and tad-pole" stages. Later the human embryo could not be distinguished from the embryo of a chicken and after that "it still remains that of a cat or dog."[36]

Higgins then posed the question of whether "the possibilities wrapped within it render it a human being," despite the fact that it was "indistinguishable from an animal." He asked: "Does not the germ of humanity it possesses render it human?" Countless medical men from Percival onward had answered these questions in the affirmative. Higgins' answer differed:

By either the Darwinian or biblical theory of the origin of things, until the embryo has reached the human point of development it has animal life only. The divine element is an inspiration which appears when the vessel is fully prepared for it. Literally, as well as figuratively, man springs from the dust of the earth. Until the individual has ascended above the plane of animal life in which he originated, he forms but a part of it.[37]

Higgins then discussed possible implications of his view. He denied that it would lead to an end of childbearing. He saw no change in the number of abortions but they would be performed more safely and the woman would obtain needed bed rest following the operation. "As at present practiced," he continued, "the danger to human life and health outweighs in importance the foetal destruction." He concluded with the claim that if a woman desired not to bear her child to preserve her "reputation, which is as much as life," or for "some other as strong motive," she had a right to an abortion early in her pregnancy.[38]

Two months after Higgins' paper was published, J. Milton Duff gave the "Chairman's Address" to the Section of Obstetrics and Diseases of Women of the American Medical Association. His speech covered numerous topics, including criminal abortion, and Duff probably had Higgins in mind when he spoke:

> The alarming increase in the number of criminal abortions with all the physical, moral and social evil it entails is a subject which demands the serious attention of the profession, of moralists and humanitarians. It has been suggested that in order to reduce the physical wrongs engendered by the performance of this operation by irresponsible incompetents, that the regular profession engage in it in a scientific manner.
>
> Let the blush of shame mantle the cheeks of those who suggest this prostitution of our noble profession in the furtherance of such a pernicious crime against God and society. As a profession we have no right to assume the position of lukewarmness and of masterly inactivity in this matter. It is our duty to be aggressive and as far as in our power educate the public up to a thorough appreciation of the pernicious results of this evil. Whenever opportunity offers to detect in this fiendish work those whose names blacken the lists of our profession we should see that they are stamped as villains, and as speedily as possible brought to justice.[39]

Higgins' call for expanded indications for abortion offended Duff, but they did not make Higgins a pariah to most of his colleagues. His obituary indicated he was vice-president of the New York State Medical Association and a member of the American Medical Association. Ironically, he was scheduled to present a paper, "The Treatment of Heart Disease," to his Cortland County Medical Association on the same day, December 18, 1903, that he died from a heart attack at the age of 45.[40]

CHAPTER **24**

FREQUENCY OF CRIMINAL ABORTION— WHAT DECREASE?

William Henry Parish read a paper on criminal abortion before his Philadelphia County Medical Society on March 22, 1893 that was published a month later in the *Medical and Surgical Reporter*. It also was published in the *Proceedings* of that Society for 1893, the *New York Medical Journal* (April 29, 1893), and perhaps other medical journals. Parish's specific theme was the legal responsibility of the physician when he is called to treat the after-effects of a criminal abortion. As to the morality and criminality of unnecessary abortion, Parish said:

> The medical profession looks upon this crime as one of the most heinous, and as closely allied to infanticide. He who is believed guilty of such a crime could never be received into membership in this or any other medical society; or if a member should so far forget his high calling as to be guilty of this crime, his expulsion would quickly follow upon the presentation of adequate evidence of his guilt.[1]

Parish indicated that abortions were rarely performed by physicians of "recognized professional standing." On the other hand, a few "graduates of the best medical schools have proved false to their noble avocation, and have brought dishonor upon themselves and, to a certain degree, discredit upon the profession of medicine." He went on to describe persons without medical training who induced abortions and women who aborted themselves. He indicated women were aware that it was criminal to produce an abortion on another, but did not view self-abortion as a crime.[2]

Parish indicated it was difficult to estimate the frequency of abortion, but "probably a half-dozen such applicants call upon me during each year."[3] When James Mohr discussed this statement in *Abortion in America*, he wrote: "William Parish considered a 'half dozen' requests for abortion in a year worthy of note in 1893, although that many per week had not been unusual according to physicians' testimony at mid-century."[4] Mohr's "testimony at mid-century" for a "half-dozen" "per week" was O.C. Turner's paper. However, Turner was discussing the number of abortions *performed* by a physician *abortionist* that he knew, not the number of *requests* Turner received (See Turner's quote in Chapter 18).

Parish then provided advice to the physician who suspected the abortion he had been called to treat had been induced criminally. This was to contact the authorities if the patient died or was about to die. If she recovered, it was his opinion that the physician should not become an informer, but should protect the "good name of his patient, who is usually, though not always, more sinned against than sinning."[5] "[S]inned against" suggests that Parish believed most criminal abortions were for illegitimate pregnancies and this is reinforced by his recommendation for preventing criminal abortion. He called for means to preserve "the purity of the morals ... of the youth of both sexes."[6] Parish's belief that the unmarried predominated in seeking abortions may be best explained by the fact that only the unmarried were naïve enough to approach Dr. Parish for an abortion.

The January 29, 1895 meeting of the Section for Obstetrics and Diseases of Women of Boston's Suffolk District Medical Society included a long discussion of "Abortion Socially, Medically and Medico-Legally Considered." Ernest Watson Cushing described how the Amsterdam physician, Frederik Ruysch (1638-1731), would give unmarried women seeking abortion "innocuous medicines till three months were over, and they would then be ashamed to seek for it and be willing to bear the child."[7] Cushing claimed that it still was true that women stopped seeking abortions after they began to feel movements of the unborn child.

Cushing discussed how the average person, Catholics excepted, did not consider that the unborn child had any rights until it had grown to a point "where it can be recognized." They saw no wrong, or at least no possibility of punishment, if they ended an unwanted pregnancy. He indicated that as a result, "there is a great crop of abortionists in Boston and in all our cities; and one is met every day by ladies who insist that if you will not get them out of their trouble they know where they can get it done."[8]

Cushing described a sophisticated technique of the Eskimos where whalebone in a leather sheath was used to rupture the membranes and produce abortion. He lamented the fact that "all the abortionists in Boston are not so careful with their procedures." He indicated that a physician "in the South" published a description of his invention that snared and extracted the fetus from the dilated uterus. To his knowledge, no medical society had expelled the physician for this.[9] This obviously was Charles Harris whom Mary Amanda Dixon Jones had already condemned.

Other Society members discussed the medical and moral aspects of abortion. A Dr. Forster indicated 34 cases had been admitted to the City Hospital in the previous three years where the specified reason for admission was criminal abortion and that there were many others admitted for the same reason although the specified reason was something else such as septicemia or pelvic cellulitis. He indicated that more than half were married women.[10]

Dr. Charles M. Green claimed that criminal abortion was increasing in the community and that married women were among those seeking abortions. He had dissuaded many married women and "some of them have thanked me afterwards."[11]

A Dr. Twombly described how the temptation was great for younger physicians "who have learned antiseptics and can do the operation perfectly well with the best results" to take the large sums offered to procure abortion. Twombly probably fit the definition of young physician able to effect abortion "with the best results," since he added, "but we should not be tempted by the offer of money to do any such thing."[12]

James Mohr may not have been aware of these multiple claims that there were more married than unmarried women obtaining abortions when he claimed physicians at the end of the century believed unmarried women were having more abortions than married women.[13] Mohr cited Mary Amanda Dixon Jones cases and Denslow Lewis's 1895 *Chicago Clinical Review* data in support of his assertion that the unmarried again were the primary abortion seekers. However, at least half of the women Dixon Jones counseled were married and Lewis was reporting on the patients at a public Chicago hospital devoted to the care of "the pauper, the friendless, and the *unfortunate.*"[14]

Other physicians in the 1890s were claiming that abortions were increasing and that married women obtained most of them. Joseph Taber Johnson, Professor of Obstetrics at the University of Georgetown, did this in a paper read before the Washington D.C. Obstetrical and Gynecological Society on June 7, 1895.[15] Johnson first discussed the effects of the 1859 AMA Report on Criminal Abortion and Storer's *Why Not?*:

> The effect for a time was salutary, and its author received letters innumerable from good people and from mothers made happy by the possession of healthy offspring, whose habit it had previously been to resort to abortion.
>
> 　The public conscience was aroused, and the promoters of the move in the Association no doubt congratulated themselves that they had accomplished a great good for society and the state, for morals, law, and religion. Secular, medical, and religious journals approved, clergymen preached, and a sense of security probably settled down upon the virtuous public that another growing evil had been boldly met, the battle against it successfully waged, and the victory won; but the sequel in this generation proves that it was no more of a victory than was gained over his creditors by the impecunious Micawber when he gave them his note of hand and thanked the Lord that his debts were paid.[16]

Johnson added that "abortion is now fully as frequent as it ever was in this country, and, moreover, that it is alarmingly on the increase." The reasons he gave for this were largely the same as when Storer and the American Medical Association first became active. Most important was the public belief, supported to some extent by law, that there was little or nothing wrong about abortion if performed at early stages of pregnancy. Johnson strongly emphasized the absurdity of these distinctions in the criminality of abortion at different stages of development of the unborn child. This, plus the stark legal difference between "killing" before birth and after, were noted in the following:

> It must kick very decidedly and unmistakably for several months before its killing constitutes a felony, and, as one judge has held, should it be knocked on the head with a hammer or strangled with a garter after its head is born, but before it is wholly delivered and separated from the

mother, it is not sufficiently alive in the eye of the law for its killing to constitute murder.[17]

Johnson claimed it was physicians' fault that such "dense ignorance longer exists in the minds of our people and that it so hinders the proper and just administration of the law." "There is not a household in the land or in the civilized world which is not more or less permeated by the influence and teaching of the noble science which we practise," he continued, "and this ignorance of the law of life, or of the fact of life, before quickening, could, if we were sufficiently alive to its importance, be utterly done away with and wiped off the face of the earth in a single year."[18]

Johnson also emphasized the medical dangers to the woman associated with criminal abortion and made the claim that for gynecologists like himself, "a majority of the patients that we are called upon to treat in our offices or in the fine residences of their fair owners are the outcome of abortions or of the preventive measures against conception." He concluded with a reemphasis of physicians' teaching role:

> Much has been said of late of the greater mission of our science in the prevention than in the cure of disease. How can a better field of labor be found than in the direction I have indicated? Where and how can medical men save more lives or prevent more suffering than by teaching women the dangers of abortion and thus saving their bodies, and perhaps their souls, from ruin in this life and in the life to come?[19]

At the same meeting, James Foster Scott, Obstetrician to the Columbia Hospital in the District of Columbia, read a paper that began:

> While *many* claim that these times are not so impure as they were in past generations, I will oppose this assumption by asserting that abortions are more frequent, whore-houses more numerous, diseases of a venereal nature more prevalent, and he who runs may read the advertisement in the daily press of our large cities of abortionists, baby-farmers, and even brothels under the disguise of "baths and massage."[20]

James Mohr quoted only part of Scott's sentence as evidence for a *decline* in criminal abortion. Mohr wrote:

> Even those physicians who remained intensely committed to the anti-abortion cause had to admit with James F. Scott in 1896 that *most* of their colleagues "claim that these times are not so impure as ... past generations."[21]

Mohr almost certainly was wrong in his claims of a decline in abortions and that the unmarried again dominated in obtaining abortions by 1900.

Scott continued:

> When I tell you of the great prevalence of the crime of criminal abortion many of you may at first think that I have gone mad. There is no darker page in history than this sin. Countless millions of human lives have been thus sacrificed, and probably at no period of the world's history has the slaughter been greater than in our own times.[22]

Scott claimed there was an abortionist "in every town and village." He described their thinly veiled newspaper advertisements and also discussed the advertisements for drugs that were claimed to end pregnancies. "Very few of the remedies advertised are efficient," he echoed Cox of Michigan, "but the mind of the woman becomes poisoned; she becomes desperate after their failure to act, and perseveres until she succeeds in her undertaking."[23]

Scott discussed the fine example of Catholic teaching on abortion and their very low rates of criminal abortion. Scott concluded that Protestant clergy, "with the assistance of the press and other auxiliaries," could greatly reduce criminal abortion among Protestant women as well. He called on Congress to create a National Bureau of Health "to disseminate knowledge and bring about many much-needed reforms."[24]

Scott then reported the belief of many physicians that married women accounted for "fully seventy-five to ninety per cent of the criminal abortions." He continued:

> Some married women give as an excuse the "demands of society," or that they are going to "take a trip to Europe" and cannot put it off, or that they shrink from the disfigurement of childbirth, or that "they have not the means to support a larger family." Could they not share what they have with the poor, innocent babe? If a woman with children were to ask me to perform an abortion on her, I would say to her: "Madam, let us kill one of the children already born, if you cannot support any more; it will be far safer to your health to allow the babe in your womb to go to full time and be delivered naturally, and the crime will be precisely the same." Such a statement usually drives it home to the woman's mind with force.[25]

Scott may have been writing his 1898 book, *Heredity and Morals as Affected by the Use and Abuse of the Sexual Instinct: Essentials to the Welfare of the Individual and the Future of the Race*, when his and Johnson's papers were presented in 1895. In subsequent editions, it was called *The Sexual Instinct: Its Use and Dangers as Affecting Heredity and Morals: Essentials to the Welfare of the Individual and the Future of the Race*. His 76-page chapter, "Criminal Abortion," began by discussing criminal abortion as a frequent consequence of "illegitimate sex."

Bad in the beginning, the crime of venery is often rendered worse by the shedding of blood; and any sophist who defends the slaughtering of the innocent child, at any period of its existence, is held in the deepest contempt by every member of repute in the medical profession, and by every one who is not so dull as to be deceived by impotent conclusions. One must abhorrently spurn such a sacrifice if he will but make the effort to inform himself in regard to the wonderful truths of embryonic development which the following pages attempt to explain clearly.[26]

Scott followed with 30 pages of description and discussion of the reproductive process and of the development of the unborn child at a level of detail that probably would have been instructive for most physicians then and even for most physicians today. The long section concluded with an unusual example of active life in a fetus prior to quickening.

[I]n one foetus, born during an accidental abortion between the third and fourth month, life was observed in a most striking manner. After the mother had given birth to it in the hospital, the nurse placed it in a jar of water, where it remained immersed for more than two hours. Not realizing that there was life in it, it was pinned to a board for the purposes of dissection in order to study the foetal circulation. Upon laying open its thorax and abdomen the operators were astonished to see violent respiratory efforts, though the lungs were incapable of expansion at this early date.

It being recognized that the foetus was at a non-viable age, and that it was insensitive to pain, the dissection continued, until finally the pericardium was laid open and the beautiful physiological demonstration of a beating human heart was afforded. The auricles and ventricles were then laid open, showing the mechanism of the action of the valves of the heart, and even then the contractions did not cease for almost two hours.

At the risk of the reader misunderstanding how one could make such a dissection on a human being, it is, nevertheless, here mentioned as a valuable example of the wonderful pertinacity of life, a point of the utmost importance.[27]

Scott repeated much of what he had said about the prevalence of abortion in his earlier paper including a claim that "probably at no period has the slaughter been greater than in our own times."[28] He also discussed the grave dangers to the woman undergoing the abortion and echoed Storer and many others in claiming that this was the only information that would deter some women.[29] He mentioned various valid and less valid excuses given by women for abortion and repeated the "Madam let us kill one of the children already born ..." passage he had provided for his physician audience.[30]

Scott ended the chapter with "The Glories of Maternity." He was a firm believer in evolution, and he described the very different roles of the parent or parents in protecting offspring as one ascended the evolutionary scale. Only the birds and mammals were seen to protect young that resemble the parents. Egg protection by fish and reptiles was a feeble comparison, while the offspring of most organisms were entirely on their own. He quoted Henry Drummond's claim in *The Ascent of Man* that mothers were the crowning achievement of "Nature."[31] Scott concluded this discussion and the chapter:

> Ages have been spent in the evolution of the Mammalia, and the culmination of this indefinitely prolonged extension of time has been the masterpiece—Man, or rather the Mother. Nature has made nothing superior, and Man is but the crown of Woman's glory.
>
> Criminal abortion is thus seen to be the most abhorrent crime against Nature which could be conceived of, and the man who permits the mother and her offspring to struggle through the long and bitter years of illegitimacy, without honoring the family relationship in the *natural* capacity of a father, refusing to provide food and shelter, and cravenly withholding his protection, is the product of a corrupt civilization so much below the gorillas and the sparrows that we can only classify him as a Monster. No mother who understands her position at the summit of Creation, or who has any of the natural instinct of love, can connive at the destruction of her babe, unless she be deranged, without abdicating her lofty and holy position of sovereignty in Nature; and if the dumb brutes could speak they would plead with her to ignore public sentiment at any cost, and to listen to the voice of instinct, of pity, and of love.[32]

The various editions of *The Sexual Instinct* reside in scores of libraries and the book is available for purchase at dozens of used book outlets. Scott's treatment of criminal abortion rivals any physician treatment of the subject for the public and his unique arguments probably dissuaded many women from ending their pregnancies.

Joseph Waggoner read a paper, "Criminal Abortion and Its Relation to the Medical Profession," to his Portage County Ohio Medical Society on October 3, 1895.[33] The 73-year-old physician and Civil War veteran noted that he had observed the crime of criminal abortion for "nearly half a century." He claimed it "exists among all classes of society" and "nothing I have met with in my professional career that has so shocked my sense of justice and mercy." He claimed that physicians were frequently and persistently requested to commit the crime "as though there is nothing wrong in its commission."

He continued:

> How it can be reasoned less a crime to destroy a youth instead of a man, or an infant instead of a youth, or a foetus in utero instead of the infant, passes all my reasoning in the conception of crime. Why, sirs, were you

to go out into the street and kill the first child or youth you met, the parents of that child or youth, with the populace, would be for arresting you and hanging you to the first lamp post, or at least prosecuting you to the utmost extent of the law, and to an ignominious death, and all would say—Amen! Yet some of these same people would urge you, yea, insist that you should enter their dwellings in the dark, plunge the dagger into the foetus in utero, and feel happy that they have got rid of a life that would have given them some care and solicitude. What a strange phase of humanity! How horrible to contemplate!

Thomas Jefferson, in the contemplation of slavery, is said to have exclaimed: "I tremble for my country when I think there is a just God." How much more ought we to tremble when we know that murder is a greater crime than robbery. Altogether, the loss of life by this crime is as much or more than by all the diseases flesh is heir to. This you may think is a strong statement, but of the fact I feel reasonably well assured.[34]

Waggoner claimed the physician was "smirched and tainted and classed with the abortionist" when he completed the abortionist's work. He also faulted physicians for their silence:

We have our societies, county, district, state and national, in which we meet and discuss the best means to check disease and prolong life. Yet how silent we are on this one question. So long as I have been a member of medical societies, I have not, with one exception, ever heard a paper which referred to this subject, and that exceptional paper only referred to the crime so far as physicians are concerned.

The same also may be said of those agents of reform and progression, the medical press. When, where and by whom do you see an editorial on this subject or a contribution from the[ir] many writers referring to this matter? We, in our society meetings, have been frittering away our time as to the best means of treating disease, while this floodgate of death is rushing on, and by our silence giving consent to this wholesale destruction of life. We are thus, in a measure, made partakers with the more guilty.[35]

Waggoner reported the stated belief of several members of the Society that at least half of pregnancies were terminated prematurely. He noted that there had been 390 births and 295 deaths in Portage County for the year. Using a figure that half of gestations ended without a birth and that three-quarters of these were from criminal causes, he concluded that there were as many deaths from criminal abortion as from all other causes.

A Brooklyn physician, William McCollom, published "Criminal Abortion" in the *Journal of the American Medical Association* for February 8, 1896. He called attention to a practice of physicians of which Frederik Ruysch, Henry Orlando Marcy, and no doubt many others were "guilty." McCollom wrote:

When a physician prescribes medicine or give advice and allows the party to believe, or gives her reason for believing that it is given for the destruction of embryo life, though he does not intend such destruction, [he] is little better than a criminal. I have heard physicians confess to such deception without seeming to realize that they were seriously compromising honesty and integrity and countenancing sin and crime.[36]

As will be described in Chapter 28, Henry Orlando Marcy gave a placebo to a young wife who requested an abortion. She had a spontaneous abortion shortly afterwards and Marcy was approached by a succession of her pregnant friends seeking a similar pill. If, as McCollom indicated, this were a fairly common practice, it probably was a significant factor leading women to think that their physicians were not opposed to abortion and that they need not be either.

McCollom discussed the "frightful prevalence" of criminal abortion and its apparent increase "among professed Christian women." He noted the much better behavior of Catholics and questioned whether the Protestant clergy were taking adequate steps to convince their parishioners about the "enormity of this sin."[37]

McCollom called on physicians to tell abortion seekers about its criminality. He noted that ignorance was a factor, "but it is not ignorance alone but a downright lack of moral sense as well, which greatly needs educating."[38] He described a stillborn child that had had its brain punctured via a sharp instrument prior to birth. "I bluntly charged the mother with murder in the presence of her husband and friends," McCollom continued, "pointing out the evidence of it, and there was no denial." He repeatedly encountered women falsely denying that they were pregnant who requested restoration of menstruation. He indicated that the physician who produced miscarriage under these circumstances was as criminally liable as the requestor. "Sometimes" he was more culpable:

Sometimes the ordinary physician who may be a member of a regular medical society violates his duty; and the distinguished college professor without the fear of God or of sufficient fear of human law takes his large fee for the criminal act. I am not drawing on the imagination, but state what I know to be true. Such statement does not sound well, but this fearful immoral destructive practice can not be checked unless facts are stated and proclamation is made of this great evil.[39]

McCollom called on physicians to "make complaint in all cases when it comes to their knowledge that physicians or other persons are violating the law in the destruction of human life." He cited his own threats to physicians that he would report them to the authorities if they did not cease performing illegal abortions. "Parties have responded," he noted, "pleaded for mercy and given solemn promise never to again produce the miscarriage of a pregnant women for any reason until they had held a consultation with a reputable physician, and its necessity was advised."[40]

McCollom's objection to giving a placebo as a presumed abortifacient was quoted almost verbatim and without credit to McCollom by H.B. Smith of Olio, Indiana in a May 1898 paper with the same title. Smith also copied McCollom's: "Criminal abortion is frightfully prevalent, and the practice is apparently on the increase even among professed Christian women."[41] However, Smith did provide a unique estimate of the number of abortion requests received by physicians and some graphic descriptions of abortion's effect on the population:

> I have asked a number of physicians how often they are approached by persons desirous of having them produce abortion. The average is twice a month. If this be the average of the country over (and I am satisfied it is below the average), it would mean that the physicians of this country are asked over 3,100,000 times a year to produce abortion. The same person may ask twenty doctors before finding one to do the work. But it is estimated, and upon good authority, too, that this vast Moloch of destruction gathers in his burning bosom one-half of the increase of humanity in this glorious republic.[42]

With 31,578 babies born in the state of Indiana in 1895, Smith concluded that there were "31,578 murders, if you please, every year in this beautiful, civilized, Christian State of ours that we all love so well." He mentioned a doctor indicted for criminal abortion who confessed to having produced more than 5,000 abortions and indicated that if half of these aborted children had survived to adulthood they would constitute a city of 2,500 inhabitants. He noted that if a person were to purposely open a reservoir and drown those 2,500 residents, "the newspapers, with double headlines, would denounce him; ministers would denounce him and tell from the pulpit of the awful, tragic death by the hand of one man of an entire city of human beings."[43]

In June 1896, the Ellsworth, Maine physician, George A. Phillips, read a paper, "Criminal Abortion: Its Frequency, Prognosis and Treatment," before the Maine Medical Association.[44] Phillips reported the results of a questionnaire he sent to 100 Maine physicians. When a pair of very low estimates were dropped, an average of 70.5 percent of abortions were criminally induced. Only from two to four percent of criminal abortions were reported to have produced death of the woman. An average of 49.5 percent of women were reported to have suffered "more or less" permanent health impairment following criminal abortions. Averages for death and health impairment following non-criminal abortion were in the same ranges as for criminal abortion.[45]

Phillips noted that "[h]undreds of women, of morals unquestioned," did not view abortion as a crime. He continued:

> It goes on with increasing frequency, and no man's hand is against it unless it is the reputable physician and the Catholic priest. Certainly I know of no other direct influence worthy of the name. The state, properly, spends hundreds of dollars annually for the protection of fish and game. Yet this wholesale slaughter of human life goes on all around us,

and no power outside the church of the Catholic and our own profession enters a protest against it.[46]

Phillips then discussed exceptions in "our own profession."

This crime goes on in the bright light of day, with no fear of punishment, no danger of conviction. Nor, so far as I am aware, does it affect the doer's social or professional standing with the public; his practice does not suffer, but for obvious reasons is increased. If his other attainments, social and professional, are good, no man turns from him on account of this. Wise and good men honor and employ him, and he wields an influence not lessened by the knowledge that countless children would have been born but for his skill in the use of that valued instrument, the uterine sound. He makes money, makes reputation, keeps the friendship of the community, is honored by the wise men in it, smiles at our poverty, and sleeps the sleep of the just, surrounded by all the blessings and comforts that $25 a head will bestow.[47]

Phillips concluded with measures to prevent criminal abortion and his belief that physicians were saving "infants," despite abortion's prevalence:

I can only emphasize the old treatment, that with no uncertain sound we should proclaim the woeful waste of life in this inhuman practice. We are apt to grow sluggish. We are apt to go a little with the tide. It is so easy to send them somewhere else and attend to them afterward, to at least grow indifferent in a toil that has no thanks, no money, the toil of teaching those who will not listen. And yet there is no other right way, and the responsibility presses the more heavily when we remember that almost alone we stand against the wholesale slaughter of infant life. Take that bulkhead out of the way and give this practice the free run that would follow, and the results can hardly be conceived.[48]

Phillips' presentation was praised by Dr. Alfred Mitchell, Dean of the Medical School of Maine. However, Mitchell but did not agree that habitual abortionists retained their social standing. Mitchell also indicated that the uterine sound now was obsolete: "The operation has become one of scientific procedure, of dilatation and curetting, with all possible antiseptic surroundings, and this fact doubtless finds an easy excuse for many who want only the excuse to warrant the procedure."[49]

Another discussant, Dr. Israel Thorndike Dana, who had written the 1866 Maine Association Report on Criminal Abortion, noted the dulled moral sentiment of communities, despite the fact that criminal abortion was a clear "violation of the divine command, 'Thou shalt not kill.'" Dana saw little effect of "restrictive measures, unless behind them there shall first be a corrected moral sense, and it is the duty of our profession to foster this."

Dr. J.M. Jonah, of Eastport, was surprised to learn of the great number of abortions in the state. He called for more stringent laws against criminal abortion and suggested a committee be appointed by the Association "to investigate the matter, and suggest legislative action."[50]

Phillips closed the discussion. He indicated in response to Dean Mitchell that other sections of the state might hold different sentiments toward "regular physicians who practice the procuring of abortions." He indicated that in his district they "were the best paid."[51]

Phillips' paper was briefly mentioned in The *Boston Medical and Surgical Journal* in their report of the annual session of the Maine Association. It included: "A motion that a committee be appointed to memorialize the Legislature failed of consideration."[52] This failure to appoint the committee recommended by Dr. Jonah stands in sharp contrast to the same Association's actions in 1858 when they quickly seconded the Buffalo Medical Association's motion to oppose the "great and growing evil" of criminal abortion. Phillips' admission that "regular physicians" in his district of Maine were openly performing abortions is additional evidence that Maine physicians viewed abortion very differently in 1896 than in 1858. However, unlike Phillips, most physicians in the 1890s, like Mary Amanda Dixon Jones and William Henry Parish, were still denying that criminal abortion was practiced to any extent by regular physicians.

Horatio Storer actively returned to his campaign against criminal abortion in the summer of 1897. He presented a paper, "Criminal Abortion: Its Prevalence, Its Prevention, and Its Relation to the Medical Examiner ...," to the Rhode Island Medico-Legal Society on August 12, 1897, and presented it again to the Newport Medical Society on August 18. Horatio first discussed the stimuli that returned him to the fray:

> A recent failure to obtain conviction in a trial for criminal abortion in Rhode Island, the case having been thought a clear one, is said to have carried such discouragement to several of the members of this Society that they are unwilling to have even the general subject referred to. Upon the other hand, if we acknowledge the frequency of the crime, and of this there can be no question, one would suppose that the time was peculiarly appropriate for attempting to ascertain the real cause of what may have been an exceptional instance of failure of justice and if possible, to find its remedy. Towards that a brief summary of the medical anti-abortion movement, comprised within the past half century, may perhaps be of aid.[53]

Horatio began this history, not with his 1857 Suffolk District Medical Society commencement of the crusade, but with his American Academy of Arts and Sciences paper of December 1858, possibly because the Academy paper was his first effort *outside* the medical profession. Much of his long paragraph describing this 1858 paper was reproduced in Chapter 7. Horatio followed this with a discussion of how "quickening," a "technical cloudiness of idea, of expression had crept into medical language and that of the law" and had made many believe that early abortion was not the destruction of an independent life. Hodge in 1839, Thomas Radford in 1848, and his father in 1855 were cited as refuting this notion and showing "conception as the true beginning of foetal life." Horatio also noted that it was his father who had first pointed out the diseases associated with criminal abortion. Horatio then described what he viewed as his own original contribution:

> None of these gentlemen, however, seem to have entered the at that time somewhat thorny path that connects induced abortion with political economy. I have always frankly acknowledged that it was from my father's recognition of the effect of abortion in producing pelvic disease that my attention was first drawn to the subject. Had it been otherwise I might never have pursued the inquiries which led me to appreciate the frequency of the crime.[54]

Horatio discussed in detail his initial efforts as they began at the Suffolk District Medical Society in 1857 and then shifted to the American Medical Association:

> In 1857, at its meeting at Nashville, the subject was presented to the American Medical Association, which I had joined in 1856, a committee was appointed, and its report was made at the meeting at Louisville in the ensuing year. My associates upon the committee were: Drs. Blatchford, of New York; Hodge, of Pennsylvania; Pope, of Missouri; Barton, of South Carolina; Lopez, of Alabama; Semmes, of District of Columbia; and Brisbane of Wisconsin. Their standing in the profession was guarantee of their conservatism and their faithfulness in the inquiry. It interested them all, and they personally contributed towards the general decision.[55]

Horatio went on to discuss the 1865 American Medical Association prize essay, its publication as *Why Not? A Book for Every Woman*, and the large distribution of this popular tract. "It was found, as the Association had anticipated," he observed, "that where religion and morality had failed, the fear of resulting physical lesions exerted a wonderfully deterrent influence, and hundreds of women acknowledged that they were thus induced to permit their pregnancy to accomplish its full period."[56]

Horatio decried the fact that the abortion-inhibiting effect generated by the physicians' crusade was now overcome by a new generation who were no longer aware that abortion was morally wrong or physically destructive.[57] He claimed that apathy of physicians and even complicity of some physicians were problems. He stated that defects of the laws related to criminal abortion still existed, making convictions difficult or impossible. He then mimicked his efforts in the 1858 paper to the American Academy of Arts and Sciences, showing the current sharply lower birth rates in New England compared to those of foreign countries while marriage rates were similar. The implication was that New England married couples were not having children and Horatio indicated that prevention of conception was not the only reason. He viewed the high rate of illegitimacy in foreign countries compared to New England as indicating that unmarried women also were much more likely in New England to abort their pregnancies. Horatio's strongest statistics supporting a high rate of criminal abortion in New England in 1897 were the same he had used in 1858, namely the abnormally high rates of stillbirths.

Storer noted the differences in the size of Catholic and Protestant families and indicated that this reflected little or no abortion among the Catholics. A footnote following this claim read:

> Since the present paper was read, it has been stated to me by a physician that, in his experience, Catholic women have proved equally guilty. I cannot believe that this can be so, save in his exceptional instance. Were it true, however, it would furnish the most cogent *a fortiori* evidence that the moment has come for renewed and earnest action by the physicians of America.[58]

Horatio concluded with the following recommendations:

> That these facts are true should be the greater reason for a Society like our own to exert itself anew, for surely such obstacles as we know exist can be overcome. All medico-legal societies and state organizations of examiners can combine towards improvement in the statutes regarding the crime. Offenders in our own profession can be discovered and pursued with greater rigor; and the measures towards enlightening the ignorance and awakening the conscience of the community, which have been pronounced legitimate by the American Medical Association, can be renewed. Now, as formerly, the well founded dread of the physical consequences of abortion can be brought home to every pregnant woman. Such procedures cannot but secure success. How perfect this may prove will depend upon the persistence and earnestness of your movement. There can be nothing, you may all be certain, that individually or collectively you may undertake, that will more deserve the blessing of Almighty God.[59]

The paper was well received by his Medico-Legal Society audience and Horatio was asked "for suggestions as to what could be done by this and similar societies." His answers paralleled his recommendations in 1859 to the American Medical Association. He recommended that the Medico-Legal Society form a Committee to identify the problems with abortion statutes and with the help of "friendly lawyers," identify solutions. He also indicated the need to overcome the ignorance "of judges, juries and advocates" regarding fetal development.

> A stream cannot rise above its source. If the belief of these men, who are but representatives of the community at large, rests upon popular ignorance of the true character of the crime, and if prevention of abortion is better than attempts at conviction of foetal murder after it has

been committed, and if it can be prevented only through awakening woman's consciences, arousing her maternal instinct, and exciting her fear of physical peril to herself, then your course is clear.[60]

Another recommendation by Horatio was to bring "the subject directly to the attention of the profession at large." He called for a "circular, judiciously worded," to be sent to the American Medical Association, to "State Medical Societies and, indeed, to all medical organizations in the country, of whatever nature, with the request that they cordially endorse the movement." He noted that there was evidence that "professedly reputable physicians" were performing abortions. "It is the duty of every honorable practitioner," he continued, "for the good name of our profession, and for humanity's sake and our national prosperity, to assist in detecting, exposing and punishing these villains."[61]

Although actions of the Medico-Legal Society as a result of Horatio's paper are not known, the following indicates that the Newport Medical Society was aroused to action three days after Horatio presented the paper to them.[62]

NEWPORT MEDICAL SOCIETY
Newport R.R.,
August 21, 1897.
Dear Sir:

At a regular meeting of the Newport Medical Society, held on August 18th, 1897, a paper previously communicated to the Rhode Island Medico-Legal Society, on August 12th, was, by request, read by Dr. H.R. Storer, Honorary President, in which it was shown that the induction of unnecessary abortion is probably now as prevalent in this country as when the subject was brought to the attention of the American Medical Association by him forty years ago in 1857.

The Society thereupon unanimously appointed the undersigned a Committee "to obtain through correspondence with medical societies and otherwise such action by the profession as may tend to lessen the occurrence of criminally induced abortion."

We accordingly ask you, through such measures as you may think most proper, to join in what should be an universal movement by physicians to check the present decrease of the rate of increase of our population.

We shall be glad to be informed of such action as you may find yourself able to take in this matter.

This letter, signed by five Newport Medical Society members other than Horatio, was printed and apparently mailed widely, since, in the next few months, several medical journals around the country made mention of this appeal to physicians in editorials condemning criminal abortion. Another tactic in Horatio's resumed crusade was to distribute a flyer advertising his books on the topic, including his 1897 paper that was published as a pamphlet. This flyer indicated that *Why Not?* was still available, as was *Is It I?* and Horatio's 1868 book with Franklin Fiske Heard.

The flyer also included a number of favorable "medical press notices" for Horatio's 1897 address.[63]

CHAPTER 25

PROTESTS AGAINST "RACE SUICIDE"

No decade produced more physician articles decrying criminal abortion than the first decade of the twentieth century. This probably reflected increased criminal abortion, but it also may have reflected more medical journal outlets for these physician protests.[1] Another factor may have been President Roosevelt's 1902 criticism of "race suicide," the reduced birth rate in what he viewed as key segments of the population. Roosevelt's first public discussion of race suicide occurred in a letter he wrote to Bessie Van Vorst that was published as a preface to the popular book, *The Woman Who Toils*. His comments included: "But the man or woman who deliberately avoids marriage, and has a heart so cold as to know no passion and a brain so shallow and selfish as to dislike having children, is in effect a criminal against the race, and should be an object of contemptuous abhorrence by all healthy people."[2] References to "race suicide" quickly followed in physician articles. Roosevelt may not have recognized criminal abortion as a factor, but this was the conclusion of these physicians.

Denslow Lewis read a paper, "Facts Regarding Criminal Abortion," at a meeting of the Physicians' Club of Chicago on March 26, 1900. An introductory paragraph made the claim that only 20 percent of pregnancies were welcome:

> If the woman has one child she is apt to think it is too soon to have another. If she has never been pregnant, it is too soon after marriage, it interferes with a trip somewhere or some social engagement, or else she is too delicate, or her husband can not afford it. Some excuse is usually found for dissatisfaction, and in most cases some attempt is made to re-establish menstruation.[3]

Lewis discussed the various means these women used in these attempts:

> The old ladies of the community are prolific in advice. Hot drinks, hot douches and hot baths are recommended. Violent exercise is suggested and jumping off a chair or rolling down stairs is a favorite procedure. Certain teas are given, especially an infusion of tansy and pennyroyal. Cathartics are supposed to be useful, and the different emmenagogue pills are too easily procurable. As a last resort ergot may be taken, or, if the woman is ignorant, arsenic, metallic mercury or other mineral poison may be used, often with a fatal result.[4]

Lewis found it remarkable that women rarely perceived that anything was wrong with attempts to end pregnancy at this early stage and saw it resulting from their belief that no life was present prior to the beat of the fetal heart. He saw the teaching of the Catholic Church as the only current restraint on the practice of abortion and called for development of "some systematic effort to teach the truth regarding all matters connected with the reproduction of the species." He included education of children on sexual matters and for education of "some eminent members of the profession" on the importance of this. Howard Atwood Kelly of the Johns Hopkins Hospital and School of Medicine opposed sex education for children and was singled out by Lewis as one such "eminent member" needing education.[5]

Much of Lewis' paper dealt with the incredible resistance of the fertilized ovum to the jumps, falls, and other assaults recommended by the "laity" for ending pregnancy. He claimed that when these measures failed, she consults "her family physician, a midwife, or some physician recommended as an expert by the ladies of her acquaintance." Lewis continued:

> I can not refrain from saying in this connection that the induction of abortion is, to my mind, the most reprehensible of medical practices. I wish I could truthfully add, that none but disreputable men could be persuaded to undertake it. I know from my experience of twenty-two years as a medical man in this city and from the observation of many cases of criminal abortion in private, hospital and medicolegal practice, that the public, and many physicians as well, look upon the induction of abortion as a matter of routine. I have been told by prominent men that they expected their physicians to take care of them. I have lost the patronage of well-known society women because I refused to "help them out," as they expressed it. I have noticed that pregnancy, in some of these women, did not go on to term, and I know who is their physician now.[6]

Perhaps Lewis paused to stare at some member or members of his Physicians' Club audience after that sentence.

Lewis discussed the various means used by abortionists to induce abortion and their various undesirable results, including death. He concluded with another consequence of criminal abortion and a plea for physician manhood:

> Among other women who have suffered abortion during the early years of their married life, it is often observed that pregnancy is impossible when the time comes for a child to be most ardently desired. Pitiable, indeed, is the condition of such a woman. Regrets are useless now. There is only remorse and perhaps indignation that the medical men who, in her youth, acceded to her request had not the manhood to tell her of her folly and to warn her of her danger.[7]

The Denver physician, Minnie C.T. Love, read a paper, "Criminal Abortion," before the Colorado Medical Society that was published in December 1903.[8] She gave credit to Horatio Storer for his *Why Not?* and his 1868 book. "I do not, either now, or in the future, in the least presume to do for the early twentieth century what Dr. Storer did for the nineteenth," she continued, "but it has occurred to me that after the lapse of so many years, there must be much valuable data which could be collected, and if this society were to offer an adequate prize for a paper which should give us that data, it would surely stimulate the profession to be more aggressive, and to try more than ever to educate the laity as to their right attitude towards this truly degrading and disgusting crime."[9]

Love reported the results of a questionnaire she mailed to 25 Denver physicians. Her first question about who obtained criminal abortions led most to claim it was middle-class married women with rich married women in second place. The unmarried, "prostitutes or unfortunates," were seen as accounting for relatively few abortions. Fourteen of her 16 respondents indicated that there had been an increase in criminal abortion over the last 50 years.[10]

Her third question asked the percentage of women's diseases that were the result of criminal abortion. There was a wide range of responses with eight seeing it as 25 percent or higher. One indicated 60 percent. Love claimed that making women aware of this high probability of subsequent disease would strongly deter abortion.[11]

Her final question dealt with whether the woman seeking the abortion, should be punished as an accessory. All answered, "Yes."[12]

Love then turned to the "perpetrators of the crime." She included women who aborted themselves and indicated that these were the worst abortion cases that she encountered. As to the professional abortionists, "there is nothing to say, language cannot do justice to their criminality, about which there is no dispute in our profession."[13]

Love uniquely related frequent spontaneous abortions to the fact that some parents viewed intentional abortion as no crime.

A significant fact which I have noticed is that the vast majority of parents consider this a fortunate accident, with no thought of the wasted life of the child, but only of the possible danger to the mother. May not this familiarity account in some measure for the failure on the part of the laity to appreciate the seriousness of such an accident? To some minds it is but a step from the unaccountably interrupted pregnancy to the one purposely terminated.[14]

Love discussed the need to educate the public on the unborn child's right to life and on the criminality and physical dangers of abortion. Other recommendations for reducing criminal abortion were to encourage "greater love of home and family ties, through religious and ethical teachings," and to improve laws against abortion so that they would convict abortionists and deter the crime. One of her solutions to the problem of criminal abortion reflected her strong eugenics views. She would prevent the birth of "moral degenerates" by "separating or sterilizing the feeble-minded and idiots, and those hopelessly insane or epileptic," and by keeping confirmed male and female criminals imprisoned for life.[15]

In the discussion of Love's paper, "Dr. Wiest" indicated that married women of the "middle or even the better class" obtained the criminal abortions in his country town. He also claimed that "a good many" members of the medical profession were producing criminal abortions and called for "this Society [to] take active steps toward throwing them out of the practice of medicine in the state of Colorado."[16]

Another discussant, "Dr. Stuver," claimed that with President Roosevelt condemning race suicide, it was physicians; duty to try to convince the patient requesting abortion "that it was a crime of the deepest die." He admitted some would seek a doctor "with a more elastic conscience," but implied that others would continue their pregnancies.[17] Stuver's may have been the first physician reference to Roosevelt's condemnation of "race suicide."

The North Branch Philadelphia County Medical Society meeting of April 14, 1904 included a paper on the "Medicolegal Aspects of Criminal Abortion."[18] The paper was by a lawyer, Thomas W. Barlow, who made reference to the 1870 paper of the earlier Society President, Andrew Nebinger, and its call for the clergy to dissuade women parishioners from abortion. Barlow indicated that Pennsylvania laws were adequate, but there was a failure of execution of these laws "by those on whom the obligation rests." He noted that it was impossible for everything to be accomplished by the "police power," and that "the work against the professional abortionist rests entirely within the medical profession itself." He proposed that the Society appoint a committee to take charge of the matter.[19]

Dr. Richard C. Norris, Professor of Gynecology at the University of Pennsylvania, saw more benefit from teaching patients about the "moral wrong and great danger of the procedure" than from appointing the committee the lawyer recommended. Dr. A.M. Eaton agreed and described how he deterred three women from seeking abortion by impressing upon patients the "moral turpitude of the crime." They followed his suggestion and moved "to a secluded part of the city" until the child was born.[20]

Norris also indicated the "confidential relation that existed between physician and patient" caused problems for prosecuting abortionists. It "deters the physician from reporting the case to the authorities, particularly, as is frequently the case, when a physician is called in after an abortion has been committed and one or both of the parties are of high social standing."[21] Another physician agreed and claimed he had refrained from giving evidence against an abortionist because the girl he treated after her abortion was of "very high standing socially."[22]

Norris' colleague at the University of Pennsylvania, Dr. Henry W. Cattell, recommended a committee of the Society maintain a "black list" of abortionists. He claimed that physicians would be willing to provide information about criminal abortions to this committee that they would not report to the authorities, since the information would not be made public. Physician sanctions against members on the black list presumably would discourage the practice of abortion.[23]

Lawyer Barlow ended the meeting by claiming it was the duty of physicians to report to the authorities "every case" of criminal abortion of which they had knowledge. He then contradicted himself, indicating it "must be decided by the physician in the individual case" "whether the relations with the patient were such as to deter such action."[24]

The New Orleans physician, Louis G. LeBeuf, presented a paper, "The Attitude of the Medical Profession Towards Race Suicide and Criminal Abortion," to the Louisiana State Medical Society. He began:

> Our attitude on this question is the same in our profession from the mouth of the Rio Grande to the mouth of the Danube, that is to say throughout the civilized world, and, though few of us have even read the Hyppocratic Oath, we all live up consistently to the letter and spirit of its teachings, on this subject. Still, when we have condemned and endeavored to arrest race suicide and criminal abortion we have not done our whole duty. Our mission is a higher one still, our education, our training, our studies, our whole life's preparation for the care of man's body, makes us also altruistic students of mankind, morally and sociologically. It is then as humanitarians, that we can do most good.[25]

LeBeuf blamed the "lack of proper maternal sentiment" for the high rate of criminal abortion. Poverty provided the excuse for the poor and "deteriorating influences of what is called refinement and civilization" provided the excuses for those with more resources. Among these "deteriorating influences" were "the Opera, the Teas, the Concerts; the husband has his clubs, his cigars, his friends, his little game of cards." If there were children or additional children, "some of these pleasures would have to be sacrificed."[26] LeBeuf continued:

> Whatever the motive this is the place for the high minded physician to attempt his influence, and his warning against this glaring desire to limitation and criminal thirst for destruction. Let us tell them of the harm they do, let us inform them of the crime performed and try and explain that humanity is not a cereal nor a plant, which can be limited and destroyed as we limit our cotton or corn acreage to protect the market.[27]

An editorial, "The Writhing of a Scotched Snake," was published in the November 19, 1904 issue of *American Medicine*. It discussed the efforts of a Maryland abortionist to obtain clemency and release from his 10-year sentence following the 1901 conviction for the criminal-abortion-related death of a woman whose dying statement, secured by a physician who attended the dying woman, was key to the conviction. The editorial focused on the numerous prominent citizens "who either signed the petition or made individual intercession for the prisoner." Their names were made public by the Governor and they were reported to include:

> a member of Congress, an ex-congressman, a candidate for Congress, an ex-governor of Maryland, a very distinguished United States senator, the president of the First Branch of the Baltimore City Council, 7 clergymen, 8 physicians, one of them a health officer, fourteen State senators (one of whom died several months ago), 86 members of the Maryland House of Delegates, and about 100 other persons of influence. Of

these intercessors the first two mentioned promptly denied both action and interest in the case. Their denials were followed up at once by the publication of their letters, typewritten on the note paper of the House of Representatives of the United States, addressed to the late governor of Maryland, and dated, one in November, 1901, the other in February, 1902, asking for pardon when the prisoner's term was scarcely more than begun. The other side of the case was everybody's business and therefore nobody's. Three daily papers printed editorials opposing the pardon. A few Methodist ministers made formal objection, and some 15 physicians wrote individual notes of protest. On the date fixed for a final consideration of the case, the friends of the prisoner appearing in force and spoke well, quoting Scripture. It was a moving appeal, acutely punctuated once or twice by a faint sob of a woman. At the end the woman said she was the mother of the girl slain. Whatever else she meant to say, sufficed unsaid. The judgment of the court stands.[28]

Abortionists like this that used their wealth (and possibly information about abortion-related wrongdoing) to influence officials who might convict or who might parole following conviction date at least to the 1840s when Madame Restell frequently avoided imprisonment. Numerous physicians discussing abortionists and abortionist rings in the early twentieth century described similar activities. Theodore Roosevelt would make reference to a similar incident in his autobiography where he described his anger at such "requests for leniency" and where he himself made public the names of the prominent petitioners.[29]

CHAPTER 26

ABORTION SYMPOSIA AND A SCOTTISH VIEW

A major Symposium on Criminal Abortion was held by the Chicago Medical Society on November 23, 1904. It was widely reported in the medical press and most fully covered in the *Illinois Medical Journal*. Charles Sumner Bacon presented the first paper, "The Duty of the Medical Profession in Relation to Criminal Abortion." Bacon estimated that there were from 6,000 to 10,000 induced abortions in Chicago each year with a large majority of these on married women. He described the committee to investigate criminal abortion that he had persuaded the Society to create. It was made up of Bacon, Rudolph Wieser Holmes, and Charles B. Reed.[1]

Bacon stated the committee's view "that the child is a human being while still unborn just as much as it is after its expulsion from the uterus." He then provided a unique attempt to show the fetus' independent existence: "The fact that the fetus is an intrauterine parasite does not prove that it is a part of the mother any more than that the intraintestinal parasitic existence of a tape worm proves that the worm is not an independent existence." "We can draw no line in the life history of a human being," Bacon continued, "from its beginning to its death when it has not the fundamental right to existence and the help of its fellows in this right."[2]

Bacon noted that accusations of criminal abortion and indictments for the crime rarely occurred unless the women died or became seriously ill and, even then, "her relatives generally try to prevent any investigation in order to shield her reputation." Bacon claimed the law still was useful when death or injury to the mother did occur and "for the restraining effect it may have." Bacon urged each physician to use his influence "to persuade his injured patient and her relatives and family or in case of her death her surviving relatives to prosecute the venal offender."[3]

Bacon noted that physicians often wrote certificates for abortion-related deaths in a way that avoided coroner notification. They did this because of the time lost in criminal proceedings, the unpleasant attacks in court from the defendant's attorney, the "enmity of the friends of the accused midwife or physician," and the pleadings of the relatives of the deceased. "Only a clear conception of the enormity of the crime and the duty that one owes to the community to prevent a like desolation of other homes," Bacon continued, "can counteract these deterring elements and keep one true to himself."[4]

A Catholic priest, Peter J. O'Callaghan, followed Bacon. He made the case that the fetus could not be killed, even if it meant the death of the mother would otherwise result. His brief discussion of the history of abortion included the claim that the Catholic Church had practically eradicated the crime of abortion in past centuries. He indicated that recent pronouncements of the Church had maintained the same doctrine: "If one or the other must die, or both die, and if both die without act of ours, responsibility is not ours."[5]

Charles B. Reed was next and he "rejoiced" that the fetus had no such unimpeachable right to life.[6] Reed indicated that, when both would otherwise die, the child should be sacrificed to save the life of the mother whose value to the state was "far greater than that of the unborn babe." Reed described various health conditions that he claimed justified destruction of the child and these included "certain cases of beginning and advanced pulmonary tuberculosis, cardiac disease, insanity, severe nephritis or serious and irreducible uterine displacements with dense adhesions."[7] He saw the Caesarean operation as an alternative in situations of severely contracted pelvis and tumors blocking the birth canal.

Reed strongly condemned abortions performed for social reasons and noted that the typical lay attitude also was "that the practice of abortion is bad, that only depraved and desperate characters engage therein." However, "when an instance arises in an unmarried daughter, the layman rushes to his family doctor with the story of his distress and prospective humiliation."[8]

Reed concluded with a plea for "justice and charity" for the unmarried woman faced with childbirth. He complained of the double standard that pilloried the woman and left the father of the illegitimate child unscathed. He called for "homes and places of refuge for the woman awaiting confinement" which would prevent her from seeking abortion as a way to avoid exposure and humiliation.[9]

Rudolph Wieser Holmes' Symposium paper, "Criminal Abortion; A Brief Consideration of Its Relation to Newspaper Advertising. A Report of a Medico-Legal Case," was actually a wide-ranging "consideration" of the issue. Holmes was more than a little contemptuous of the women who approached physicians seeking abortions:

> It is a sad parody on the high virtue and purity of women that they do not see the evil they do when they seek, and only too often secure, a criminal destruction of their unborn children. You all know the naive way, the insinuating manner with which our modern woman attempts to consort with her doctor in gaining her point: with one it is beginning connubial incompatibility, another has too many children already—this too many children includes one to a full dozen progeny, another had such a difficult labor last time that her doctor told her it would kill her to have another, again it is "money," and the particularly candid woman will openly declare she hates children, and then finally the unfortunate turns up with her pitiable tale. The most deplorable part of this question is that these requests do not come from the wanton, the women who really are carrying burdens beyond their strengths, or the poor, but [it is] the better educated, the women of society, who are the most persistent transgressors.[10]

Holmes claimed that physicians were the people most able to influence women to change their minds about ending their pregnancies. "Well directed arguments concerning the dangers of having the operation done are to my mind more effective than too strong presentations of the moral aspect," he continued, "so soon as we present to the woman that she is doing a criminal offense, is breaking a moral law, we arouse her enmity from the suggestion implied that she is immoral or a criminal."[11]

Holmes criticized the Illinois law that made abortion much less of a crime when the mother survived than when she died: "Such a law is discriminative; as infanticide is murder, so should foeticide be murder; the abortionist directly, maliciously, with 'malice aforethought' deliberately kills the fetus, while it is far from his intention to kill the woman."[12]

Holmes decried the numerous advertisements in nearly all newspapers for drugs and instruments for producing abortion, and for the abortionists themselves. He indicated that one Chicago daily paper "nets a clean (or better unclean) profit of over $50,000.00 a year," and he noted that this paper carried fewer such ads than some of the others. He claimed that existing State and Federal statutes and "an aggressive prosecuting attorney, backed by a strong, active organization as the Chicago Medical Society," could make the advertising pages of the newspapers "present the same purity" as their news columns.[13]

Holmes was followed by the Cook County Coroner, John E. Traeger, who claimed that midwives were responsible for many of the city's abortions. Prior to his tenure, there had been very few convictions for the crime. However, he had succeeded in sending four midwives to Joliet prison and two more had recently been convicted. He gave details of one case where a midwife's abortion caused the woman's death. She was waiting for him when he arrived at his office the next morning. Traeger continued:

> She told me of the case, that she was a midwife, that she had been attending the woman and that her patient had died, also that the authorities had charged her with performing an abortion, but she protested her innocence, saying she had been charged with the offense before, but had always been able to fix herself with the coroner—But Mrs. Jahnke is now a resident of Joliet and if the Pardon Board does not interfere she will be there for the next fourteen years.[14]

At the same Symposium, J.M. Sheean, Attorney for the Medico-Legal Committee of the Chicago Medical Society, briefly discussed the history of laws on criminal abortion from the common law adopted early in the country's history to the present Illinois statutes. He noted how the law's exception of abortion "for *bona fide* medical purposes" was changed in 1867 to "as necessary for the preservation of the mother's life." He also indicated that mental depression or a threat of suicide was not a basis for abortion only "an actual physical condition which renders improbable the continued life of the mother."

Sheean concluded:

> The law itself is as far advanced as the public conscience. Indeed, the law as it stands is further advanced than apparently the pubic demand for its enforcement would require, and so if anything is to be accom-

plished, it is not to be done by appeals to the legislature for modifica-
tions of the law at this time; it is not by making appeals for more stringent laws, but it is by so stimulating the public conscience as to require
and demand that the law as it stands today should be strictly enforced.[15]

The final Symposium paper dealt with the question of whether patient communications to physicians should be privileged and thus not subject to investigation by the courts. Harold N. Moyer, M.D., claimed every "practicing physician,
has at some time been the bearer of a medical secret in relation to abortion," and
"the privileged communication or medical secret has stood in the way more
largely than any one factor in the prosecution of the abortionist." Part of the problem was that many physicians were ignorant of the fact that Illinois did not recognize such privileged communications and were unsure of their duty to the State
and to the patient. "The courts can prevent misuse of medical evidence, and an
abuse of it for wrongful purposes" he concluded, "and the matter can be safely left
in their hands. Let us have no privileged medical communications."[16]

Following the formal papers, Mr. Fletcher Dobyns, the Assistant State's Attorney, discussed the large problems in convicting abortionists. He called on physicians to become better versed in obtaining full and complete evidence when they
encountered a case of criminal abortion. This included proof of pregnancy, proof
that the operation was for abortion, proof that it was not necessary to save the life
of the mother, and proof that she died as a result of the abortion. Dobyns concluded with a discussion of how these evidentiary hurdles were met in a case
where a conviction was obtained following death of the mother.[17]

Two women physicians added their comments during the discussion. Dr.
Lucy Waite, Head Surgeon of the Mary Thompson Hospital for Women and
Children, reinforced Dr. Reed's concerns about charity for the unmarried victim
of seduction. She called for "justice" as well:

> I believe there is only one measure which can effectually solve this
> problem. Make parentage constitute a legal marriage contract and one
> of the principal temptations to commit criminal abortion will be abol-
> ished. This will protect the life and future good name of the innocent
> one of the three, the child, and will give to the mother an honored posi-
> tion in society and, incidentally, the father also. It may be objected that
> this law would put some men in the position of bigamists, but we have
> a law covering bigamy and I think these cases would be very interesting
> ones to bring before the State's Attorney.[18]

Dr. Rosalie M. Ladova was concerned that the evening's discussion gave a
false impression of who were performing criminal abortions.

> Anyone who listened to the discussion this evening, who does not know
> the facts, might carry the impression that it is only the midwives who
> are guilty of criminal abortion. To be frank with ourselves and square
> with others, we want to admit that we have black sheep in the family.

Some of our professional brethren are buying apparent professional success at the cost of their manly honor. Why not clear our society which stands for the highest and the best where we gather for instruction and inspiration of these hypocrites.[19]

Ladova also discussed the duty of physicians to dissuade women from criminal abortions.

It has been my experience that many of the people who come to us with the request of having the operation performed do not know nor realize the gravity and dangers of it, either to themselves or to the physicians. By pointing out to them the risk of infection and fatal hemorrhage, as well as the gravity of the crime they ask us to perpetrate, we can get them reconciled to their condition, and persuade them to leave well enough alone.[20]

Her successes in getting parents "to leave well enough alone" undoubtedly provided the ancestors of scores of people alive today in the Midwest.

A less-noticed symposium on criminal abortion took place at the Nebraska State Medical Society in May 1905. Inez C. Philbrick, a physician and women suffragist from Lincoln, presented a paper, "Social Causes of Criminal Abortion."[21] She began by noting the alarming prevalence of criminal abortion, citing the 1881 Michigan estimate that one-third of pregnancies ended in criminal abortion. "No more startling than its prevalence," she continued, "is the universal indifference, lay and professional, with which it is regarded."[22]

Philbrick then discussed the conflict of strong sexual appetites with the need for small families. In the majority of instances when she received requests for abortion, the requesting woman stated that it was at the insistence of the husband and Philbrick could "conceive no lower depths of selfishness and brutality to which humanity can descend than is revealed in such a statement."[23]

Philbrick noted the church's failure to stem abortion and the Catholic Church's exception to this. She went on to vilify the American press and contrasted its actions in an earlier day when editors provided "dignified and ardent championship of moral issues." However her strongest criticisms were for the medical profession:

It is a matter of common knowledge that in every community members of the profession live by its induction. Not infrequently one learns of those in high places who have their price. But far greater than sins of commission are those of omission. That the profession has failed to assume the responsibility of speaking in certain tones and with an authority founded upon supposed fitness of training and adequacy of knowledge on the vital questions of sex which vex our civilization is, in the light of its history, explicable. Traditions long surrounding medical schools were not those exalting chastity. Not infrequently professors counseled students to libertinism rather than virtue, and lent the force of

example to that of precept. The name of medical student was a syno-
nym for license. ... For sins of commission an over-crowded profession
containing a large percentage of the unfit, intellectually and ethically, is
responsible. With poverty confronting not alone the physician, but his
helpless wife and children, we cannot expect that he will be scrupulous
in his choice of work.[24]

Philbrick's references to the libertinism of medical professors and medical students, to medical school graduates who were "unfit, intellectually and ethically,"
and to the poverty resulting from an overcrowded medical profession may largely
explain why some regular physicians were undercutting the efforts of most other
physicians to end unnecessary and illegal abortions.

Another Symposium paper, "Measures for Prevention of Criminal Abortion," was by A.B Somers, M.D., of Omaha. Somers indicated that the law as it
existed should suffice to prevent criminal abortion, "but from some cause or combination of causes, the law is inoperative."[25] He called for elimination of the
newspaper advertising for abortion-producing drugs and abortion services and
asked for a resolution by the Association "asking all newspapers in this state, in
fact all advertisers, including druggists, to keep their advertisements within the
limits of the criminal code."[26]

Another Somers' recommendation was "enlightenment" of girls and women
who did not recognize the danger to life or the large amount of invalidism that
resulted from criminal abortion. He noted that the abortionists were highly aware
of these dangers, but

the loss of life of a life or two does not hinder these men from continuing their nefarious practice. Why should it, as the whole business is a
life-taking process, the life of the child not being considered in the least,
and it is only an added risk the mother takes when she decides to take
the life of her offspring. A few lives of mothers, more or less, do not
count so much when we consider the large destruction of infants constantly going on.[27]

Somers concluded:

Abortionists are known to the medical fraternity, and while many of
them are not in good medical standing and cannot gain admission to our
medical societies, others are quite prominent in our society meetings
and social gatherings. Such should be made to feel, by an overwhelm-
ing medical sentiment, that all illegitimate measures of this kind are
discountenanced by the profession as a whole, and that criminals have
no place in our deliberations and councils. ... A few expulsions of
members in good standing in this society would also doubtless have a
salutary effect. I am not satisfied that we need all the evidence required
in a court of justice to do this."[28]

Other papers presented at the meeting included "The Pathology and Treatment of Criminal Abortion," by W.O. Henry;[29] "Criminal Abortion—The Nebraska Law," by William A. De Bord;[30] and "The Ethics of Criminal Abortion," by William B. Ely.[31] Ely's paper concluded: "To sum up the whole subject in a word, then, the ethics of criminal abortion is the ethics of degradation, the ethics of degeneration, of impurity, of unchastity, of bestiality and lechery."[32]

What may have been the first symposium on "therapeutic abortion" was held by the St. Louis Medical Society on October 6, 1906. Dr. Henry Schwarz began with a paper, "Diseases of the Kidneys as Indications for the Interruption of Pregnancy."[33] Schwarz took a conservative approach, noting that it was very rare that the fetus needed to be sacrificed for kidney problems. Even a condition such as chronic nephritis did not call for interruption, although it was recognized that fetal death was not uncommon and "the mother must be given the benefit of any doubt about the fetus being alive, when the advisability of inducing labor is under discussion."[34]

Tuberculosis was considered at the symposium by another St. Louis physician, Louis M. Warfield. Tuberculosis of the larynx was seen always as an indication for pregnancy interruption, but rarely tuberculosis of the lungs. Since children born of mothers with far advanced "phthisis" often were healthy, "the child should receive the first consideration."[35] Early tuberculosis "might" justify interruption if the disease is advancing, if she is losing weight, "and if she can be put under the most favorable surroundings" after the operation.[36]

W.H. Vogt, M.D., of St. Louis, discussed heart disease as an indication and he claimed that only in very rare instances did the condition justify interrupting pregnancy.[37] Bernard W. Moore, M.D., indicated the same for persistent excessive vomiting. He claimed most was of neurotic origin and with proper treatment "should never result fatally." Moore noted that it was prevalent when the pregnancy was "unwelcomed." He described a case where a woman lost 37 pounds during four weeks of constant vomiting. "After the induction of abortion, which seemed necessary to save her life," Moore continued, "she confessed that she had vomited at will, in order that the pregnancy might be ended."[38]

The St. Louis gynecologist, Frederick Joseph Taussig, also was a contributor and it is possible he organized the symposium, given his likely role as abortion provider for area physicians when abortion was judged necessary. His paper, "The Ethics and Laws Regarding the Interruption of Pregnancy," may have been his first published work on the subject of induced abortion.[39] Taussig would become the major American authority on the subject of abortion over the next four decades, including authorship of two major books on the subject.

Taussig began by discussing the appropriateness of abortion when essential to save the life of the mother. He indicated that some worried that this provided "a loophole of escape to all those who desire to interrupt pregnancy for their own personal gain." He claimed that this killing was justifiable, even as killing by soldiers was justifiable in the defense of their country, but "we must in our laws and code of ethics set down certain rules for the protection of society so that this privilege accorded the physician is not abused."[40] He advised that the medical profession, "to protect its good name," "define as accurately as possible the special conditions under which the interruption of pregnancy is permissible and require that in every instance these special conditions really exist." In addition, pregnancy interruption should follow consultation with one or more physicians and the consultant should be "some person of note in the community."[41]

Taussig then suggested that "a board of consultants" be appointed by the municipality to determine when abortion was appropriate and legal. "The success of the advisory board of three physicians on questions of insanity, recently appointed in this city," he continued, "leads me to believe that a board of three persons similarly appointed from a list of those specially qualified to serve in this capacity would be a means of protecting the community in a matter vital to its interests."[42]

A Scottish friend of Horatio Robinson Storer, Sir Alexander Russell Simpson, presented the Inaugural Address to the Forfarshire Medical Association at Dundee, Scotland on October 6, 1905. His paper, "Criminal Abortion," was published in *The Scottish Medical and Surgical Journal*.[43] It reflected an awareness of history, literature, and science that was generally absent in the writing on criminal abortion by American physicians. Its appreciation by the American medical audience is reflected in the fact that it was republished in the United States in the *Clinical Review* as "Criminal Abortion from the Ethical Point of View."[44]

Simpson began by explaining his consideration of the topic, noting "the crime of procuring abortion is all too common, and the suspicion of its occurrence gives rise to delicate and difficult enquiries."[45] He continued with a historical discussion of the high prevalence of abortion in Greece and Rome. He saw Hippocrates prohibition as evidence of the prevalence of abortion in Greece. His paragraphs showing its prevalence in Rome read:

> Seneca, writing from his exile in Corsica to comfort his mother Helvia, calls to mind her many virtues; and among the rest he says: "You were never ashamed of reproduction as if it were an unbecoming burden, according to the fashion of others who want to be admired for their figure; and you never destroyed the germ of life that had begun to develop in your womb."
>
> When a son could congratulate his mother on the score of her never having been guilty of abortion, we can see how prevalent the practice must have been in their social circle, and can understand how needful it was that laws should be passed sentencing those who were guilty of it in varying degrees to fine, imprisonment, and death.[46]

Simpson discussed the fact that France, Germany, and Great Britain had many cases of criminal abortion with very few leading to conviction of abortionists. "Our Transatlantic colleagues deplore the extent which the evil practice has attained in America," he continued, "where the number of men and women who are known to make a business of abortioning seems to be greater than in Europe."[47] He provided references to Dixon Jones' 1894 article and T. Gaillard

Thomas' book in support of both the American deploring and the American frequency of criminal abortion.

Simpson discussed three classes of applicants for abortion: women desiring to conceal their illicit intercourse; married couples wishing to avoid children or additional children who fail in attempts at contraception; and "women of ample means who shirk the duties of maternity, because the restraints attendant on pregnancy and parturition interfere with their round of society pleasures, or because they wish to avoid what they regard as a disfigurement of their person." Simpson also discussed the providers of abortions and he viewed women as most numerous. They covered up their abortion practice with the practice of midwifery, maintenance of "private lying-in homes," or "baby-farming." "Most of all to be reprobated," he continued, "are those members of our profession who sell themselves and degrade their diplomas."[48]

Simpson discussed methods for producing abortion and discussed the ineffectiveness of drugs, including ergot. He indicated that attempts to jar the system such as jumping from high places and "rude manipulations of the abdomen" rarely produced abortion, although some women prone to abortion would abort even with such minor provocations. He finally discussed "immediate interference with the uterus" and this included injections into the uterus of various liquids and puncture or separation of the membranes with instruments ranging from knitting needles to the "better adapted instruments that belong to the equipment of the general practitioner, or even of the specialist in gynecology."[49]

He noted that in some instances the patient was unharmed physically by the induced abortion, but "mischief" frequently followed. He discussed injuries to the uterus that caused "hypertrophy, displacement, or inflammatory processes which impair the health and comfort of the woman, who may find further on in life when she would fain become a mother, that she has doomed herself to sterility or to recurrence against her will of the abortion she once too willingly induced." Not infrequently more serious immediate effects occurred including hemorrhage and "septic processes" with some of these fatal. He described the "pathetic" instances where women died or were seriously injured after subjecting "themselves to abortive procedures, when, after all, they had not been pregnant."[50]

Simpson's next section was "The Essence of the Criminality." He cited three reasons that abortion needed to be regarded as criminal. The State suffered since abortion opposed "the object and intention of marriage, which is the legal institution for the propagation of the race and the upkeep of the population." The woman was subject to danger to her health and life. He continued with the third:

> Above all it implies the destruction of a life at whatever stage of pregnancy the attempt is made. The life of the infant, the foetus, the embryo is ruthlessly sacrificed. Modern science gives no space for metaphysical and juridical discussion as to a date of quickening supervening during the course of pregnancy, as if the developing being became animated so many days or weeks or months after conception took place. It recognizes that from the hour that a fertilized ovum was lodged in its uterine nest, the woman carried within her a new life

that was on the way to develop into a man. As during its intra-uterine existence it is dependent entirely on the mother, so for a time after birth it is mainly dependent upon her for its continued sustenance. Later, its dependence is on the protection of the paternal roof, and later still on the conditions of the city or country of which it has become a citizen. And from beginning to end it has a claim upon the justice of the State for freedom to live and develop. This is the essence of the crime: it destroys a human life. The life, to be sure, was very young and very tender. The more need it had to be sacredly guarded. For it had all the untold possibilities of humanity in prospect.[51]

As for the remedy, Simpson claimed "correct ideas as to the real meaning of marriage" needed to be diffused "throughout the community."[52] He provided a quote from Mr. Coulson Kenrihan's *A World without a Child* as one of the "correct ideas." It included:

"It is in Fatherhood, in Motherhood, that men and women become likest God, since, in a sense, they are permitted to share with Him the joy and the mystery, the majesty and awe and wonder of creation. For this were they born into the world, born as it were in the purple. When man and woman, youth and maiden, love each other purely and truly, then, be their place high or humble, they become princes and princesses by right of succession and by right of royal birth; then to them comes naturally the voice and the manner of courts; and when they marry, be their home cottage or be it castle, they shall enter it as prince and princess into a palace.

"But they shall come to higher estate than this. There be they who maintain that love and life are consummated by the coming together in marriage of those who love; but so to speak is to misread the sacred mysteries. Is the means to an end of more moment than the end itself? Is it the scattering of the grain in springtime or the reaping of the ripe corn at harvest which crowns the husbandman's year? When a man becomes a father, a woman a mother, then is he a king and a creator indeed, then is she a queen, and crowned with the rarest diadem that womanhood may wear."[53]

This novelist's view of marriage was supplemented by that of Dr. Woods Hutchison, a "student of evolution" who "traces the evolutionary development of man from a group of monogamous apes." Simpson quoted the following from Hutchison's article in the September 1905 issue of *The Contemporary*:

"[Marriage's] universal sway over the minds and hearts of men rests not upon the fiat of any prince, pope, or godlet; but upon its own inherent superiority over every other form of mating, as sternly proved by the experience of millions of past generations, human and prehuman. The right of one man to choose one woman to love and to protect all his life long, of the woman to choose her knight and worshipper, and of both to expect of the other unswerving faithfulness and comradeship until death do them part, is founded on the life of all the ages.

"Nor is this evolutionary sanction in any sense a low or selfish one. Far from it. It is ennobling and altruistic in the highest degree, for it looks to the benefit not of the individual, but of the race, not of the life that now is, but of that which is to come. Marriage is neither for the pleasure of the man nor the protection of the woman, but for the welfare of the children, and neither of the parties thereto has any individual rights which are entitled to half the consideration of those of the children. No institution, of course, can promote the good of the race and seriously antagonize that of the individuals composing it; and marriage adds enormously to the effectiveness, the dignity, and the pleasure of life, both for husband and wife. Yet to contract a marriage on any of these grounds without giving chief regard to the mental and physical vigour, the sanity, and the efficiency of the probable offspring thereof, is far more profoundly immoral upon biological grounds than upon religious or legal."[54]

After thus showing how novelist and evolutionist agreed to the "necessity of wholesome marriage ideals for the race and nation," Simpson noted the rarity of criminal abortion among the Jews. He quoted various biblical references that trained the Jews "to anticipate for their progeny a glorious future," and showed how these fit with the total absence of references to abortion in the bible.[55]

He concluded by discussing other anticipations of progeny success:

John Trebonius, learned, of agreeable address, something of a poet, and one of the masters in St. George's High School in Eisenach, every time that he entered his class-room took off his barret-cap and bowed to his pupils. Poor enough lads many of them were; among them a miner's son named Martin Luther. Challenged by his colleagues for the unusual courtesy, he replied: "There are among these boys men of whom God will one day make burgomasters, chancellors, learned doctors, and magistrates. Although you do not yet see them with the badges of their dignity, it is right that you should treat them with respect." It is with something of that sentiment that we should welcome into the world the children of the mothers we attend in labour. We may, long ere his birth, have heard the first beating of the heart of one who will be the hero of an after generation. And no mother could dream of abortion who thought it possible that her child might be a William Wallace to deliver his country from a foreign yoke, or a John Knox to win for his nation the yet higher boon of spiritual freedom, a Robert Burns to sing her songs, or a Walter Scott to tell her stories.

Let no man, above all, let no woman, think lightly of the life that is still at home in a mother's womb, and when it comes to a wider home, let it be welcomed with a song.[56]

The friendship of Sir Alexander Russell Simpson and Horatio Storer dated from 1854-1855 when Alexander was a medical student at the University of Edinburgh and Storer was assisting Alexander's uncle, James Young Simpson. One hopes this unique tribute to unborn human beings by Simpson was read by Storer. It probably was, since Storer himself provided a letter to Simpson that became an article in the same journal, although by 1911 when it was published the journal had changed its name to the *Edinburgh Medical Journal.*[57]

CHAPTER 27
CUSHING'S WOMB STRIKE, CATTELL'S CRUSADE, AND SANDERS' "BIRTH"

An article in the *Annals of Gynecology and Pediatry* showed a sharp increase in criminal abortion in France from 1898 to 1904.[1] This was attributed to an increase in use of contraceptive techniques. When these failed, women took the next step and had their pregnancies interrupted. An editorial in the same journal by Ernest W. Cushing dealt with a similar increase in criminal abortion in the United States "and perhaps especially in New England."[2] One reason Cushing cited for the increase was "a general slackening of respect for religious authority which has condemned abortion as a sin and as murder of an unborn child." In conjunction with this, Cushing indicated that few people possessed the required "imagination to consider an ovum as a human being." Another reason for the increase was the "general feeling that the world is getting too full of people." He also included economics: "people are forced, as by the iron hand of fate, to limit their families or go under in the struggle for survival."[3]

Another factor was a "'strike' of the womb."

> It is a part of the emancipation of woman, and like divorce it has come to stay.
>
> It is no use to say to woman that God says, "in sorrow shalt thou bring forth children." She answers that it is rubbish, that God never said it and that she *won't*, there now.
>
> The woman's point of view seems to be that she has been enslaved long enough. That now she is free, and that her body belongs to herself and no one else. That no woman ought to endure sexual intercourse unless she is disposed thereto, that if she does not love a man she ought not to live with him and is justified in getting a divorce, that if "by mistake" she gets pregnant, her physician ought to immediately "help her" out of her "difficulty." That there ought to be no children born who are not wanted in the family; that it is vulgar and indecent to have more children than can be properly brought up and educated or more than three at any rate; that the function and duty of a husband is to pay bills and make money and have an automobile and take his wife about and dress her well and not bother her with "nasty" allusions to his sexual desires, on pain of her divine displeasure.[4]

Cushing at least did not see this "strike" as universal:

> We would humbly suggest to young doctors contemplating matrimony, however, that in a forgotten part of a neglected book they will find a de-

scription of the kind of woman they would do well to find, even the virtuous woman of the book of Proverbs, for although she is not like the
"new" woman, there are still such women to be found in the world, and
now as in old times their price is far above rubies.[5]

A paper by the Brooklyn physician, William P. Pool, marked a sharp change
from the strict positions on pregnancy termination of his Brooklyn colleagues,
Mary Amanda Dixon Jones and William McCollom.[6] In the case of a contracted
pelvis, Pool recommended that the uterus be emptied early in the pregnancy rather
than using the Cesarean operation. However, if the mother wanted her child to
survive, the obstetrician should respect her wishes and go with the Cesarean.[7]
Early abortion also was recommended in most cases when the mother had nephritis, pernicious vomiting, heart disease, and tuberculosis. In the case of a woman
with diabetes, Pool claimed: "It is best to terminate pregnancy as soon as it is discovered."[8]

The Boston physician, Frank A. Higgins, probably was referring to Pool
when he welcomed "a strong tendency generally in the medical profession toward
a broadening of the indications for the termination of pregnancy."[9] Higgins did not
believe this broadening of indications would lead to any appreciable increase of
unnecessary abortions "as the great majority of physicians are undoubtedly honest
in this respect as in other things, and are no more likely to go astray than formerly."[10]

Higgins then described chronic diseases that he believed justified abortion in
early pregnancy. These were tuberculosis, heart disease, and nephritis. He also
mentioned less common chronic diseases: grave anemia, diabetes, and chorea,
which usually indicated the appropriateness of termination of pregnancy. For acute
diseases that threatened the "special senses, such as the eyesight in Bright's disease, or the mind in melancholia or other nervous affections," Higgins claimed
"there should be no question of the propriety of terminating the pregnancy."[11]

The paper led to considerable discussion. C. Lester Hall, from Kansas City,
Missouri, indicated "the objection to the induction of premature labor is held not
only by the Roman Catholic church but by us all." He continued:

> It is dangerous to discuss this question before the general profession,
> and it is particularly dangerous for the public to have the impression
> that labor can be induced prematurely without danger. As operators, we
> know it can be done, and we are prepared to do it in certain cases, but
> those who deal with women and their weak husbands know that there is
> a constant outcry, even among good people, for the bringing about of
> this very thing.[12]

Other discussants included Charles Sumner Bacon who disagreed about the
necessity to induce abortion for several of the chronic conditions Higgins mentioned. If the woman had excellent care "she may go through her pregnancy very
well." He claimed vomiting also could usually be treated without the need for
abortion.[13]

The strongest objections to Higgins' call for such broadening of indications came from the Philadelphia physician and medical professor, Henry W. Cattell. Cattell made his objections in a letter to the *Journal of the American Medical Association* expressing regret that the *Journal* had published Higgins' paper. Cattell mentioned 33 autopsies he had performed as the senior coroner's physician of Philadelphia on women who had died as a result of accidental abortions, self-induced abortions, and abortions induced "by others for money." He indicated that 18 abortionists had been "brought to the bar of justice" and there were others who were "under police surveillance or whose records are being looked up by a Committee recently appointed by the Philadelphia County Medical Society."[14] Cattell, the Chairman of the new Committee, continued:

> With this short preface, and now that the subject is under discussion, it would be interesting to have Dr. Frank A. Higgins of Boston, the author of the above paper, answer the following questions: How many induced abortions have you performed and at what period of gestation? What was the reason for so doing in each case? Have you induced abortion on the same woman more than once? How many of the patients were married women and how many were single? How many patients applying for this form of treatment were rejected by you? Of those rejected, did any one else perform the operation? Have the rich or the poor been the more prone to seek relief? Have you ever had to revise your diagnosis after performing the operation; like those who have stated that a cesarean section had to be undertaken to save the life of the mother and before the hour set for the operation have had her give birth to a living child without instrumental aid? Do you usually perform the operation in a hospital, at the home of the patient, or in your own office? Do you perform the operation only after consultation with a confrere? Would you consider pregnancy from rape a proper indication for the prompt termination of pregnancy? If you had a death following the operation, would you state on the certificate that you had induced abortion?[15]

Higgins replied to Cattell in a letter published a week later.[16] He provided a description of nine cases where abortion was induced "before the viable period," and, despite his earlier long list of chronic and acute conditions that justified therapeutic abortion, these nine were indicated to be the total induced before seven months. Most of these involved continued vomiting and this included one woman who had two pregnancies ended for this reason. All cases but one followed consultation with one or more physicians and all were married women. Higgins mentioned that two of his patients died, one "of exhaustion" and one of "tubercular meningitis." Higgins did not answer Cattell's questions about the location of the operation, about rape as an excuse, about whether any patients requesting abortion were rejected, and about whether the induced operation was mentioned on the death certificates. Cattell probably was not happy with Higgins' incomplete answers, but no further Cattell response to Higgins was located.

Cattell did provide a letter to the Medical Society of the State of Pennsylvania giving more results of his Committee.[17] Cattell noted that they had investigated over 30 persons "making a practice of performing criminal abortions" in Philadelphia. As a result, these abortionists had either left the city, were under police surveillance, were fugitives from justice, were awaiting trial, or were serving prison sentences. Cattell noted that a drive to rid Boston of its abortionists had led many of the Boston abortionists to take up residence and practice in Philadelphia. He called on the State Medical Society and the American Medical Association to take up the matter so that abortionists flushed from one city would not move to another.

Cattell also read a wide-ranging paper before the American Academy of Medicine. He discussed the current high incidence of unnecessary abortion and claimed that some were performed by "scoundrels, too many of whom are members of our profession."[18] Others were carried out by the women themselves using instruments and drugs. He discussed the "Sunday newspapers," "polluted with advertisements, the true purpose of which is unmistakable."[19] He made reference to a recent paper of the St. Louis physician, John M. Grant, where Grant claimed that 96 percent of the criminal abortion cases he attended were married women.[20] However despite this gloomy picture of the state of society, Cattell claimed that progress was being made against criminal abortion as a result of the combined efforts of physicians, the legal profession, and the laity:

> Every conviction of an abortionist brings home to a section of the public the fact that abortion is abhorrent to right thinking, antagonistic to right living. Women are learning that the trouble of bearing a child is nothing compared with the lifetime of misery which may follow an abortion; they are coming slowly but surely into the realization that as the foetus lives from the moment of conception, abortion is murder.[21]

Cattell then provided the information that one of the principals in "the notorious dress-suit case of Boston" was a Philadelphia abortionist who had escaped arrest and he again stressed the need for cooperation among different cities.[22] He concluded with a general plea for action against criminal abortion:

> And will not every member of this great Association which touches the national life at so many points and with such peculiar power, himself a believer in the Hippocratic oath to give no woman an abortive pessary except in those rare instances where the life of the mother is at stake, do all that in him lies in this hour of our highest physical, moral, and intellectual development, to check the growth of this abortion evil, so potent with peril to the individual, the home and the State?[23]

The discussion of Cattell's paper dealt largely with the problems physicians faced when moving to another state where they not infrequently failed the licensing examination. However, Vermont's Henry D. Holton returned the discussion to the subject of criminal abortion that had occupied his attention at least since 1866 when he proposed the Resolution thanking Horatio Storer for declining the $100 prize for his Prize Essay. Holton began by discussing the difficulties he had faced in securing convictions of known abortionists. He then discussed prevention of criminal abortion:

> There are two things that have helped me out wonderfully in this matter. I have one method which I employ for my Catholic patients and another for my Protestant. The method for my Protestant patients is a little book called "Why Not?" This is an explanation why we should not take the life of the unborn child. I say to them "Are you familiar with the reasons for not having this operation?" When they answer "No" I say: "Here is a little book I wish you would take home and read carefully and when you are through with it bring it back to me." I have kept these books circulating in that way for a good many years. I don't remember any case in which a person brought the book back again, but they always sent it back and I heard nothing more about it. With my Catholic friends, after hearing their story, I say: "Have you talked with the father about this?" "Oh no; oh no" is the answer. "Well," I say, "please go over and talk to him, and when you come back, stop and let me know what he says." They invariably went to the priest, but never stopped to talk to me.[24]

Henry Cattell commented: "I certainly congratulate Dr. Holton upon his novel method of preventing race-suicide and I hope it may be given wide publicity. It should certainly be known as Dr. Holton's method of preventing abortion!"[25]

The "notorious dress-suit case of Boston" that Cattell mentioned was found floating in Boston Harbor in the fall of 1905. It contained the torso of a young woman. Autopsy disclosed that she was recently pregnant and that the uterus had been punctured, either by the instrument used to produce abortion or by the sharp bones of the mutilated fetus. A month later another suitcase with her limbs was found floating in the harbor. Rings on her fingers identified the woman and this led to the arrest of two men who confessed to disposing of the suitcases. The men took authorities to the location of the head which was submerged in a leather traveling bag with about fourteen pounds of lead shot. They pleaded guilty and were sentenced to seven years in prison. They implicated two physicians in the woman's abortion. One stood trial, but was acquitted. The other became a witness for the government in the case.[26]

In July 1905, the Health Officer of Alabama, William H. Sanders, M.D., read a paper, "The Physiologic and Legal Status of the Fetus in Utero," before the Section on Obstetrics and Diseases of Women at the Annual Meeting of the American Medical Association.[27] Sanders made a strong case that "a self-acting and, in a qualified sense, a self-sustaining human being" was created at conception. "The cardinal postulate I desire to emphasize," he began "is that the vitality, the life-force, and the physiologic functions of the new being reside within itself and not in the hostess." He indicated that "the new being eats because it is hungry and breathes because it feels the need of oxygen, both acts being vital efforts of its own." Shortly after settling down "in its velvety and temporary home" the "new comer" "proceeds to differentiate itself into bone, sinew, tendon, muscle, blood vessels, viscera, brain, and nerve, and with the skill of a consummate artist fashions these in miniature of an adult human being, the highest type of animal life."[28]

Sanders then made the case that this creature had already been "born."

> At the end of nine months the silent and unseen artist has filled his temporary home with his living self, whereon the hostess by means of forces marvelously scientific and practical ushers him into the outside world as a plump and rosy baby. When was that baby born, a few minutes ago or nine months ago? Science and logic give one and the same answer. If birth means the act of coming into life, as the dictionaries tell us, unquestionably the baby under discussion came into life nine months ago, and at the end of that period simply changed its domicile.[29]

Sanders wanted to abolish the term conception "and substitute for it the more scientific and correct term, birth." This would help "to clarify the entire subject of fetal life and would lead to the enunciation of definite, inflexible, and absolutely correct principles of jurisdiction applying thereto." Sanders then asked: "[D]oes not the new being, from the first day of its uterine life, acquire a legal and moral status that entitles it to the same protection as that guaranteed to human beings in extrauterine life?" He answered that it actually deserved "greater protection for the reason that to the nature of a human being it adds the condition of utter helplessness, a condition that should appeal in mute, but sublime eloquence to the manhood, the womanhood, and above all, to the motherhood, of those who can shield and protect it."[30]

Sanders admitted that there would be objections to substituting *birth* for *conception*. One was the date of birth would not be precisely known and another was it would be several months after birth before birth would be known for certain. He claimed the following advantages outweighed these problems:

> 1. It would be essentially and scientifically correct to locate birth where and when it actually occurs, in spite of the fact that several months would usually elapse before it could be known that a birth had certainly taken place.
> 2. It would place a pregnancy, from the first day of its probable occurrence to its termination, on the high legal and moral grounds it deserves to occupy.
> 3. It would dignify the position of the *foetus in utero*, and would establish beyond all doubt or confusion the right of the fetus to the same protection, moral and legal, as is accorded to human beings who have completed the period of their uterine existences.
> 4. It would unify the terms, fluxion, abortion, and miscarriage, under the one term, premature delivery; then, two expressions, premature delivery and delivery at full term, would cover the entire subject.

5. It would enable lawmakers to enact clear and definite laws for the protection of the *foetus in utero*, which laws, jurists and juries could administer without doubt or confusion.

6. It would have a strong tendency to promote virtue and to prevent crime, and to build up in every community a positive demand for the protection of human life at its tenderest and most helpless period; it would tend to educate the people on a subject in reference to which they stand in great need of education and would thereby save the lives of many innocent and undelivered babies.[31]

Later physicians would also call for legal recognition of the onset of pregnancy and Taussig and others made reference to Sanders' paper (See Chapter 28). However, the first known reference was critical. Thomas G. Atkinson, M.D., the editor of the Chicago-based *Medical Standard*, provided an article that he claimed refuted Sanders' position.[32] Atkinson's competence to do this may be indicated by his calling Sanders "Saunders" throughout.

Atkinson began by noting that Sanders was one of many who claimed the unborn child had the same status as the born child. Atkinson thought that these repeated assertions sounded like the man who repeatedly claimed he was sober and who thus produced the suspicion in his audience that he was not quite sober. "The fact of the matter is," he continued, "and we might as well confess it, that we are not, and the public especially are not, satisfied as to the precise status of the fetus in utero."[33]

Atkinson then described Sanders' claim that "birth" should be used to describe the event of conception. He complemented Sanders for having "the courage and the logic to carry his premises to such clear cut conclusions, because it enables us to see something of where the defect lies which we have all more or less 'felt in our bones.'"[34] Atkinson began by examining "some of the author's more definite utterances." According to Atkinson one of these was

"The conjunction of spermatozoon and ovum, ... endows the newly formed unit with physiologic functions and psychologic attributes; indeed makes it in a qualified sense, an independent human being."

As a journal editor, Atkinson should have been an unlikely candidate to misquote a writer that is being criticized, but the closest thing to this by Sanders was: "In contributing the germs they respectively furnish, the male and female have done all they can do toward the creation of the new unit and toward its endowment with physiologic and psychologic functions similar to their own."[35] Sanders was referring to the future endowment of "psychologic functions" not to their endowment in "the newly formed unit."

Atkinson claimed that the "the attributes of living bioplasm" did not distinguish the embryo "from any other piece of bioplasm contained within the maternal organism—a tumor for example."[36] He continued:

And when the doctor asserts that the new being grows and develops "not as the passive result of the work done by the physiologic forces of the female," and "emphasizes as his cardinal postulate that the vitality, the life force, the physiologic functions of the new being reside in itself and not in the hostess," one cannot help wondering what species of hallucination has blinded him to the facts.[37]

However, Atkinson then admitted that this organism did "take hold of and appropriate the food brought within its reach," but this "is a histological and a physiological function, common to all protoplasmic structure."[38] Although unsaid, he might have added: "a tumor for example."

Atkinson next claimed "the fetus has from an organic point of view, no physiological status at all." He continued:

> The three cardinal functions constituting the vital trio upon which its physiological entity as an animal (to say nothing of a human being) rests, namely, circulation, respiration, and cerebration, are utterly wanting, and, so far as it is concerned, play no part in its development. And as the suppression of any one of these three functions, after delivery, will result in its "going out of life" it is hard to understand how it can "come into life" until these functions are established, as they are at the time when Dr. Saunders tells us the baby "simply changes its domicile."[39]

The denial that the fetus had circulation raises additional questions about Atkinson's medical training. And his claim that respiration was a prerequisite for the being to "come into life" suggests that Atkinson would not oppose abortion until birth. As it turns out he was not quite that willing to countenance abortion. Atkinson even ended his section, "Physiological Status," by claiming that the "human fetus has no more and no less value or status than other fetuses."[40] This certainly was a step up from equating it to a tumor.

Atkinson then contrasted Sanders' claim that the fetus "is entitled to 'the same protection, legal and moral, that is accorded to human beings who have completed their uterine period of existence," with Sanders' claim that the fetus should not be sacrificed "without carrying the case to the nearest and wisest medical supreme court possible." Atkinson indicated that if the former claim were true "no fetus may under any circumstances be destroyed, to save maternal life or for any other end, and the loss, however accidental, of the product of conception, however early, must be followed by a coroner's inquest and a trial by jury."[41]

Atkinson then provided his explanation of why "society" limited destruction of the fetus to situations where there was "physical danger to the mother." He not only mentioned the mother's greater right to life than the fetus, but indicated there was a second reason: "the chances of adding to the race are greater if the mother is saved than if the fetus survive [sic]." "Manifestly, then," Atkinson continued, "the real legal status of the fetus, i.e., its value to and claims upon society are determined by and precisely commensurate with the potential acquisition by society of a new member—just that and nothing more." "The protection accorded the fetus in utero is not accorded as the inalienable right to its own life and person, such as inheres to an individual who has completed the uterine period of his existence," he elaborated, "but as a safeguard to the physical perpetuity of the race."[42]

Atkinson saw a need for additional indications for abortion:

If, as has been demonstrated, sociology regards the fetus sheerly in the light of a potential addition to society, and recognizes physical conditions under which an abortion, at the discretion of a council of medical men, is not only permissible but imperative, it is only a pious cant which will shrink from the suggestion that there may possibly be other conditions which, at the discretion of a council of intelligent laymen (a jury for instance) might render an abortion, properly performed, a legitimate and even laudable act.[43]

Like Sanders, Atkinson provided a summary with numbered items. Number 7 through the final Number 10 all dealt with society's need for additional indications for abortion and "for a readjustment of the whole sentiment and legislation on the subject." He claimed "no such scientific or moral barriers stand in the way of such readjustment as we are popularly taught to believe."[44]

Atkinson thus can be considered a pioneer in calling for non-medical indications for induced abortion. He was listed as "Associate Professor of Physiology and Neurology, American College of Medicine and Surgery, Chicago." His later publications dealt primarily with testing and correction of vision. These specialties suggest he was not inducing abortions for medical or non-medical reasons and it remains a mystery why he made this "bald violation of prevailing sentiment" as Atkinson himself proudly referred to his position four years later.[45]

Charles Sumner Bacon undoubtedly had Atkinson in mind when he made the case that despite lacking some functions like respiration that occur after birth, the unborn child "is still a living being and as much an independent existence as, for example, an intestinal parasite which depends on its host for protection and nourishment."[46] This was in Bacon's Chairman's Address to the Section on Obstetrics and Diseases of Women at the Annual Meeting of the American Medical Association in May 1906.

Bacon admitted that the unborn child did not have the same legal protection as "human beings *ex utero*." The laws in most states and countries allowed the taking of the unborn's life under certain circumstances, particularly when it was necessary to prevent the death of the mother. Although the physician would not face prosecution if he believed abortion was necessary to preserve the life of the mother, Bacon recommended he "fortify his opinions by consultation with a reputable colleague."[47] His conclusion echoed his comments at the November 1904 Symposium:

It is difficult to deny to the human fetus the innate right of every human being the equal right to life. On the protection of this moral law the child *in utero* must chiefly rely for its preservation. The moral responsibilities of the physician for the child *in utero* are greater than his legal responsibilities.[48]

CHAPTER 28

MORE CONDEMNATIONS OF ABORTION AND ABORTIONISTS

Albert VanderVeer, Professor of Surgery at Albany Medical College, read a paper, "Spontaneous and Criminal Abortion From a Medico-Legal Point of View," in April 1906. The thrust of his paper was that abortionists needed to be convicted but that evidence against them was difficult to obtain. He presented three cases where instruments used for criminal abortion had passed through the uterus into the peritoneal cavity. Two involved bougies inserted months or years prior to the surgery that finally removed these sources of pain and other symptoms. A glass rod was used in the third case and peritonitis led to the woman's death, despite the surgical efforts to save her.[1]

VanderVeer discussed the difficulty of obtaining evidence to convict abortionists.

> Take for instance, Case I, where it was absolutely impossible to secure an admission from the husband or wife as to what had been done. They would not even admit that an attempt had been made to bring on an abortion.
>
> Again in Case II, until the evidence was presented to the husband and wife they would not admit in the slightest degree having unlawful treatment; but when confronted with the fact they were sufficiently overcome to tell all, even the name of the physician, a man living in an adjoining State. While the State laws are fairly severe in reaching such cases yet in this case there was no evidence presented, and the physician's testimony in defending himself was taken on the same basis as that of the party who wished to incriminate him.[2]

VanderVeer also discussed the huge risk that women subjected themselves to with "each effort to bring about a criminal abortion." He indicated that the most skilled treatment of these self-induced abortions frequently was insufficient to save the women. He then discussed the use of aseptic surgery by some abortionists for women of "the middle, and particularly the wealthy classes." Although these women typically did not die, VanderVeer claimed they were subject to serious illnesses, ectopic pregnancies, and habitual abortion that prevented a later desired full-term pregnancy.

He concluded:

> Beyond a doubt, men in our profession, and lay women who are possessed of skill in this practise, and professional abortionists, however they may have acquired their knowledge, should be prosecuted, when-

ever they are under suspicion, with the utmost severity. From a medico-legal standpoint they are criminals, and the members of our profession cannot be too thorough in obtaining evidence to fasten this crime upon the guilty parties.[3]

Another call for ridding the profession of abortionists came from the Kansas physician, R.H. McDonnell, in a paper presented on April 26, 1906.[4] McDonnell began by showing how the rate of increase in population in the United States had dropped sharply after 1880. He indicated that Abraham Lincoln in his message to Congress on December 1, 1862 predicted on the basis of the rate of increase up to that point that there would be 103,208,415 inhabitants in the country in 1900. The actual 1900 census figure was 76,303,387. McDonnell next noted that Kansas showed an annual increase of only three-tenths of a percent from 1890 to 1900.[5] He continued:

> I have submitted my figures to you for the purpose of demonstrating how often the crime of abortion is committed and what it means to the State and Nation. If some means are not found to prevent, or at least check it, the downfall of the Republic is certain. Because of the diffi-culty to convict, the law seems unable to reach the men who daily mur-der unborn infants, not only in the State, and Nation, but here at home as well, and I am convinced that a large percent of these crimes are committed in the inner rooms of the physician's office.[6]

McDonnell discussed physicians' noble mission and the praise that was due the man who "lives a life and does a work that makes him an honor to the profes-sion." On the other hand, the physician who produced criminal abortions was "worthy only of contempt, and should be forced out of the profession, even if the law can not hunt him out and give him the imprisonment he deserves."[7]

Another call for ridding the profession of abortionists was the editorial, "AMONG OURSELVES WE FREELY DISCUSS IT," in the *Journal of the Michigan State Medical Association*.[8] It began:

> One evening during the past month, there appeared in the *Detroit Jour-nal*, a shameful paragraph, which purported to be the statement, made to the police, by a certain physician in Detroit, who had been appre-hended for performing a criminal abortion. The physician is quoted as follows:
>
> "There is nothing out of the way about that. It may be legally wrong, but morally there isn't anything the matter with it, as long as there is no life at stake. We do that kind of thing right along and while we physicians may publicly deny it, among ourselves we freely discuss it and admit our work along that line."
>
> One statement in the above is as true as the others are damnably false. "Among ourselves we *are* freely discussing it;" we are discussing

what shall be done with just such criminals as this physician is alleged to be. But are we doing anything to prevent it?[9]

The editor's answer was "No," despite the high and increasing rate of abortions he claimed were occurring. He called for "the great weeklies, such as *Colliers* and *The Ladies' Home Journal*," to take on the problem of criminal abortion as they had recently taken on "its little sister evil, the use of patent medicines." The *Detroit Free Press* was criticized for a dozen advertisements for abortionists and abortifacients and other advertisements with more veiled descriptions for the same services and items.

The editor claimed that there were physicians in every city of the state that "habitually perform abortions." He continued: "We keep them—usually—out of our medical societies, but thereafter wash our hands of them and let them go their own way, plying their nefarious trade, unmolested. 'Among ourselves we freely discuss it,' and that is all."[10] He claimed it was physicians' duty to correct this and called for a committee of the State Society to study the problem and to appoint sub-committees throughout the state. These sub-committees would oversee symposia on criminal abortion in county societies and request local papers and post office authorities to end the objectionable advertisements. The editor concluded: "In these and in other ways, some good might perhaps be accomplished. Anyhow, we ought to do more than 'to freely discuss it among ourselves.'"[11]

Henry Orlando Marcy, provided a paper, "Education as a Factor in the Prevention of Criminal Abortion and Illegitimacy," at the American Medical Association's Annual Meeting in 1906. Marcy called for teaching young men and women about the dangers of premarital intercourse and the dangers to the woman's health if abortion were induced. Marcy claimed married women were frequent seekers of abortion and echoed the claim of scores of physicians that "this type of wrong in the community is greater in the so-called higher classes of society."[12]

He described the case of one married woman who requested abortion and the subsequent similar requests of her friends:

> My reasoning with the young wife was fruitless. "If I did not care for her there were others whom she knew whose services would avail." Thinking a little delay might bring about a better reasoning, I gave her a placebo with very careful instructions how she should take her medicine. On her way home she met with a slight railroad accident, the jar and fright inducing a miscarriage. She showed her gratitude by sending to me one after another of her friends, I think seven in number, who insisted in having the same prescription that I had given Mrs. X., and not one of them could be convinced that, if I only would, I could [not] easily produce a similar safe result.[13]

Marcy claimed the case illustrated that "the average women" viewed termination of an undesired pregnancy "of so little importance that it will not be seriously estimated as a criminal offence."[14]

Marcy's admission that he had administered a placebo instead of totally rejecting the young wife's abortion request no doubt led her to conclude that unnecessary abortion was legitimate. At least seven other women learned the same lesson from Marcy's action. This supports William McCollom's decade-earlier claim that such physician behavior was contributing to the prevalence of criminal abortion. Marcy's experience also shows the power of word-of-mouth advertising of abortion providers. The abortionist would undoubtedly become widely known and heavily patronized without the need for newspaper advertisements. Competition *between* abortionists for the lucrative trade may have been the reason such advertising was prevalent.

An Illinois physician, H.A. Pattison, read a paper, "Abortion," to the Macoupin County Medical Society on April 25, 1907.[15] Pattison made a positive reference to William H. Sanders' "The Physiologic and Legal Status of the Fetus in Utero," apparently agreeing to have the child "born" at conception and only "delivered" at birth.[16] He claimed that abortion at any period after conception was "a crime against life and against society." Pattison cited as "proof" the hypothetical case of "an obscure family named Lincoln" living in a Kentucky log cabin.

> The mother of this family had many duties and cares. At a certain time she became pregnant. Suppose that for some reason she felt it too much to go through the long period of gestation, the perils of maternity, and the cares of motherhood, and had submitted to an abortion. Abraham Lincoln would never have been born, and that obscure woman would have committed the greatest crime ever perpetrated against this republic.[17]

Pattison then discussed the more typical applicant for abortion, his reaction to one of these, and a suggestion to prevent a *second* criminal abortion:

> These women are intelligent, educated. They are kind, thoughtful, unselfish. They will protect a child or an animal. They are never cruel. Yet they will murder or permit to be murdered the child *in utero*. It is because they do not realize the enormity of their wickedness. They must be taught. It is largely through the family physician that this instruction must come. The teaching will often fail to produce immediate results. A single success is worth the required patience.
>
> During the first months of my practice a young woman, recently married, came to me with a request that I terminate a pregnancy. After pointing out the dangers and the moral factors involved, I told her I hoped she would call upon me again in about seven months, when I would gladly help her. I forgot the incident. Some months after, I received a note from a woman in a neighboring town, asking me to attend her in confinement. When I called upon her, her face seemed familiar and I finally recalled her previous visit to my office. I had the satisfaction of delivering a large healthy boy of whom his parents are justly proud.

A young married woman of culture and refinement suggested to me that in all cases of criminal abortion where the fetus is large enough to show the form of the child it should be shown to the mother who permitted the crime. This, my friend believes, would serve to deter the woman from committing the same crime again.[18]

J.H. Lyons gave the President's Address, "The Moral Qualifications of the Physician," to the Washington State Medical Association at its September 1907 meeting. He began by pointing out the physician's important role as a provider of moral guidance and claimed that the medical schools were not preparing physicians to provide such guidance.[19] He quickly moved to craniotomy and abortion and admitted that the physician had the legal authority to sacrifice the life of the unborn child. "But no one, I hope, will have the temerity to claim that the mere fact of being permitted by law to do an act," he continued, "makes that act morally right."[20]

Lyons claimed that "thousands of innocent lives" were "sacrificed every year." He indicated these lives were ended "not in wantonness, but in pity, and from the purest though mistaken motives, because the physician does not recognize the application of the law which says 'Thou shalt not kill.'" "The mere fact of the existence of a human being carries with it the right to a continuance of that existence," he continued, "and this is an inalienable right, a natural right which is incorporated in every fiber of our being, and no one, not even the physician, can justly deprive a human being of that right."[21]

Lyons described the unique role and duty of the physician "to aid in overthrowing this evil." He claimed the "lecturer on the platform" and clergyman could "declaim against the crime," but the "special application" was "rarely made."

With the physician, however, the conditions are different. In the privacy of the chamber, or the seclusion of the doctor's consultation room, with none but the guardian angels of the unborn child to hear, the physician as her trusted friend has the opportunity to explain the great physical wrong contemplated, and then to reinforce it with the oral reasons which she cannot assail. But he should go farther. It is his duty to give her a new idea of life and its duties. He should explain to her her duty to society, to humanity, and to herself. She needs to be taught that life is no longer a time for play or mere pleasure, that she has entered upon the serious duties of life, and that the discomforts, or even the dangers incident to the pregnant state are inseparable from her position in life.[22]

Lyons admitted that sometimes "interruption of gestation" was necessary, but in his "more than twenty years" the necessity never occurred. He also had never seen a woman who died because an abortion was not performed, "though I have seen many, very many, who lost their health and their lives because of such procedures."[23]

He concluded:

> No woman, however, goes to the professional abortionist first. She always consults her family physician first. The opportunity, then, is his to place her on the right road. Show her the physical danger as well as the moral wrong, and if he but will, he may impart a lesson which will never be effaced. True, he will fail in some cases, but in many, very many cases, he has the opportunity of saving the young woman for her home and for herself.[24]

Lyons surely was wrong that no woman ever went to the abortionist first. Most married women were aware of who would provide abortions and who would not. The "young woman" he referred to may not yet have learned where *not* to go to get an abortion.

At the same meeting, C.N. Suttner presented "A Plea for the Protection of the Unborn." He discussed the high prevalence of criminal abortion and claimed "we are daily asked to perform the crime. Often they come asking about a fee, saying Dr. W. will do it for so much, and so forth."[25]

He reported that he had kept a record of 97 women who had come to him requesting abortion "during the last nine years." He had advised them "correctly." The unmarried should marry or if that were not possible go to "a foundling asylum conducted by the sisters." The married should "abide by their vow." Only 21 followed his advice.

> The others—what became of their unborn babes? Some of these women I found in hospital, when I was naively told by the nurse, "Oh! They had a currettement." Or others, when stopped and quizzed, would say: "I did not need one of you doctors," and haughtily walked away. One young lady of the upper class consented to go to a maternity, and hid her shame for seven months; when her brother found out her condition, he promptly got the doctor! But where is the child? She is again in society.[26]

Suttner discussed another married woman whose contraception failed. She consulted one of the "hyenas with the title of M.D." who supported her abortion request with the claim that her pelvic diameter was too small to bear a child. He and a colleague intervened and "by facts and threats" convinced her to go to term. "I believe that we should be as proud of saving a child from the modern Herod," he continued, "as of curing it of the rabies, or of cerebro-spinal meningitis." He also indicated that the profession's "accomplishments of pathology, surgery, etc." were less important than opposing "by word and deed" "the murder of the innocents, and the prevention of their conception."[27]

A Milwaukee physician, Wilhelm Becker, provided a unique discussion of abortion, abortionists, and public attitudes toward abortion in a paper presented to his State Medical Society on June 24, 1908.[28] Becker included a history of abortion and indicated that American Indian tribes practiced abortion. "Some of the 'medicine men' enjoy a considerable reputation as abortionists," he continued, "even among white people."[29] Becker also claimed the Hippocrates of the Hippocratic Oath "once performed an abortion upon an actress."[30] This was in error, although the error may not have become known by American physicians for a few more decades. As was discussed in Chapter 2, the gynecologist, Alan F. Guttmacher, was fully aware that a different physician than Hippocrates of Cos was involved in the entertainer's miscarriage, but still made the erroneous claim in the 1950s.

Becker discussed "three distinct varieties of habitual abortionists." First was the family physician, "forced into abortions by sheer necessity." He claimed physicians lost "family after family because of their stand against performing abortions." Following the refusal, the woman "shows no increase in her rotundity" and "when Bobbie, her first-born is taken with the whooping-cough, Dr. Y, another highly esteemed general practitioner, has charge of the case." "It requires a character of adamant," Becker continued, "and an ample supply of the necessities of life to withstand these temptations."[31]

The second variety was the professional and he came in two types:

A, the "ethical" one, is a member of the various medical societies but is careful not to put in a personal appearance, particularly after his reputation as an abortionist has become well established. Everyone knows him as an abortionist but there is no documentary evidence against him. In the meantime he is building flats and, owing to his financial standing, is never at a loss for a friend to help him out of scrapes by operative skill or writing a death certificate. ...

Sub-division B is the full-fledged, professional, out-and-out abortionist. ... He has a standing "ad" in the paper that he will "relieve ladies in trouble." He has his agents all over the state. He belongs to a well-organized association, the "Abortion Trust," and furnishes the majority of the fatal cases—he and the midwife. He performs not only real abortions, but imaginary ones. His female agent, usually a young semi-prostitute, "ropes in" an unsophisticated young man of good family at a dance hall or similar resort; later she shams a pregnancy and prevails upon him to take her to a doctor of whom she has heard, to take away the product of conception. The young man is thereby fleeced of a hundred dollars, more or less. I know of one instance in which a young man employed in a public office was blackmailed out of town by this procedure.[32]

Becker noted that these men often had memberships in "respectable, secret, protective societies." This fact would be mentioned to juries when they came to trial and prevented convictions. He also noted that one of these abortionists was attempting to obtain a political position in the city Health Office. "His avowed aim is the investigation of abortion cases," Becker continued, "and the subsequent exoneration of the perpetrators of the crime, providing they are *personae gratae with him*."[33]

Becker continued:

> The third variety is the midwife, the directress of the lying-in hospital. The proportion of fatalities in consequence of abortions performed by midwives, is comparatively small. Owing to their cheap rates these women are in great demand and do an enormous business. The respectable middle classes, especially the married women, are their patrons. These midwives are solicited by doctors, eminent and obscure, surgeons and internists, to give them their work when they get into trouble. The author, who once cured one of these "ladies" of a case of constipation, was offered, in grateful return, the lucrative medical attendance of her cases in trouble. Heretofore, she volunteered, she had given all of her cases to Dr. So-and-so, and only once in a great while one of her patients died. Are we sincere in our endeavor to exterminate the practice of abortion?[34]

Becker discussed economic pressures that produced abortion throughout the world and throughout the ages and he included "our latitude and age." In addition, there was the "disgrace fixed upon unwedded maternity" that was causing most of the deaths of women following abortion.[35] Next came the current "moral attitude and its development."

> Are not abortions a very common theme of drawing-room conversation? Do women hide the fact of their having been performed on them? When they related these miscarriages, do they hesitate to answer whether they were "brought on" or spontaneous? The following incident, which is based upon fact, may give you an idea. After the conviction of a certain abortionist, in which case I was one of the witnesses, an unmarried woman, a school-teacher who was being treated by me, took me to task in the name of a number of her colleagues for having been instrumental in convicting the "poor benefactor of womankind." At my surprise and wonderment, which I manifested in the question whether the young woman needed a benefactor of that kind, she merely shrugged her shoulders. Stimulated by this incident, I canvassed the opinion of all the women with whom I came in contact, and with the very few exceptions of some old women beyond child-bearing age, they were, one and all, eager to express their sympathy for the convicted abortionist.
>
>   This brings us to the difficulty of convictions of abortionists. The first great factor is the moral anesthesia of the public toward abortions. It is my firm belief that even his lordship, the King's high prosecutor, should he get a decent girl into the family way, would appeal to his friend the doctor, to interrupt that pregnancy. And what can be expected of a jury composed of mere men, burdened with human frailties, and above all under the influence of their wives?[36]

Becker concluded with a recommendation that society drop its condemnation of illegitimate pregnancy and provide strong support for these women. This included teaching "wives and daughters to regard their less fortunate sisters as their perfect equals."[37] Following the supportive discussion of his paper, Becker returned to this theme:

> If it were not for these customs, bred by hypocrisy, and fostered by selfishness of those safely harbored in the haven of wedlock, most of these girls would carry their pregnancy to term. Negotiations would then be opened with the relatives of the father, which would frequently end in the consummation of lawful marriage.[38]

Another article claiming current increases in criminal abortion and, if anything, decreases in physician opposition, was "Criminal Abortion in Its Broadest Sense."[39] This was Walter B. Dorsett's Chairman's Address before the Section on Obstetrics and Diseases of Women of the American Medical Association. Dorsett noted that physicians were the ones who became aware of criminal abortions. "Possessing the information that we undoubtedly do," he continued, "should it not be our duty as citizens, as well as physicians, and members of this important branch of the great American Medical Association, to suggest some means for the suppression of an evil that threatens such an onslaught to our civilization?" He indicated that clergymen also were aware of the "enormity of the crime" through their bedside visits to the victims of the abortionist. Despite this knowledge, Dorsett claimed they were unwilling to shock "the delicate feelings of a fashionably dressed congregation."[40]

Dorsett described the "fashionable or fad doctor" and his work:

> This fad doctor is one with a lucrative practice, and is often "the lion" at social functions. He it is who empties the uterus in cases of emesis gravidarum without first racking his precious brain in trying all recognized remedies and methods to check the vomiting. He it is who finds so many cases of contracted pelvis, where it is utterly impossible to do anything but an early abortion to save the woman's life. He it is who finds so many cases of retention of menses, that require dilatation and curetment. He it is who finds the urine "loaded with albumin," necessitating an immediate emptying of the uterus to prevent death from Bright's disease. Such men and women prostitute the profession of medicine and should be exposed.[41]

Dorsett claimed the medical schools were failing to teach medical ethics and specifically the enormity of the crime. He contrasted "the Hippocratean teaching of the ancients" with current schools' "utter disregard as to the morals of their students." The graduate faced with little or no income eventually succumbed to the requests to procure abortion "and often drops into the practice."[42]

"Much has been said by the chief executive of our nation on race suicide, and much has been reiterated by other right thinking people;" Dorsett continued, "still, little has been done toward the enactment of new laws or the enforcement of those already on the statute books to punish those guilty of the crime."[43] Dorsett then cited various estimates of the high prevalence of criminal abortions, including 100,000 in New York, and 6,000 to 10,000 annually in Chicago. He continued:

> With feticide among our best element, and with a constantly increasing influx of degenerates from foreign countries, what can be expected of us as a nation a few generations hence? We, physicians, above all others, are best prepared to answer the query.
>
> It is not my purpose to institute utopian plans, through or by which criminal abortion can be suppressed, still some suggestions may be in order.
>
> 1. The obligatory teaching of medical jurisprudence and medical ethics in its true sense in our medical colleges. This should be statutory, and medical examining boards should be empowered to enforce the laws of their states, and declare all schools not requiring a full course in medical ethics not in good standing and their graduates ineligible to practice medicine.
>
> 2. The enactment of good and sufficient laws and the amendment of insufficient laws now on our statute books.[44]

Dorsett then described research a lawyer had conducted for him which showed that women seeking or performing self-abortions were guilty of no crime in 35 of the states and territories, that 30 states had no laws prohibiting selling of abortive drugs, that one fifth of the states and territories made the crime of abortion depend on the age of the fetus, that there was a wide range of penalties when the woman died as a result of abortion, that 32 states had no law that took a physician's license away for performing an abortion, and that only one state, Missouri, had a law that allowed a physician to testify about an abortion he had discovered in a patient. He claimed these laws were "inefficient and inadequate in most, if not all, of our states." He called on the American Medical Association to take steps to improve them:

> Let us, the members of this section through our representative in the House of Delegates appeal to this body and request the president of the American Medical Association to appoint a committee to be known as the Committee on Criminal Abortion, whose duties shall be to see that the state societies have appointed similar committees, whose duty it shall be to enlist the interest of their state legislatures in the enactment of good and sufficient laws against criminal abortion, and that this committee of the House of Delegates report annually as to the status of laws on criminal abortion in the different states, as well as what suggestions they may have to make in the prosecution of the crime.[45]

There is a striking parallel between Dorsett's and Horatio Storer's recommendations for national and state society action to improve abortion statutes. However, Dorsett did not mention Storer, whose major efforts were a half-century in the past.

The following Resolutions of Dorsett's Section were presented to the House of Delegates at the same Annual Meeting:

> *Resolved*, That the subject of the Chairman's address be referred to the House of Delegates, and that this body be and is hereby requested to appoint a standing committee which shall be called the National Committee on Criminal Abortion, whose duty shall be to investigate the laws on criminal abortion as they now appear on the statute books of the different states and territories of the Unites States, and to request all state and territorial medical societies to appoint like committees whose duty shall be to confer with the attorneys general of their states and territories, in the enactment of new and adequate laws governing criminal abortion. Be it further
>
> *Resolved*, That the state and territorial committees shall confer with the said National Committee on Criminal Abortion, in cooperation with the National Committee on Medical Legislation, shall report annually to the House of Delegates what progress has been made in the several states and territories toward the suppression of criminal abortion, as well as what suggestions they may have to make as to prosecution of the cause.[46]

The House of Delegates referred them to the Reference Committee on Hygiene and Public Health.[47] This Committee provided a Supplemental Report recommending that no action be taken to establish this National Committee on Criminal Abortion, since "it is within the purview of the Committee on Medical Legislation." The Association concurred with this recommendation.[48] This failure to generate a new Committee on Criminal Abortion may indicate that even those physicians who were active in the American Medical Association were losing fervor in their opposition to criminal abortion.

The Milwaukee physician, E.F. Fish, discussed the pressures to perform abortion that the young physician faced.[49] His article included the following reference to claims that "fifty percent of the profession are abortionists" and to a "hypnotic influence" that Fish himself appears to have experienced:

> He tells her to "go" and meets her a couple of weeks later on the street, only to learn that somebody had done the deed. This thing occurs three or more times during the first months of his practice. When finally, hungry, penniless, his clothing threadbare, his rent due, a case presents itself and he yields to the temptation—because he needs the money; because he is told that unless he takes it another will, and he has learned this is too true, because he has heard that a large percentage of the profession is more or less tainted; because he has read the transactions or been present at a meeting of the Wisconsin State Medical Society where it was freely and publicly said that fifty percent of the profession are abortionists; and

finally, he sometimes yields because he simply cannot help it on account of hypnotic influence difficult to describe.[50]

No other estimate of the fraction of physicians who were abortionists has been located that approached this "freely and publicly" announced estimate that this was true of half of Wisconsin's physicians.

A "largely attended meeting of the Medical and Chirurgical Faculty" in Baltimore on May 15, 1909 included a series of Resolutions on Criminal Abortion. These were offered by the renowned gynecologist, surgeon, and co-founder of Johns Hopkins Hospital, Dr. Howard Atwood Kelly, and "after several earnest speeches, were unanimously adopted with great applause." They included:

> "Resolved, That we to-day, believing that there exists an increasing laxity in public morality and an increase in the crime of abortion, do further declare that we consider the act to be equivalent to murder in the first degree when not imperative to save the prospective mother from death or extreme illness. We hereby express our extreme abhorrence of the act at the same time that we hold the man or the woman, whether in high or low social position, as a criminal fit only for the penitentiary. Furthermore, be it
>
> "Resolved, That we request each member of the Medical and Chirurgical Faculty to take all possible means to stamp out this vile practice and to assist in bringing every abortionist to the bar of public justice.
>
> "Resolved, That we request all our members not only to refrain from any and every act by any possibility to be construed as complicity, but to abandon a merely negative position and sedulously strive to quicken the public conscience until the people themselves take an aggressive attitude toward infant murder in all its forms."[51]

A Columbus, Ohio physician, A.B. Davenport, read a long paper, "Criminal Abortion," before the Columbus Academy of Medicine on May 29, 1909.[52] Davenport echoed the traditional medical condemnation of criminal abortion claiming it was a crime against "the child," "the mother," "the relatives, and last, but not least, against the commonwealth."[53] He estimated the frequency of criminal abortion to be as high as one for every five or six pregnancies and noted its prevalence in all classes of society but "particularly the upper classes."[54] He was personally aware of a woman who had ten criminal abortions in five years. He saw the crime "constantly increasing in our cities, and to a less extent in the villages."[55]

On excuses given by women for criminal abortion, he cited the usual "save the honor" of the unmarried and noted that this was "ignoring the fact that the pearl of great price has already been lost."[56] For the married there were the too large family, too little income, social demands, travel plans, etc.[57] He indicated there were legitimate health reasons for induced abortion and cited the contracted pelvis, excessive vomiting, and threatened kidney disease. "While some of the conditions enumerated *may* be sufficient to justify interference," Davenport continued, "they are too often made to serve as an excuse for what is simply criminal practice."[58] He indicated that in his nineteen years of practice had never needed to terminate a pregnancy for any of these reasons.

Davenport emphasized that regular physicians were "the most active of all in committing the crime." "These are the men we must reach in our own profession,' he continued, "and after we have done so we may rest assured the law will take care of others engaged in criminal work."[59] He called for prosecution of physician abortionists and, if they were members of medical societies, "utterly cast them out, for they deserve nothing better at your hands." "They have trailed the garment of our profession in the dust," he continued, "and have soiled it with innocent blood."[60] Davenport's and scores of other physicians' condemnations of such regular physician abortionists clearly contradict modern claims that physicians were opposing criminal abortion largely as a means to eliminate those who did not have regular medical degrees.

Like McCollom, Davenport decried the giving of placebos to women requesting abortion.

> The law considers the intent, no matter what the methods or results may be, and he who gives a placebo in order to gain time in which to convince the patient of the error of her ways is treading upon dangerous ground; besides, the effect upon the patient is such that she thinks that the physician is willing to commit the crime, and if he fails it is through no fault of his; for lo! hath he not tried?[61]

Davenport then described the proper means for dealing with the woman requesting an abortion:

> The only thing to do is to have a heart-to-heart talk with her, and make clear your position in the matter, and impress upon her the moral and physical wrong she would inflict upon herself and her unborn child. ... He should clearly indicate the present as well as the future dangers attending the commission of the act. Often those deficient in moral sense are keenly alive to the proper presentation of the physical dangers awaiting them in thwarting nature's laws.[62]

Davenport praised the Catholic clergy for their "clear and emphatic" teaching about criminal abortion and contrasted "the seeming indifferent attitude" of most Protestant ministers.

> It is rare, indeed, to hear a single word directed from the pulpit toward this great social and moral evil. It is not because the ministry is in ignorance of the prevalence of the crime, for their ministrations at the bedside have brought them full knowledge; or that it is not in violation of secular, moral and divine law—none of these. The most charitable construction I can place upon their silence is *ministerial cowardice*.[63]

Canada continued to have its share of criminal abortions. An editorial, "Does

It Pay? No!," in the May 1909 *Canada Lancet* gave several reasons why physicians should not perform criminal abortions.[64] Most dealt with lowering oneself in the eyes of the profession, the public, and the doctor's "own estimation." In addition, the clientele was undesirable and one was apt to be turned in to the authorities by the very persons who employed the doctor to perform the abortion. And when a good family persuaded the physician to procure an abortion for an errant daughter, they were apt to lose confidence in the physician who would do wrong and find another family physician. One suspects that this was received skeptically by his physician audience, given the many contradictory claims that physicians lost families when they *refused* to perform a requested abortion. Similar doubts may have greeted the editor's final reason for avoiding abortions. This was that one could obtain as much money from legitimate services.[65]

The Canadian physician, John Hunter, M.B., also stressed the disadvantages of being a physician abortionist in an article published in February 1910.[66] Hunter began with a glowing account of the medical profession and by noting the universal condemnation of criminal abortion by "reputable scientific medicine." He elaborated:

> The attitude of scientific medicine is now, and always has been, this, viz., that foetal life is never to be interfered with unless morbid physical conditions imperatively demand such interference. The destruction of the human embryo for selfish or mercenary purposes takes rank with the most cowardly and debasing of murders. Murder is usually committed, under abnormal conditions. The perpetrator is frenzied by passion, or drink. But criminal abortion by a physician is a deliberate plot, concocted by at least two, and often with others accessory to the crime.[67]

Hunter blamed the medical profession for its lenient treatment of abortionists.

> The abortionist performs the act, and then tells his victim: "Now, if anything goes wrong, call in your family physician. If he does suspect anything he won't say much about it, as you can tell him what a disgrace it would be to your family, etc., etc." Let the criminal abortionist find that his acts are altogether outside the bounds of professional sympathy, and he will soon recognize that his work is of an extremely dangerous character.[68]

Hunter pointed out how the young physician occupied a unique role in providing wise counsel. Young patients would be more apt to accept his advice than the advice of their minister or others. When this new physician was cultured and revered "Christianity, character, race and profession," there was no greater influence in the community for good. On the other hand:

The intemperate, immoral, foul-tongued, unscrupulous physician is as deadly a poison to the moral and physical well-being of society as septic matter is to the structures of the body. What is there in the life of the criminal abortionist to entice any reputable young physician to it! The crime is a cowardly, heinous, dangerous one. The pay is no compensation for such a crime and for such risks. He implicates others in a crime, the stain of which they can never wash away. The end of the abortionist's life is usually closed in poverty, disgrace and imprisonment.[69]

Hunter called on the older physicians to help make young physicians aware that "the act of criminal abortion is never the 'dernier resort' for even unmarried persons." He continued by indicating that all experienced physicians "can easily multiply instances where sympathy, tact and wise instructions—in the case of the married—have sent these women to endure their pregnant state bravely, and to give birth to children for whom in after years they would gladly lay down their own lives." Similar counsel by physicians to the unmarried "has brought about many a happy marriage, or the girls have met their fate heroically, and have made homes for themselves and their children."[70] These "multiple instances" of births that occurred because of physicians' "sympathy, tact and wise instructions," no doubt provided ancestors for a substantial proportion of the Canadians alive today.

Frederick Joseph Taussig published a book, *The Prevention and Treatment of Abortion*, in 1910.[71] It dealt primarily with clinical aspects of abortions of all types. However, he included a chapter, "Prevention of Criminal Abortion," that described the high frequency of criminal abortions and how the crime was "practically never punished." He claimed the high rate of criminal abortion was producing "one of the most serious sociological problems," and that "every community must in self-preservation enact laws and exert its utmost influence to stem this tide that will otherwise sweep it to destruction."[72]

Taussig recommended education and legislation as the means to "stem this tide." Education was essential to counter the "myth" that life began when the woman felt movements of the fetus. He continued:

A forceful treatise on the "Moral and Legal Status of the Fetus in Utero" was written by W. H. Sanders a few years ago, in which just this error was emphasized. Women of all classes should know more concerning the processes of gestation. They should be shown how early the fetal heart begins to pump blood through its vessels. They should be taught that in the first weeks, if not sooner, the sex is already determined.[73]

Taussig had arranged medical lectures for women "in one of the social settlements" of St. Louis and he indicated the women were amazed to discover the six-week embryo had discernible features. Taussig believed that such information "will keep many women from having an abortion." Women also would be discouraged from seeking abortion if they were made aware of the high dangers to health and life of induced abortion "even under modern antiseptic methods."[74]

Taussig next discussed the reasons current laws were not preventing the crime. Problems of obtaining evidence prevented some cases from reaching trial, and, when tried, prevented convictions. He believed that most abortions were performed by "disreputable" doctors and midwives and called for more stringent requirements for medical and midwife practice. He then proposed another requirement:

> I am firmly convinced that if every abortion, no matter what the cause, would have to be officially reported, it would prove a long step ahead in the way of correcting present evils. Moreover, independent of its effect upon this question, the government is entitled to know of the death of any living being, whether that being has advanced to full-term development or not. It is time that the antiquated ideas of modern law as to when life begins be modified in accordance with our present knowledge. Life begins with conception.[75]

Taussig also discussed therapeutic abortion. He claimed heart and kidney disease often were indications as was pulmonary tuberculosis. Persistent vomiting was an indication, but only after the patient showed signs of severe debilitation. He continued:

> Vomiting is at times brought on by the patient so as to influence the physician to hasten the emptying of the uterus. If this is suspected, the patient must be removed to a hospital and kept under constant watch. Fritsch mentions a patient who by persistent vomiting and by abstaining from food lost thirty-seven pounds in four weeks. After the doctor had finally felt compelled to do an abortion, she laughingly remarked to him that she could have refrained from vomiting if she had cared to.[76]

Taussig indicated marked narrowing of the birth canal was an indication, although the woman should be persuaded to have a Caesarian section instead.[77] Taussig's concern for the unborn child reappeared strongly when he discussed pelvic obstructions to birth:

> Where a fibroid or ovarian cyst, associated with pregnancy, is incarcerated in the pelvis, there is no reason for induction of abortion, but an indication for the operative relief of these tumors. At times the pregnancy will have to be sacrificed. Where the obstruction is an inoperable cancer of the cervix there is also no justification for interference, since here the mother's life is lost anyway and every effort must be made to get a living child by Caesarian section.[78]

The same general view about the importance of preserving the unborn child would be included in 1916 and 1931 articles by Taussig.[79] However, when he wrote a major book, *Abortion, Spontaneous and Induced, Medical and Social Aspects*, published in 1936, Taussig recommended much easier access to abortion and made little reference to his earlier strong antiabortion views. He would even refer to "the growing embryo" as "but a shapeless mass of cells," and claim that it wasn't "fair that the health of the mother or her usefulness in the social order be undermined by the development of this new being whose continued existence is so precarious and whose value to the world is relatively of such dubious importance."[80]

Taussig's change of perspective on the unborn child was one example of increased physician calls for liberalization of the indications for therapeutic abortion. A few physicians even called for outright legalization after 1910. Physician condemnations of abortion and abortionists continued, but at a lesser rate and they were more apt to come from the central and southern states. It is doubtful, however, that this reflected any decrease in criminal abortion and it may have reflected a further increase and increased physician awareness of the practice may have led to it being tolerated if not embraced. However, although Taussig would recommend consideration of socioeconomic factors in abortion decisions in the 1930s and 1940s, he at the same time was persuading his married patients who were seeking abortions to continue pregnancies and was successful at least half of the time.[81] He was not alone in trying to convince women to avoid abortion and it is probable that the fraction of children born as a result of such physician persuasion remained as high as it had been in the nineteenth century. Some *living* physicians of your mother and grandmother may deserve thank you notes.

AFTERWORD

Hopefully the book has made it clear that most physicians in the nineteenth century and first decade of the twentieth strongly opposed unnecessary abortion and opposed it primarily because of their concern about its unborn victims. In almost all of their papers and articles these physicians described the unnecessary destruction of the fetus as "murder" and many called for it to be punished as such.

We also hope to have successfully identified the key role that Horatio Robinson Storer played in making the medical profession aware of the new epidemic of unnecessary abortion and in motivating the strong physician lobbying that produced stringent laws against abortion in all of the states and territories. The other goal of the physicians' crusade was to make the public aware that a human being existed from conception, and Hugh Lenox Hodge, both Storers, and scores of later physicians emphasized that this was physicians' duty. The "public" for most physicians became the women, typically wives, who requested abortions. Numerous physicians wrote about their successes in convincing these women to bear their children. Birth certificates served to document the successes of thousands of their colleagues. Millions of children were added to the population that would have died in the womb without the new laws and the successful persuasion. If the reader with Protestant roots is not aware of the debt he owes to these physicians, he or she should return to the final paragraphs of Chapter 1.

Abortions still were common and physicians typically were perplexed that many of the women who sought and obtained abortions were not only married, but were compassionate and caring individuals in every other way. Several physicians claimed that the maternal instinct was proportional to the length of pregnancy. We noted a few contrary examples, but they probably were correct. It took the indoctrination of the Catholic confessional, the physicians' inner-office "confessional," or, for a few women, medical school, to make them consider an unwanted embryo or tiny fetus equivalent to a baby. On the other hand, when the pregnancy was welcomed such consideration no doubt was automatic.

The reader of this book also will be aware of the high rate of abortion for more than a century before *Roe v Wade*. One implication is that abortion surely would continue at substantial levels even if unnecessary abortions again became illegal. The pressure to avoid pregnancy, and if unsuccessful, to eliminate pregnancy, has so far shown itself to be too great. Education of the public to the value of all human life was proposed as the solution to the problem of unnecessary abortion by scores of physicians over more than a century and it still is a valid proposal. As H.A. Pattison put it in 1907: "A single success is worth the required patience." And as Horatio Storer noted four decades earlier: "every life saved is, as a general rule, the precursor of others that else would not have been called into existence."

After 1910, physicians' condemnations of abortion and abortionists were increasingly mixed with calls for reduced restrictions on abortion and even with a few pleas for total legalization. This reduced opposition to unnecessary abortion culminated with the 1967 calls for fewer restrictions on abortion by the American Medical Association and the American Psychiatric Association. However, neither Association asked for the virtual abortion on demand that followed *Roe v Wade* and the major pressure for that decision did not come from physicians.

Despite this later waning of the crusade against abortion, there were a number of bright spots. One was Seale Harris, the son of abortion-snare-defender Charles Harris, who provided a 1934 article that was one of the strongest condemnations of criminal abortion and abortionists ever written.[1] Another was the New Jersey obstetrician and hospital director, Samuel A. Cosgrove, who, in the 1940s and 1950s, embarrassed the nations' hospitals into sharply reducing their unnecessary "therapeutic" abortions.[2] Even the physicians like Frederick Joseph Taussig who supported liberal indications for abortion continued to persuade their married patients to continue unwanted pregnancies and many readers with births prior to the 1973 *Roe v. Wade* decision can be thankful that there still were significant remnants of the "physicians' crusade against abortion."

SELECTED BIBLIOGRAPHY

Banton, John Floyd. *Revolution in the Practice of Medicine* (Chicago: Review, Printing and Pub. Co., 1885).

Bedford, Gunning S. *The Principles and Practice of Obstetrics* (New York: William Wood & Co., 1874).

Brodie, Jane Farrell. *Contraception and Abortion in 19th Century America* (Ithaca: Cornell University Press, 1994).

Browder, Clifford. *The Wickedest Woman in New York: Madame Restell, The Abortionist* (Hamden, Connecticut: Archon, 1988).

Cooke, Nicholas Francis. *Satan in Society: By a Physician* (Cincinnati: C.F. Vent, 1876).

_____. *Licensed Foeticide* (Detroit: American Observer, 1879).

Cowan, John. *The Science of a New Life* (New York: J.S. Olgivie, 1918).

Cox, Edward, Homer O. Hitchcock, and Simeon S. French. "Report of the Special Committee on Criminal Abortion," *Report of the State Board of Health, Michigan 1881* (Lansing: W.S. George, 1882).

Coxe, A. Cleveland. *Moral Reforms Suggested in a Pastoral Letter with Remarks on Practical Religion* (Philadelphia: J.B. Lippincott, 1869).

Dworkin, Ronald. *Life's Dominion* (New York: Alfred A. Knoph, 1993).

Dyer, Frederick N. *Champion of Women and the Unborn: Horatio Robinson Storer, M.D.* (Canton, Massachusetts: Science History Publications/USA, 1999).

_____. "Autobiographical Letter from Horatio Robinson Storer, M.D., to His Son, Malcolm Storer, M.D., Discussing the "History of Gynaecological Teaching," *Journal of the History of Medicine* 54 (July 1999): 439-58.

Ellinger, Tage U.H. *Hippocrates on Intercourse and Pregnancy* (New York: Henry Schuman, 1952).

Fishbein, Morris. *History of the American Medical Association, 1847 to 1947* (Philadelphia: Lippincott, Grambo & Co., 1947).

Fowler, Orson Squire. *Creative And Sexual Science: Or, Manhood, Womanhood, And Their Mutual Interrelations; ... Etc., As Taught By Phrenology And Physiology* (Cincinnati: Cincinnati Publishing, Co., 1870).

Gardner, Augustus Kinsley. *Conjugal Sins Against the Laws of Life and Health and Their Effects upon the Father, Mother and Child* (New York: J.S. Redfield, 1870). Reprinted by (New York: Arno Press, 1974).

Hale, Edwin Moses. *On the Homoeopathic Treatment of Abortion* (Chicago: Halsey & King, Homoeopathic Pharmacy, 1860).

_____. *A Systematic Treatise on Abortion* (Chicago: C.S. Halsey, 1866).

_____. *The Great Crime of the Nineteenth Century, Why Is It Committed? Who Are the Criminals? How Shall They Be Detected? How Shall They Be Punished?* (Chicago: C.S. Halsey, 1867).

_____. *A Systematic Treatise on Abortion and Sterility* (Chicago: C.S. Halsey, 1868).

Hitchcock, Homer O. "Report on Criminal Abortion," *Fourth Annual Report of the Secretary of the State Board of Health of the State of Michigan* (Lansing: W.S. George & Co., 1876).

Hodge, Hugh Lenox. *An Introductory Lecture to the Course on Obstetrics and Diseases of Women and Children* (Philadelphia: Lydia R. Bailey, 1839).

_____. *Introductory Lecture* (Philadelphia: T.K. and P.G. Collins, 1854).

_____. *Fœticide, Or Criminal Abortion : A Lecture Introductory To The Course On Obstetrics And Diseases Of Women And Children, University Of Pennsylvania, Session 1839-40* (Philadelphia: Lindsay and Blakiston, 1869). Reprinted in *Abortion in Nineteenth Century America* (North Stratford, N.H.: Ayer, 1974).

Howe, Elijah Franklin. *Ante-Natal Infanticide* (Terre Haute: Allen & Andrews, 1869); Reprinted in *Abortion in Nineteenth Century America* (North Stratford, N.H.: Ayer, 1974).

Intrikin, Franklin Wayne. *Woman's Monitor* (Cincinnati: C.F. Vent, 1871).

Kass, Amalie M. *Midwifery and Medicine in Boston: Walter Channing, M.D. 1786-1876* (Boston: Northeastern University Press, 2002).

Kellogg, John Harvey. *Plain Facts For Old and Young* (Burlington: I.F. Segner, 1889).

_____. *The Home Hand-Book of Domestic Hygiene and Rational Medicine* (Battle Creek: Modern Medicine, 1903).

Kinney, Janet. *Saga of a Surgeon: The Life of Daniel Brainard, M.D.* (Springfield, Illinois: Southern Illinois School of Medicine, 1987).

Luker, Kristin. *Abortion and the Politics of Motherhood* (Berkeley: Univ. of California Press, 1984).

Mauriceau, A.M. *The Married Woman's Private Medical Companion,* ...(New York: 1847).

Mohr, James C. *Abortion in America: The Origins and Evolution of National Policy, 1800-1900* (New York: Oxford University Press, 1978).

_____. *Doctors and the Law* (New York: Oxford University Press, 1993).

LeProhon, Edward P. *Voluntary Abortion, or, Fashionable Prostitution, with Some Remarks upon the Operation of Craniotomy* (Portland: B. Thurston & CO., 1867).

Morantz-Sanchez, Regina. *Conduct Unbecoming a Woman* (New York: Oxford, 1999).

Napheys, George Henry. *The Physical Life of Woman: Advice to the Maiden, Wife and Mother* (Philadelphia: David McKay, 1890).

National Committee on Maternal Health, Inc., *The Abortion Problem* (Baltimore: Williams & Wilkins Co., 1944).

Nebinger, Andrew. *Criminal Abortion; Its Extent and Prevention,* (Philadelphia: Collins, Printer, 1870). Reprinted in *Abortion in Nineteenth Century America* (North Stratford, N.H.: Ayer, 1974).

Olasky, Marvin N. in *The Press and Abortion, 1838-1988* (Hillsdale, N.J.: Lawrence Erlbaum, 1988).
_____. *Abortion Rites: A Social History of Abortion in America* (Washington, D.C.: Regnery, 1995).
Percival, Thomas. *Medical Ethics* (Manchester: S. Russell, 1803).
Reagan, Leslie J. *When Abortion Was a Crime* (Berkeley: Univ. of California Press, 1997).
Ross, Ishbel. *The Life Story of the First Woman Doctor* (New York: Harper and Brothers, 1949).
Roosevelt, Theodore. *An Autobiography* (New York: Macmillan, 1913).
Ryan, Joseph Glennon Pierce. *Wrestling with the Angel: The Struggle of Roman Catholic Clergy, Physicians, and Believers with the Rise of Medical Practice, 1807-1940*, Ph.D. dissertation, American University, 1997.
Ryan, Michael. *A Manual of Medical Jurisprudence and State Medicine* (London: Sherwood, Gilbert and Piper, 1836).
Scott, James Foster. *The Sexual Instinct: Its Use and Dangers as Affecting Heredity and Morals: Essentials to the Welfare of the Individual and the Future of the Race* (Chicago: Login Brothers, 1930).
Smith-Rosenberg, Carroll. *Disorderly Conduct: Vision of Gender in Victorian America* (New York: Oxford, 1985).
Spalding, Martin J. *Pastoral Letter of The Most Rev. Archbishop ... May 1869* (Baltimore: John Murphy & Co., 1869).
Stockham, Alice B. *Tokology: A Book for Every Woman* (Chicago: Sanitary Publishing Co., 1885).
Storer, David Humphreys. *An Address on Medical Jurisprudence* (Boston: John Wilson & Son, 1851).
_____. *Address Delivered at the First Medical Commencement of the Massachusetts Medical College* (Boston: John Wilson and Son, 1855).
_____. *An Introductory Lecture before the Medical Class of 1855-56 of Harvard University* (Boston: David Clapp Printer, 1855).
Storer, Horatio Robinson. *On Criminal Abortion in America* (Philadelphia: Lippincott & Co., 1860).
_____. *Why Not? A Book for Every Woman* (Boston: Lee and Shepard, 1866). Reprinted in: *A Proper Bostonian on Sex and Birth Control* (New York: Arno Press, 1974).
_____. *Is It I? A Book for Every Man* (Boston: Lee and Shepard, 1867). Reprinted in: *A Proper Bostonian on Sex and Birth Control* (New York: Arno Press, 1974).
_____ and Franklin Fiske Heard. *Criminal Abortion: Its Nature, Its Evidence, and Its Law* (Boston: Little, Brown, and Co., 1868).
Taussig, Frederick J. *The Prevention and Treatment of Abortion* (St. Louis: C. V. Mosby, 1910).
_____. *Abortion—Spontaneous and Induced: Medical and Social Aspects* (St. Louis: C. V. Mosby, 1936).

Thomas, T. Gaillard. *Abortion and Its Treatment, From the Stand-Point of Practical Experience (*New York: Appleton and Company, 1892).

Todd, John. *Serpents in the Dove's Nest* (Boston: Lee and Shepard, 1867).

Van de Warker, Ely. *The Detection of Criminal Abortion and a Study of Foeticidal Drugs* (Boston: James Campbell, 1872). Reprinted in *Abortion in Nineteenth Century America* (North Stratford, N.H.: Ayer, 1974).

Wright, Henry Clarke. *The Unwelcome Child, or, the Crime of an Undesigned and Undesired Maternity* (Boston: B. Marsh, 1858).

NOTES

Foreword

[1] James C. Mohr, *Abortion in America: The Origins and Evolution of National Policy, 1800-1900* (cited hereafter as Mohr, *AIA*) (New York: Oxford University Press, 1978), pp. 147-170. Mohr named his Chapter Six, "The Physicians' Crusade Against Abortion," and credited Storer with starting the crusade.

[2] Ibid., pp. 200-25.

[3] These claims were made in Cyril J. Means, "The Law of New York Concerning Abortion and the Status of the Foetus, 1664-1968: A Case of Cessation of Constitutionality," *New York Law Forum* 14 (Fall, 1968): 411-515. Means served as general counsel for the National Association for the Repeal of Abortion Laws when he wrote this article. It was repeatedly cited in the *Roe v. Wade* majority opinion.

[4] "Brief of 281 Historians as Amici Curiae Supporting Appellees," *Webster v. Reproductive Health Services.*

[5] Mohr, *AIA*, p. 36.

[6] Ibid., pp. 160-64.

[7] Ibid., pp. 164-65

[8] Gerald V. Bradley, "Academic Integrity Betrayed," *First Things* (August/September 1990): 10-12. Ramesh Ponnuru, "Aborting History," *National Review* 47 (October 23, 1995): 29-32, 32.

[9] For Example, Ronald Dworkin, *Life's Dominion* (New York: Alfred A. Knoph, 1993), p. 112. Kristin Luker, *Abortion and the Politics of Motherhood* (Berkeley: Univ. of California Press, 1984), pp. 27-29. Jane Farrell Brodie, *Contraception and Abortion in 19th Century America* (Ithaca: Cornell University Press, 1994), pp. 269-70. Carroll Smith-Rosenberg, *Disorderly Conduct: Vision of Gender in Victorian* America, (New York: Oxford, 1985), p. 233. Leslie J. Reagan, *When Abortion Was a Crime* (Berkeley: Univ. of California Press, 1997), pp. 10-11.

[10] Frederick N. Dyer, *Champion of Women and the Unborn: Horatio Robinson Storer, M.D.* (cited hereafter as Dyer, *Champion*) (Canton, Massachusetts: Science History Publications/USA, 1999).

Chapter 1

[1] Horatio Robinson Storer (hereafter HRS), "Contributions to Obstetric Jurisprudence: No. I.—Criminal Abortion," *North-American Medico-Chirurgical Review* (hereafter *NAMCR*) 3 (1859): 64-72, 72. The "Burke and Hare" reference refers to William Burke and William Hare who were indicted in 1828 for 16 murders they carried out in Edinburgh, Scotland within a single year. The murders were highly salient to Horatio because of his year in medical training at the same Edinburgh University Medical School that had innocently bought the bodies of the murder victims for dissection by medical students.

[2] "Memorial. To the Governor and Legislature, ..." The Indiana State Archives has a copy of the "Memorial" sent to them in 1860.

[3] HRS, *Why Not? A Book for Every Woman* (Boston: Lee and Shepard, 1866); *Is It I? A Book for Every Man* (Boston: Lee and Shepard, 1867).

[4] HRS and Franklin Fiske Heard, *Criminal Abortion: Its Nature, Its Evidence, and Its*

Law (Boston: Little, Brown, and Co., 1868).

[5] Marvin Olasky denied this in his *Abortion Rites* published in 1992 (See Bibliography). He claimed that James Mohr was incorrect in reporting high rates of abortion for the married. Olasky did accept Mohr's claim that abortion decreased by the end of the century. Almost every chapter of the current book shows the predominance of married women obtaining abortions and Chapter 24 demonstrates that both Mohr and Olasky were wrong about a decrease by the end of the century.

[6] Hugh L. Hodge, *An Introductory Lecture to the Course on Obstetrics and Diseases of Women and Children* (Philadelphia: Lydia R. Bailey, 1839), p. 17. Mohr repeatedly claimed (*AIA*, pp. 149, 272 n. 34, 283 n. 1) that Hodge did not publish his lecture until 1854.

[7] Hugh L. Hodge, *Introductory Lecture* (Philadelphia: T.K. and P.G. Collins, 1854).

[8] John P. Leonard (hereafter JPL), "Quackery and Abortion," *Boston Medical and Surgical Journal* (hereafter *BMSJ*) 43 (January 15, 1851): 477-81.

[9] Ibid., p. 478.

[10] Ibid., p. 479.

[11] HRS, "Contributions to Obstetric Jurisprudence: No. I.—Criminal Abortion," pp. 64-72, 64n-65n.

[12] David Humphreys Storer (hereafter DHS), *An Introductory Lecture before the Medical Class of 1855-56 of Harvard University* (Boston: David Clapp Printer, 1855).

[13] DHS, "Two Frequent Causes of Uterine Disease," *Journal of the Gynaecological Society of Boston* (hereafter *JGSB*) 6 (March 1872): 194-203, 198-99.

[14] "Editorial Notes," *JGSB* 6 (May 1872): 393-400, 394.

[15] "An Introductory Lecture before the Medical Class of 1855-56 of Harvard University," *BMSJ* 53 (December 13, 1855): 409-11, 410-11.

[16] Frederick N. Dyer, "Autobiographical Letter from Horatio Robinson Storer, M.D., to His Son, Malcolm Storer, M.D., Discussing the "History of Gynaecological Teaching," (cited hereafter as Dyer, "Autobiographical Letter") *Journal of the History of Medicine* 54 (July 1999): 439-58, 444.

[17] Jesse Boring, "Foeticide," *Atlanta Medical and Surgical Journal* 2 (January 1857): 257-67, 259.

[18] Ibid., p. 258.

[19] Storer's early achievements are discussed in the first four chapters of Dyer, *Champion*.

[20] James Joseph Walsh, "American Physician Converts," *Catholic Convert* 4 (March 1917): 1-2, & 17, 17.

[21] "Editorial Notes," *JGSB* 2 (May 1870): 307-20, 314. "Gynaecological Society of Boston (hereafter GSB) Proceedings, meeting of May 17, 1870," *JGSB* 2 (June 1870): 380-92, 387.

[22] Mohr, *AIA*, p. 36.

[23] Ibid., p. 165.

[24] Ibid., p. 166.

[25] Ibid., pp. 160-64.

[26] The percentage of children being born as a result of the physicians' crusade is directly related to the number of women originally seeking abortion and to the number of these women who changed their minds because of the crusade. As will be seen, as many as 25 percent of pregnancies may have been ending in induced abortion in the middle of the nineteenth century. However, assume that without the new physician-passed laws or physician persuasion it would have been only 15 percent with 85 percent of pregnancies going to term. If 17 percent (approximately 1 of every 6) of these women who would have had abortions changed their minds because of the physicians' crusade, this would leave

12.45 percent of pregnancies ending in abortion and 87.55 percent of pregnancies going to term. The ratio of 87.55 to 85 is 1.03, i.e., there would have been 3 percent more children being born as a result of the crusade.

Chapter 2

[1] Alan F. Guttmacher, "Therapeutic Abortion: The Doctor's Dilemma," *Journal of the Mt. Sinai Hospital* 21 (October 1954): 111-21, 111.

[2] Tage U.H. Ellinger, *Hippocrates on Intercourse and Pregnancy* (New York: Henry Schuman, 1952), p. 15.

[3] Thomas Percival, *Medical Ethics* (Manchester: S. Russell, 1803).

[4] Thomas Percival, *The Works, Literary, Moral, and Medical of Thomas Percival, M. D.* (London: Crutwell, 1807) Vol. 2, pp. 430-31.

[5] John Brodhead Beck, "Infanticide," T.R. Beck and J.B. Beck, *Elements of Medical Jurisprudence* (Albany: Packard and Van Benthusen, 1835), pp. 271-448, 293.

[6] Walter Channing was Horatio's professor of medical jurisprudence and Channing "relied heavily" on Beck's text. See Amalie M. Kass, *Midwifery and Medicine in Boston: Walter Channing, M.D. 1786-1876* (Boston: Northeastern University Press, 2002), p. 123.

[7] HRS, "Contributions to Obstetric Jurisprudence: No. I.—Criminal Abortion," pp. 64-72, 64n.

[8] Beck, "Infanticide," pp. 290-91.

[9] Ibid., p. 291.

[10] Ibid., p. 311.

[11] Michael Ryan, *A Manual of Medical Jurisprudence and State Medicine* (London: Sherwood, Gilbert and Piper, 1836), p. 282.

[12] HRS, "Contributions to Obstetric Jurisprudence—Criminal Abortion IV: Its Proofs," *NAMCR* 3 (May 1859): 455-65, 459.

[13] DHS, *An Address on Medical Jurisprudence* (Boston: J. Wilson & Son, 1851), p. 4.

[14] DHS, "Two Frequent Causes of Uterine Disease," p. 195.

[15] HRS, "Contributions to Obstetric Jurisprudence—Criminal Abortion VII: Its Obstacles to Conviction," *NAMCR* 3 (September 1859): 833-54, 834.

[16] Discussed in Levin Smith Joynes, "Some of the Legal Relations of the Foetus in Utero," *Virginia Medical Journal* 7 (September 1856): 179-91.

[17] William Henry Brisbane to HRS, March 19, 1859, *Scrapbook of letters on abortion, 1857-1859* [B MS b47], Boston Medical Library in the Francis A. Countway Library of Medicine [hereafter Countway Scrapbook of letters on abortion]. Brisbane was a slave-holding cotton planter who became an abolitionist, Baptist pastor, physician, political activist, public official, farmer, writer, and editor-publisher. Born of aristocratic Scots in Beaufort District, South Carolina in 1806, he died in 1878 in Arena, the Wisconsin River town he founded.

[18] HRS, "Obstacles to Conviction," p. 834.

[19] James C. Mohr, "Beck, John Brodhead," *American National Biography* (New York: Oxford University Press, Vol. 1, 1999), pp. 436-37, 437.

[20] Mohr, *AIA*, p. 27.

[21] James C. Mohr, *Doctors and the Law* (New York: Oxford University Press, 1993), pp. 80-81.

[22] James C. Mohr, "Beck, John Brodhead," p. 437.

[23] "Criminal Abortionism in New York," *New York Medical Gazette* 1 (July 6, 1850), 6. Horatio cited the data in HRS, "Contributions to Obstetric Jurisprudence—Criminal

Abortion II: Its Frequency, and the Causes Thereof," *NAMCR* 3 (March 1859): 260-82, 267.

[24] Morris Fishbein, *History of the American Medical Association, 1847 to 1947* (Philadelphia: Lippincott, Grambo & Co., 1947), pp. 24-25.

[25] Gunning S. Bedford, "Vaginal Hystereotomy," *New York Journal of Medicine* 2 (March 1844): 199-203.

[26] Ibid., p. 202.

[27] "Criminal Abortions," *BMSJ* 30 (May 15, 1844): 302-3, 302.

[28] HRS to David Humphreys and Abby Jane Brewer Storer, August 21, 1844, Horatio Robinson Storer papers. Massachusetts Historical Society (hereafter MHS). Reproduced in Dyer, *Champion*, p. 11.

[29] "Procuring of Abortion. Commonwealth v. Luceba Parker," *American Journal of the Medical Sciences* (hereafter *AJMS*) 13 (April 1847): 491-492.

[30] Mohr, *AIA*, pp. 120-21.

[31] "Punishment of Criminal Attempts at Abortion," *BMSJ* 32 (February 12, 1845): 45.

Chapter 3

[1] George E. Gifford, "The Ichthyologist Dean," *Harvard Medical Alumni Bulletin* 39 (1964): 22-27.

[2] HRS, "Observations on the Fishes of Nova Scotia and Labrador, with Descriptions of New Species," *Boston Journal of Natural History* 6 (1850): 246-70, 253.

[3] Robert Buchanan, editor, *The Life and Adventures of John James Audubon the Naturalist* (New York: G.P. Putnam & Son, 1869), p. 322.

[4] Dyer, *Champion*, pp. 23, 28-30. Several other invitations are mentioned in Storer's "Russia/Harvard Journal" located at the MHS.

[5] Hermann Jackson Warner (hereafter HJW), diary entry, 14 June 1850, HJW papers, 1835-1913. MHS.

[6] Charles Girard, Text of unidentified speech read before the Harvard Natural History Society, June 14, 1850, Smithsonian Institution Archives: Record Unit 7190, Box 1, Folder 3.

[7] HRS, "Observations on the Fishes ...", p. 254.

[8] HJW, diary entry, 25 May 1850, HJW papers, 1835-1913. MHS.

[9] For additional evidence of the frequency of such early abortions, see Mohr, *AIA*, pp. 15-16.

[10] "Criminal Abortionism in New York," p. 6.

[11] Ibid.

[12] Ibid.

[13] Ibid. The "public press" included the *National Police Gazette* that published Bedford's "Vaginal Hystereotomy" paper on November 15, 1845.

[14] Clifford Browder, *The Wickedest Woman in New York: Madame Restell, The Abortionist* (Hamden, Connecticut: Archon, 1988), p. 87

[15] Another instance of Horatio assisting his father's professional efforts was reported in Hermann's diary on May 3, 1851 when DHS went to Charleston, South Carolina for the AMA meeting in 1851. Hermann noted Horatio "looks a bit after patients." Other early examples of Horatio's assistance to his father are described in Dyer, *Champion*, pp. 14, 29.

[16] HRS, "On the Decrease of the Rate of Increase of Population now Obtaining in Europe and America," *American Journal of Science and Art (Silliman's)* 43 (March 1867): 141-55, 150. (The delay in publication until 1867 is discussed in Chapter 7.) HRS, "Its Fre-

quency, and the Causes Thereof," p. 267.

[17] Warner reported that Horatio described "how medical jurisprudence is little understood" and "how the (Court?) should settle down upon fixed rules as respects medical testimony. HJW, diary entry, 11 November 1850, HJW papers, 1835-1913. MHS.

[18] JPL, "Letter from California—Climate and Diseases of the Country—Gold Digging—The Colera," *BMSJ* 41 (August 22, 1849): 52-55; JPL, "Letter from California," *BMSJ* 41 (December 19, 1849): 394-99.

[19] "Death of Dr. John P. Leonard," *BMSJ* 44 (July 9, 1851): 461-62, 461.

[20] HRS, "The History and Resources of the Valley of the Mississippi," Courtesy of the Harvard University Archives: HU 89.165.221.

[21] Dyer, *Champion*, pp. 130-32; 312-13; 368-78.

[22] JPL, "On the Different Varieties of Diarrhoea," *BMSJ* 42 (1850): 304-9; 341-46; 401-7; 425-31.

[23] Adin Ballou, *An Elaborate History and Genealogy of the Ballous in America* (Providence: Press of E.L. Freeman & Son), p. 1216.

[24] JPL, "Quackery and Abortion," p. 479.

[25] HRS, "Medical School Journal," part of accession number Acc. 2001-063, Boston Medical Library in the Francis A. Countway Library of Medicine.

[26] HJW, diary entry, 25 January 1851, HJW papers, 1835-1913. MHS.

[27] Ballou, *An Elaborate History and Genealogy of the Ballous in America*, p. 1216.

[28] Robert T. Legge, "Note on J.P. Leonard, M.D., Gold-Rush Visitor," *California Historical Society Quarterly* 31 (June 1952): 161-62, 162.

[29] Ibid., pp. 161-62.

[30] "Death of Dr. John P. Leonard," p. 461.

[31] Ibid.

[32] JPL, "The Cases of Fever Lately Observed In Cumberland, R.I." *BMSJ* 37 (September 1, 1847): 89-96; JPL, "Case of Cyanosis, or Blue Skin," *BMSJ* 38 (May 31, 1848): 363-65.; JPL, "On Epidemic Influence," *BMSJ* 38 (1848): 431-41; 461-64; 475-78.

[33] J.V.C. Smith, "Catalogue of the Marine and Fresh Water Fishes of Massachusetts." In Edward Hitchcock, *Report on the Geology, Mineralogy, Botany and Zoology of Massachusetts* (Amherst: J.S. & C. Adams, 1833); DHS, "A Report on the Fishes of Massachusetts," *Boston Journal of Natural History* 2 (1839): 289-570. HRS, "Observations on the Fishes of Nova Scotia and Labrador, with Descriptions of New Species."

[34] HRS, "The Criminality and Physical Evils of Forced Abortions," *Transactions of the American Medical Association* (hereafter *TAMA*) 16 (1865): 709-45, 712-13.

[35] JPL, "Quackery and Abortion," p. 480.

[36] Ibid., p. 481.

[37] Ibid., p. 478. DHS joined the AMA by 1849 when the Association met in Boston.

[38] HRS, "Medical School Journal," September 2, 1850-June 9, 1851, December 10 and December 24, 1850, part of accession number Acc. 2001-063, Boston Medical Library in the Francis A. Countway Library of Medicine.

[39] Legge, "Note on J.P. Leonard, M.D., Gold-Rush Visitor," p. 161.

[40] JPL, "Quackery and Abortion," p. 478.

[41] Ibid., p. 479.

[42] Ibid., pp. 478-79.

[43] Ibid., p. 479.

[44] Ibid., pp. 479-80. "[U]nhouselled, unanointed, unannealed" was from a version of Hamlet that has not been identified.

[45] Legge, "Note on J.P. Leonard, M.D., Gold-Rush Visitor," p. 161.

[46] JPL, "Quackery and Abortion," p. 480.

[47] HRS, "The Criminality and Physical Evils of Forced Abortions," p. 731.

[48] JPL, "Quackery and Abortion," p. 481.

[49] Ibid.

[50] DHS, *An Address on Medical Jurisprudence*, p. 3.

[51] DHS, "Report of the American Medical Association Committee on Obstetrics," *TAMA* 4 (1851): 363-366, 366. The paper was "Poisoning by Ergot, in attempting Criminal Abortion; on the effects of that substance, with reflections upon some of the causes of sudden death. By Myddleton Michel, M.D., Lecturer on Anatomy and Physiology: Charleston, S.C." published in the *Charleston Medical Journal and Review* for September 1850.

[52] Another possibility that may justify further historical research is that Horatio wrote "Quackery and Abortion" or some portion of it as a section of his father's paper on medical jurisprudence. When his father refused to include this, Horatio persuaded John Preston Leonard to publish it.

[53] HJW, diary entry, 20 October 1851, HJW papers, 1835-1913. MHS.

[54] "Alleged Manslaughter by Procuring Abortion," *BMSJ* 44 (May 14, 1851): 288.

[55] "Attempt to Produce Abortion with Oil of Tansey, Followed by Death," *BMSJ* 44 (May 14, 1851): 306.

[56] Walter Channing, "Sudden Enlargement of the Abdomen During Pregnancy," *Extracts from the Society for Medical Improvement* 1 (1853): 238-40, 238.

[57] "Criminal Abortionist," *BMSJ* 50 (March 8, 1854): 128.

[58] "Procuring Abortion," *BMSJ* 51 (October 4, 1854): 224-25, 224.

[59] Ibid., pp. 224-25.

[60] Dyer, *Champion*, pp. 68-78.

[61] Hugh L. Hodge, *Introductory Lecture* (Philadelphia: T.K. and P.G. Collins, 1854), p. 18.

[62] Ibid., p. 19.

[63] Ibid.

[64] DHS, "Two Frequent Causes of Uterine Disease," p. 200.

[65] David Francis Condie, "On Criminal Abortion: A Lecture Introductory …" *AJMS* 29 (April 1855): 466-68. Walter L. Burrage described how "[t]his monthly journal has continued to be the leading medical publication of the country to the present time" in his sketch of its editor: "Hays, Isaac," In Howard A. Kelly and Walter L. Burrage, *Dictionary of American Medical Biography* (New York: Appleton, 1928), pp. 545-46, 546. However, many Boston physicians would surely have claimed that distinction for their *BMSJ*.

[66] Ibid., p. 466.

[67] Ibid., p. 468.

[68] Isaac Skillman Mulford, "On Criminal Abortion," *New Jersey Medical Reporter* 8 (April 1855): 189-91.

[69] Ibid., p. 189.

[70] Ibid., p. 190.

[71] Ibid., pp. 190-91.

[72] DHS, "Two Frequent Causes of Uterine Disease," p. 199.

[73] DHS, *Address Delivered at the First Medical Commencement of the Massachusetts Medical College* (Boston: John Wilson and Son, 1855).

[74] Ibid., pp. 12-13.

[75] Dyer, *Champion*, pp. 73, 78, 88.

[76] Francis Minot, "Morbid Adhesion of the Placenta after Abortion," *BMSJ* 53 (August 9, 1855): 35-38.

[77] "Infant Mortality," *BMSJ* 62 (December 3, 1857): 364-65, 365.

[78] DHS, *An Introductory Lecture* ..., p. 6.

[79] DHS, "Two Frequent Causes of Uterine Disease, p. 172. Stress added.

[80] Ibid., pp. 195-97.

[81] Ibid., pp. 200-1.

[82] Ibid., pp. 201-3.

[83] HRS, "Contributions to Obstetric Jurisprudence: No. I.—Criminal Abortion," p. 65n.

[84] Mohr apparently did not learn that the suppressed portion of DHS's Lecture was published in 1872, despite the fact that Mohr made reference to HRS's 1897 paper (*AIA*, p. 122) that discussed this in a footnote on page 6.

[85] Dyer, "Autobiographical Letter," p. 448.

Chapter 4

[1] Boston Society for Medical Observation. "Journal, February 4, 1856," [B MS b98.2, v. 6], Boston Medical Library in the Francis A. Countway Library of Medicine.

[2] Dyer, *Champion*, pp. 92-93.

[3] R.H. Tatum, "A few Observations on the Attributes of the Impregnated Germ," *Virginia Medical Journal* 6 (June 1856): 455-459.

[4] HRS, "Its Obstacles to Conviction," p. 834.

[5] Tatum, "A few Observations ...," p. 457.

[6] Ibid.

[7] Ibid., p. 459.

[8] Levin Smith Joynes, "Some of the Legal Relations of the Foetus in Utero," pp. 179-91. HRS praised it in his "Its Obstacles to Conviction," p. 834.

[9] Jesse Boring, "Foeticide," p. 257.

[10] John Keith to HRS, February 17, 1857, Countway Scrapbook of letters on abortion.

[11] Dyer, *Champion*, p. 96.

[12] The May publication of these Minutes apparently accounts for Mohr's statement (*AIA*, p. 152) that Storer "opened his crusade publicly in May 1857."

[13] Suffolk District Medical Society. Minutes, meeting of February 28, 1857, *BMSJ* 56 (May 7, 1857): 282-84, 283.

[14] Ibid., pp. 283-84.

[15] Ibid., pp. 282-83.

[16] Ibid., p. 284.

[17] Dyer, "Autobiographical Letter," p. 446.

[18] Countway Scrapbook of letters on abortion.

[19] James W. Hoyte to HRS, March 20, 1857, Countway Scrapbook of letters on abortion.

[20] Charles A. Pope to HRS, March 24, 1857, Countway Scrapbook of letters on abortion.

[21] William Henry Brisbane to HRS, April 6, 1857, Countway Scrapbook of letters on abortion. Stress added. Mohr (*AIA*, p, 140) reproduced much of Brisbane's response to Storer, but described it as written "to a colleague in 1857." Storer was only mentioned in the endnote. Mohr thus failed to note Storer's influence on Brisbane's effort that led to the "third state" providing sanctions against women for seeking abortion. Perhaps Mohr wanted to make it appear that there were more regulars independently seeking changes in abortion laws.

[22] C.W. LeBoutillier to HRS, March 28, 1857, Countway Scrapbook of letters on abortion.

[23] Henry Ingersoll Bowditch to HRS, April 20, 1857, Countway Scrapbook of letters on abortion.

[24.]HRS, Henry Ingersoll Bowditch, and Calvin Ellis, "Suffolk District Medical Society Report of the Committee on Criminal Abortion," April 25, 1857 [34.A.1857.1], Harvard Medical Library in the Francis A. Countway Library of Medicine. It is reproduced in large part in the *American Medical Gazette* 8 (July 1857): 390-97.

[25.]The cover letter for the Report indicates it was read at the April meeting. Suffolk District Medical Society meetings were held the last Saturday of each month.

[26.]This letter from Secretary Charles D. Homans to Society members precedes and is part of the printed Report cited above.

[27.]HRS, Henry Ingersoll Bowditch, and Calvin Ellis, "Suffolk District Medical Society Report of the Committee on Criminal Abortion" [34.A.1857.1], p. 2, Harvard Medical Library in the Francis A. Countway Library of Medicine.

[28.]Ibid., p. 4.

[29.]Ibid., p. 2.

[30] Ibid., pp. 5-6. The statutes are given in full in Dyer, *Champion*, p. 107.

[31] Ibid.

[32] Ibid., p. 9.

[33] Ibid.

[34.]Ibid., pp. 9-10.

[35] Ibid., p. 10.

[36.]Ibid., p. 11.

[37.]Ibid., pp. 12-13. The statute is given in full in Dyer, *Champion*, pp. 110-11.

[38.]Suffolk District Medical Society. "Records, Special Meeting of May 9, 1857" [B MS b75.410.1, v. 1], pp. 143-156, p. 143, Boston Medical Library in the Francis A. Countway Library of Medicine.

[39] Ibid.

[40] Ibid. Stress added.

[41.]Ibid. The Minutes of the Regular Meetings of the Suffolk District Medical Society, unlike those of the Special Meetings, apparently have not been preserved.

Chapter 5

[1.]"B." (Charles Edward Buckingham, hereafter CEB), "The Report upon Criminal Abortions," *BMSJ* 56 (May 28, 1857): 346-47.

[2.]The *BMSJ* issue for May 7 prompted a May 7 letter from Stephen Tracy to HRS (May 7, 1857, Countway Library) and Tracy lived in Andover.

[3.]"B." (CEB), "The Report upon Criminal Abortions," p. 346. Stress added. This sentence would become the focus of numerous discussions.

[4] Ibid.

[5.]"Medicus," "Communications—Suffolk District Medical Society," *The Medical World* 2 (1857): 211-12.

[6.]"Criminal Abortion," *New-Hampshire Journal of Medicine* 7 (July 1857): 208-16, 214.

[7.]"The Report of the Committee upon Criminal Abortion," *BMSJ* 56 (June 11, 1857): 386-87.

[8] "B." (CEB), "Criminal Abortion," *BMSJ* 57 (August 13, 1857): 45-46.

[9.]Mohr, *AIA*, p. 154.

[10.]"Criminal Abortion," *New-Hampshire Journal of Medicine*, p. 208. Stress added.

[11.]Massachusetts Medical Society. "Records of Meetings, Meeting of June 3, 1857" [B MS b75.10, v. 2], Boston Medical Library in the Francis A. Countway Library of Medicine.

[12] Ibid.

[13.]"Criminal Abortion," *New-Hampshire Journal of Medicine*, pp. 213-14.

[14.]Ibid., p. 216.

[15] JPL, "Quackery and Abortion," p. 481.

[16.]J. Berrien Lindsley to HRS, July 4, 1857, Countway Scrapbook of letters on abortion. Mohr misrepresents the contents of this letter (*AIA*, p. 151) claiming that Lindsley urged Storer to put the matter before the AMA when it already had been so placed. He also claimed Lindsley declined to be a member of the committee, but no such refusal was in the letter. Despite referring to this letter that clearly shows Horatio was not in Nashville, Mohr claimed that Storer was there (*AIA*, p. 154).

[17.]"The Report upon Criminal Abortions—Comments of the *New Hampshire Journal of Medicine*," *BMSJ* 56 (July 23, 1857): 503-4.

[18.]"Criminal Abortion; The Boston Medical and Surgical Journal and its Attempts at Bullying," *New-Hampshire Journal of Medicine* 7 (August 1857): 248-51.

[19] Ibid., p. 250.

[20] "B." (CEB), "Criminal Abortion," p. 45.

[21] Dyer, *Champion*, pp. 123-24.

[22.]"Abortionism, Pro et Contra," *American Medical Gazette* 8 (July 1857): 390-97, 390.

[23.]Ibid. Stress added.

[24] David Meredith Reese, "Report on Infant Mortality in Large Cities," *TAMA* 10 (1857): 93-107.

[25] Ibid., p. 97.

[26] HRS, "Contributions to Obstetric Jurisprudence—Criminal Abortion III: Its Victims," *NAMCR* 3 (May 1859): 446-455, 447n.

[27] "Criminal Abortion or Foeticide," *Atlanta Medical and Surgical Journal* 2 (August 1857): 760.

[28] "Criminal Abortions," *Peninsular Journal of Medicine and the Collateral Sciences* 5 (August 1857): 97-100, 99.

[29] Ibid., p. 100.

[30] Edmund Potts Christian, "The Abortion Case," *Peninsular Journal of Medicine and the Collateral Sciences* 5 (October 1857): 215-22, 217. The *Ohio Medical and Surgical Journal* reproduced Christian's article in their number for January 8, 1858.

[31] Ibid., p. 215.

[32] Ibid., p. 217.

[33] Janet Kinney, *Saga of a Surgeon: The Life of Daniel Brainard, M.D.* (Springfield, Illinois: Southern Illinois School of Medicine, 1987), p. 140.

[34] "Killing no Murder," *Medical and Surgical Reporter* (hereafter *MSR*) 15 (August 1871): 195-96, 195.

[35] Kinney, *Saga of a Surgeon*, pp. 76-79.

[36] Ibid., p. 110.

Chapter 6

[1] "A Class of Abortives," *BMSJ* 5 (November 22, 1831): 240-41.

[2] "Artificial Abortions," *BMSJ* 31 (September 11, 1844): 124.

[3] Ibid.

[4] "Criminal Attempt at Abortion," *BMSJ* 31 (August 21, 1844): 66-67.

[5] A.M. Mauriceau, *The Married Woman's Private Medical Companion, ...*(New York: 1847).

[6] Ibid., pp. 15-18n.

[7] Ibid., pp. 141-43n.

[8] "Abortion Advertisements," *BMSJ* 56 (October 8, 1857): 206.

[9] Ibid.

[10] "Criminal Abortions," *Buffalo Medical Journal and Monthly Review of Medical and Surgical Science* 14 (September 1858): 247-51, 247.

[11] "Criminal Abortion," *Maine Medical and Surgical Reporter* 1 (January 1858): 39-40.

[12] "Criminal Abortions," *Buffalo Medical Journal ...*, pp. 247-248.

[13] Ibid., p. 249.

[14] Ibid., pp. 250-51.

[15] Dyer, *Champion*, pp. 502-3.

[16] Ibid., p. 136.

[17] "Criminal Abortions," *Buffalo Medical Journal and Monthly Review of Medical and Surgical Science* 14 (October 1858): 309-313, 312-313.

[18] Ibid., p. 313.

[19] Dyer, *Champion*, pp. 502-3.

[20] "Criminal Abortions," *Buffalo Medical Journal ...*, p. 313.

[21] Mohr, *AIA*, p. 155.

[22] "Criminal Abortions," *Buffalo Medical Journal ...*, pp. 309-10.

[23] Ibid., p. 313.

[24] "An Early Crusade Against Criminal Abortion," *Buffalo Medical and Surgical Journal* 18 (August 1912): 51-52.

[25] "Austin Flint," *American National Biography* (New York: Oxford University Press, Vol. 8, 1999), pp. 130-131, 131.

[26] Edmund Potts Christian, "Report to the State Medical Society on Criminal Abortions," *Peninsular and Independent Medical Journal* 2 (June 1859): 129-40. Christian included a note that the report had been published earlier in the Michigan Society's *Transactions* with severe omissions.

[27] Ibid., p. 135.

[28] Dyer, *Champion*, pp. 127-30.

[29] Ibid., pp. 130-32.

[30] Spencer Fullerton Baird, Thomas Mayo Brewer, and Robert Ridgway. *A History of North American Birds, Volume II* (Boston: Little, Brown, and Co., 1874), p. 45.

[31] "Proceedings of the Councillors, February Meeting, 1858," Medical Communications of the Massachusetts Medical Society 9 (Boston: Massachusetts Medical Society), Appendix, pp. 76-77.

[32] "Massachusetts Medical Society Report on Abortion" [B MS c 75.2], Boston Medical Library in the Francis A. Countway Library of Medicine.

[33] "Report on Criminal Abortion," *TAMA* 12 (1859): 75-78, 76.

[34] Dyer, *Champion*, p. 136.

[35] HRS, "The Use and Abuse of Uterine Tents," *AJMS* 37 (January 1859): 57-62.

[36] Ibid., p. 61.

Chapter 7

[1] HRS, "On the Decrease of the Rate of Increase of Population now Obtaining in Europe and America," *American Journal of Science and Art (Silliman's)* 43 (March 1867): 141-55.

[2] American Academy of Arts and Sciences. Minutes, meeting of May 11, 1858, Boston Athenaeum.

[3] HRS, "Criminal Abortion: Its Prevalence, Its Prevention, and Its Relation to the Medical Examiner ...," Microfiche #AN 0320 in the Adelaide Nutting Historical Nursing Mi-

crofilm Collection which is a microfiche of an offprint of the article in *Atlantic Medical Weekly* (Providence, R.I.) 8 (October 2, 1897): 209-18. Page numbers of the offprint are 1-34. Quote was from p. 3.

[4.] Ibid., pp. 4-5.

[5.] HRS, "On the Decrease of the Rate of Increase of Population now Obtaining in Europe and America," p. 148.

[6] Ibid., pp. 149-54.

[7.] Ibid., p. 155.

[8.] "Contributions to Obstetric Jurisprudence," *NAMCR* 2 (December 1858): 1149-50.

[9.] HRS, "Contributions to Obstetric Jurisprudence: No. I.—Criminal Abortion," pp. 64-72, 66.

[10.] Ibid., p. 64.

[11] Ibid., pp. 64-65.

[12.] Ibid., p. 65.

[13] Ibid., p. 66.

[14.] Ibid., pp. 68-69.

[15] Ibid., pp. 69-70.

[16] Ibid., pp. 70-71.

[17] Ibid., p. 72.

[18.] HRS to the Councillors of the Massachusetts Medical Society, January 27, 1859 [B MS c75.2], Boston Medical Library in the Francis A. Countway Library of Medicine.

[19.] Massachusetts Medical Society. "Records of the Councils, February 2, 1859" [B MS b75.9, v. 5], pp. 231-232. Boston Medical Library in the Francis A. Countway Library of Medicine.

[20] Walter Channing, "Effects of Criminal Abortion," *BMSJ* 60 (March 17, 1859): 134-42.

[21] Kass, *Midwifery and Medicine in Boston*, p. 258.

[22] Channing, "Effects of Criminal Abortion," p. 140.

[23] Ibid.

[24.] HRS, "Its Frequency, and the Causes Thereof," pp. 260-82.

[25.] Ibid., p. 278.

[26.] Ibid.

[27] Ibid., p. 279.

[28.] Ibid., p. 280.

[29.] Ibid., p. 281.

[30] Dyer, *Champion*, pp. 170-2.

[31] HRS, "Its Frequency, and the Causes Thereof," p. 281.

[32] Ibid., p. 282.

[33] "Dr. Horatio R. Storer, of Boston," *American Medical Gazette* 10 (April 1859): 298-99.

[34.] Alexander J. Semmes to HRS, March 16, 1859, Countway Scrapbook of letters on abortion.

[35.] Charles A. Pope to HRS, March 18, 1859, Countway Scrapbook of letters on abortion.

[36.] Alexander J. Semmes to HRS, March 26, 1859, Countway Scrapbook of letters on abortion.

[37.] Hugh L. Hodge to HRS, March 30, 1859, Countway Scrapbook of letters on abortion.

[38.] A. Lopez to HRS, April 2, 1859, Countway Scrapbook of letters on abortion.

[39.] William Henry Brisbane to HRS, April 6, 1859, Countway Scrapbook of letters on abortion.

[40.] Thomas Blatchford to HRS, May 3, 1859, Countway Scrapbook of letters on abortion.

[41.] Edward H. Barton to HRS, April 12, 1859, Countway Scrapbook of letters on abortion.

[42] James Mohr assumed that the members had been selected when the Committee was created in 1857 (*AIA*, p. 155). Mohr claimed (*AIA*, p, 151): "In selecting his correspondents, Storer was careful to solicit the backing of those physicians who were already campaigning for anti-abortion policies in their own states." However, the only correspondent so campaigning was Brisbane and he probably began his actions after Storer wrote him in 1857. Mohr claimed (*AIA*, pp. 144-45) committee member, Thomas Blatchford, was "the man most responsible for publicizing Madame Restell's activities in 1845." Gunning S. Bedford was the Restell publicist.

[43] "Report on Criminal Abortion," *TAMA* 12 (1859): 75-78, 75.

[44] Ibid., p. 77. Horatio's quote came from *Man Transformed* (Oxford, 1653).

[45] Ibid., pp. 77-78.

[46] Minutes, 1859 Annual Meeting, *TAMA* 12 (1859): 27-28.

[47] Thomas W. Blatchford to HRS, May 3, 1859, Countway Scrapbook of letters on abortion.

[48] HRS, "The Surgical Treatment of Hemorrhoids and Fistula in Ano, with Their Result," *JGSB* 2 (April, 1870): 221-49, 223.

[49] Thomas W. Blatchford to HRS, May 5, 1859, Countway Scrapbook of letters on abortion.

[50] D.F.C. (David Francis Condie), "The Transactions of the American Medical Association," *AJMS* 39 (April 1860): 439-52, 440.

[51] Ibid., p. 441

[52] HRS, "Its Victims," pp. 446-55.

[53] Ibid., p. 449.

[54] Ibid., pp. 450-451.

[55] Ibid., p. 455.

[56] HRS, "Contributions to Obstetric Jurisprudence—Criminal Abortion IV: Its Proofs," *NAMCR* 3 (May 1859): 455-65.

[57] HRS, "Two Cases illustrative of Criminal Abortion," *AJMS* 37 (April 1859): 314-18.

[58] HRS, "Its Proofs, p. 460.

[59] Ibid., p. 463.

[60] Ibid., p. 459.

[61] HRS, "Contributions to Obstetric Jurisprudence—Criminal Abortion V: Its Perpetrators," *NAMCR* 3 (May 1859): 465-70.

[62] Ibid., p. 466.

[63] Ibid., pp. 466-67.

[64] Ibid., p. 468.

[65] Ibid., pp. 468-69.

[66] Ibid., p. 469.

[67] HRS, "Contributions to Obstetric Jurisprudence—Criminal Abortion VI: Its Innocent Abettors," *NAMCR* 3 (July 1859): 643-57.

[68] Ibid., pp. 650-51. The authority calling for the Caesarian operation rather than repetition of craniotomy almost certainly was the British physician, Thomas Radford, who did this in his 1848 "The Value of Embryonic and Foetal Life, Legally Socially, and Obstetrically Considered" that was mentioned in Horatio's January article, and which, although not designated as such, may have been another stimulus for Horatio's "thought of the present undertaking."

[69] Ibid., p. 655.

[70] Ibid., p. 657.

[71] HRS, "Contributions to Obstetric Jurisprudence—Criminal Abortion VII: Its Obstacles to Conviction," pp. 833-54.

[72.]Ibid., p. 834.

[73] Ibid.

[74.]Ibid., p. 849.

[75] Ibid., p. 853.

[76] Ibid., p. 854.

[77.]"Leading Articles," *British Medical Journal* no. 147 (October 22, 1859): 857.

[78.]HRS, "Contributions to Obstetric Jurisprudence—Criminal Abortion VIII: Can It Be At All Controlled By Law?" *NAMCR* 3 (November 1859): 1033-38.

[79] Ibid., p. 1035.

[80] Ibid., p. 1037.

[81] Ibid., pp. 1037-38.

[82.]HRS, "Contributions to Obstetric Jurisprudence—Criminal Abortion IX: The Duty of the Profession," *NAMCR* 3 (November 1859): 1039-46, 1039.

[83] Ibid., p. 1040.

[84] Ibid., p. 1043.

[85.]Ibid., p. 1046.

[86.]HRS, *On Criminal Abortion in America* (Philadelphia: Lippincott & Co., 1860).

[87.]"Criminal Abortion," *BMSJ* 62 (February 16, 1860): 65-67.

[88] Ibid., p. 65.

[89.]Ibid., p. 67.

[90] D.F.C. (David Francis Condie), "On Criminal Abortion in America," *AJMS* 39 (April 1860): 465-68.

[91] Ibid., p. 465.

[92] Ibid., p. 467.

[93] Ibid., p. 468. As noted earlier, the quote (slightly misrepresented by Condie) came from *Man Transformed* (Oxford, 1653).

Chapter 8

[1.]"Memorial. To the Governor and Legislature, ..." "To the President and Councilors of the State Medical Society." Both documents are parts of accession number Acc. 2001-063, Boston Medical Library in the Francis A. Countway Library of Medicine. The Indiana State Archives has a copy of the "Memorial" sent to them sometime in 1860.

[2.]HRS to Mr. Collins, December 17, 1859, College of Physicians of Philadelphia: Joseph Carson Collection (v. 2 [Z10c/10]).

[3.]"The New York State Medical Society," *BMSJ* 62 (February 16, 1860): 67.

[4.]"Address of Henry Miller, M.D., President of the Association," *TAMA* 13 (1860): 55-76, 56.

[5.]Ibid., pp. 57-58.

[6.]Minutes, 1860 Annual Meeting, *TAMA* 13 (1860): 41-42.

[7.]Mohr, *AIA*, p. 202.

[8.]"Proceedings, Adjourned Meeting of the Councillors, May 30, 1860," Medical Communications of the Massachusetts Medical Society 9 (Boston: Massachusetts Medical Society), Appendix, p. 103.

[9.]"Proceedings, Adjourned Meeting of the Councillors, October 3, 1860," Medical Communications of the Massachusetts Medical Society 10 (Boston: Massachusetts Medical Society), Appendix, pp. 2-3.

[10] "The Abortionists of New York," *National Police Gazette* 1 (November 15, 1845): 100.

[11] Augustus Kinsley Gardner, "Physical Decline of American Women," *Knickerbocker*

55 (January 1960): 37-52.

[12] "Gardner, Augustus Kinsley," In Howard A. Kelly and Walter L. Burrage, *Dictionary of American Medical Biography* (New York: Appleton, 1928), p. 452.

[13] Gardner, "Physical Decline of American Women," pp. 46-47.

[14] Ibid., p. 48.

[15] Ibid.

[16] Personal communication with Arlene Shaner, Reference Librarian, Historical Collections, The New York Academy of Medicine who consulted the Minutes of the Academy's meetings for 1867.

[17] "Hale, Edwin M., M.D.," *Biographical Cyclopaedia of Homeopathic Physicians and Surgeons* (Philadelphia: Galaxy, 1873), pp. 24-25, 24.

[18] Edwin Moses Hale, "Abortion: Its Prevention and Treatment," *North American Journal of Homoeopathy* 8 (May 1860): 641-57.

[19] Edwin Moses Hale, *On the Homoeopathic Treatment of Abortion* (Chicago: Halsey & King, Homoeopathic Pharmacy, 1860).

[20] Ibid., p. 5. Hale may have been the first to describe the sale to the public of mechanical devices for production of abortions.

[21] Ibid., p. 7.

[22] Ibid., p. 13.

[23] Edwin Moses Hale, *A Systematic Treatise on Abortion* (Chicago: C.S. Halsey, 1866).

[24] Hale, *Homoeopathic Treatment of Abortion*, 13-14.

[25] Ibid., p. 14.

[26] Ibid. Mohr (*AIA*, p. 77) incorrectly referred to this as an "intrauterine douching technique."

[27] Ibid.

[28] Edwin Moses Hale, *The Great Crime of the Nineteenth Century, Why Is It Committed? Who Are the Criminals? How Shall They Be Detected? How Shall They Be Punished?* (Chicago: C.S. Halsey, 1867), p. 40.

[29] Nicholas Francis Cooke, *Satan in Society: By a Physician* (Cincinnati: C.F. Vent, 1876), pp. 130-31

[30] Gunning S. Bedford, *The Principles and Practice of Obstetrics* (New York: William Wood & Co., 1874), pp. 678-79. Bedford's quote about "Jorg, of Leipsic," was taken verbatim from the footnote in Storer's "Its Perpetrators."

[31] Ibid., p. 679.

[32] Ibid.

[33] Ibid., p. 678n.

[34] HRS, "Studies of Abortion," *BMSJ* 68 (February 5, 1863): 15-20.

[35] Ibid., pp. 15-16.

Chapter 9

[1] "Infanticide," *BMSJ* 71 (August 18, 1864): 66-67.

[2] Ibid., p. 67.

[3] Minutes, 1864 Annual Meeting, *TAMA* 15 (1864): 1-53, 50.

[4] Ibid.

[5] Ibid., p. 35. At some point before the Boston meeting, Henry Ingersoll Bowditch was added to the Committee.

[6] Minutes, 1865 Annual Meeting, *TAMA* 16 (1865): 1-60, 38.

[7] Jonathon Mason Warren, "Journal," May 10, 1865, Warren papers. MHS.

[8] Mohr (*AIA* p. 158) appears to have believed that the proposal for the antiabortion essay

contest occurred at the same AMA meeting where the prize was awarded, since Mohr wrote: "The origins of that contest are unknown, but it seems no coincidence that the annual convention that approved the scheme met in Boston," and "[H]ow many physicians were likely to have had a major manuscript on that subject ready to go?"

[9] HRS, "The Criminality and Physical Evils of Forced Abortions," p. 717.

[10] Ibid., p. 711.

[11] Dyer, *Champion*, p. 176.

[12] HRS, "The Criminality and Physical Evils of Forced Abortions," p. 713n.

[13] "Philadelphia Friend" to HRS, February 10, 1866, *Why Not? A Book for every Woman*, pp. 88-89.

[14] See Dyer, *Champion*, p. 314.

[15] HRS, "The Criminality and Physical Evils of Forced Abortions," pp. 714-15.

[16] Ibid., p. 719.

[17] Ibid., pp. 720-21.

[18] Ibid., p. 722.

[19] Ibid., p. 723.

[20] Ibid.

[21] Ibid., p. 727.

[22] Ibid., p. 738.

[23] HRS, "The Causation, Course, and Treatment of Insanity in Women: A Gynaecist's Idea Thereof; Being the Report of the Standing Committee on Insanity for 1864-5," *TAMA* 16 (1865): 121-255. Also see Dyer, *Champion*, pp. 176-81.

[24] HRS, "The Criminality and Physical Evils of Forced Abortion," p. 740.

[25] HRS, "The Causation, Course, and Treatment of Insanity in Women," p. 198.

[26] HRS, "The Criminality and Physical Evils of Forced Abortion," p. 741.

[27] Ibid., p. 742.

[28] Ibid., p. 745.

[29] Ibid.

[30] "Report of the Section on Practical Medicine and Obstetrics," *TAMA* 16 (1865): 91.

[31] HRS, *Why Not? A Book for every Woman* (Boston: Lee and Shepard, 1866).

[32] HRS, "Criminal Abortion: Its Prevalence, Its Prevention, and Its Relation to the Medical Examiner," pp. 12-13.

[33] Minutes, 1866 Annual Meeting, *TAMA* 17 (1866): 41.

Chapter 10

[1] Hale, *A Systematic Treatise on Abortion*, pp. 263-89.

[2] Ibid., p. 288.

[3] Ibid., p. 284.

[4] Ibid., pp. 29-30.

[5] Ibid., p. 236.

[6] Ibid., p. 317.

[7] Ibid., p. 319. Stress in the original.

[8] William Henry Holcombe, "A Systematic Treatise on Abortion," *United States Medical and Surgical Journal* 1 (July 1866): 383-91.

[9] Ibid., pp. 387-88.

[10] Ibid., pp. 388-89.

[11] Ibid.

[12] Ibid., pp. 389-90.

[13] "Meeting, December 11, 1866," *The Hahnemannian Monthly* 3 (February 1867): 335-

336, 336.

[14] Edwin Moses Hale, *A Systematic Treatise on Abortion and Sterility* (Chicago: C.S. Halsey, 1868), p. iii.

[15] Reuben Ludlam, "Criminal Abortion," *United States Medical and Surgical Journal* 2 (April 1867): 257-73.

[16] Ibid., pp. 260-61.

[17] Ibid., p. 262.

[18] Ibid., p. 264.

[19] Ibid., p. 266.

[20] Ibid., p. 271.

[21] Ibid.

[22] Ibid., p. 273.

[23] Edwin Moses Hale, "Criminal Abortion. A Lecture …," *American Homeopathic Observer* 4 (June 1867): 288-89.

[24] Hale, *The Great Crime of the Nineteenth Century* (Chicago: C.S. Halsey, 1867).

[25] Hale, "Criminal Abortion. A Lecture …," p. 289.

[26] Ibid., p. 4.

[27] Ibid.

[28] Ibid., p. 5.

[29] Ibid.

[30] Ibid., p. 7.

[31] Ibid., p. 8. Hale probably copied this Storer quote from "Criminal Abortion," *Northwestern Christian Advocate* 15 (March 13, 1867), p. 82.

[32] Ibid., p. 10.

[33] Ibid., pp. 11-12.

[34] Ibid.

[35] Ibid., pp. 13-14.

[36] Ibid., pp. 14-15.

[37] Ibid., pp. 17-18.

[38] Ibid., p. 20.

[39] Ibid., p. 23.

[40] Ibid., pp. 24-25.

[41] Ibid., pp. 26-33.

[42] Ibid., pp. 33-34.

[43] Ibid., p. 39.

[44] Ibid., pp. 39-40.

[45] Ibid., p. 40.

[46] Hale, "Criminal Abortion. A Lecture …," p. 289.

Chapter 11

[1] "Butler, Samuel Worcester," In Howard A. Kelly and Walter L. Burrage, *Dictionary of American Medical Biography* (New York: Appleton, 1928), p. 184.

[2] "Criminal Abortion," *MSR* 13 (November 4, 1865): 306.

[3] "A Social Evil—Infantiphobia," *MSR* 14 (February 10, 1866): 114.

[4] Ibid.

[5] Ibid.

[6] "Infantiphobia and Infanticide," *MSR* 14 (March 17, 1866): 212-13.

[7] Ibid., p. 213.

[8] "Infanticide—Criminal Abortion," *MSR* 14 (April 7, 1866): 276-77, 277.

[9] Ibid.

[10] Ibid., p. 276.

[11] "Infanticide—Criminal Abortion," *MSR* 14 (May 19, 1866): 397.

[12] Ibid.

[13] Thaddeus A. Reamy, "Report on Obstetrics," *Transactions of the Ohio State Medical Society* 21 (1866): 55-84.

[14] Ibid., p. 65.

[15] Ibid., p. 66.

[16] Ibid., pp. 67-68.

[17] Ibid., p. 68.

[18] Ibid., p. 69.

[19] Ibid., p. 83.

[20] *The Journal of the Senate of the State of Ohio ...., 1867* (Columbus: L.D. Myers & Bro., State Printers, 1867), p. 233. "Many of the facts presented" dealt with the inappropriateness of quickening as a marker of the beginning of life.

[21] Israel Thorndike Dana, "Report of Committee on the Production of Abortion," *Transactions of the Maine Medical Association for the years 1866 through 1868* (Portland: Stephen Berry, 1869), pp. 37-43.

[22] Ibid., p. 39.

[23] Ibid., pp. 40-41.

[24] Ibid., p. 42.

[25] Ibid.

[26] "The Mutual Relations of the Medical Profession, Its Press, and the Community," *JGSB (Supplement)* 4, no. 6 (June 1871): 1-20, 8.

[27] HRS, *Why Not? A Book for every Woman*, pp. 10, 87-91.

[28] "Review of *Why Not? A Book for every Woman*," *MSR* 15 (July 21, 1866): 74.

[29] "Review of *Why Not? A Book for every Woman*," *BMSJ* 75 (August 30, 1866): 104.

[30] See Dyer, *Champion*, pp. 210-19.

[31] "Review of Why Not?," *BMSJ*, p. 104.

[32] "Review of *Why Not? A Book for every Woman*," *New Orleans Medical & Surgical Journal* 20 (July 1867): 111-15, 112.

[33] Ibid., pp. 112-13.

[34] HRS, "On Self Abuse in Women, Its Causation and Rational Treatment," *The Western Journal of Medicine* 2 (August 1867): 449-57, 452.

[35] Caroline Dall to HRS, June 5, 1866, *Is It I? A Book for Every Man*, p. 139.

[36] HRS to Caroline H. Dall, 18 June 1866, Caroline Wells Healey Dall papers, 1811-1917. MHS.

[37] "'Why Not? A Book for Every Woman.' A Woman's View," *BMSJ* 75 (November 1, 1866): 273-76.

[38] Ibid., p. 275.

[39] Ibid., p. 276.

[40] "'A Woman's View' of 'Why Not?'" *BMSJ* 75 (January 10, 1867): 490.

[41] Henry Orlando Marcy, "The Early History of Abdominal Surgery in America," *JAMA* 54 (February 19, 1910): 600-5, 602.

Chapter 12

[1] HRS, "The Abetment of Criminal Abortion by Medical Men," *New York Medical Journal* 3 (September 1866): 422-33.

[2] Ibid., p. 433.

[3.]Massachusetts Medical Society. "Records of Meetings: Annual Meeting, May 30, 1866" [B MS b75.10, v. 2], Boston Medical Library in the Francis A. Countway Library of Medicine.

[4] "The Criminality and Frequency of Abortion," *Medical Record* 1 (July 16, 1866): 240.

[5] HRS, "Letter from Dr. Storer, of Boston," *Medical Record* 1 (July 16, 1866): 244-45.

[6] Edmund Potts Christian, "The Pathological Consequences Incident to Induced Abortion," *Detroit Review of Medicine and Pharmacy* 2 (April 1867): 145-55.

[7] Ibid., p. 145.

[8] Ibid., p. 154.

[9] Ibid., p. 155. Stress added. As will be seen, other physicians viewed the physician's office as comparable to the Catholic confessional.

[10] Ibid.

[11] William McCollom, "Criminal Abortion," *Transactions of the Vermont Medical Society* (1865): 40-43, 42.

[12] Morse Stewart, "Criminal Abortion," *Detroit Review of Medicine and Pharmacy* 2 (January 1867): 1-11.

[13] Ibid., p. 1.

[14] Ibid., pp. 2-3.

[15] Ibid., p. 6.

[16] Ibid., p. 7. The quotes are from Psalm 109.

[17] Ibid., p. 11.

[18] Edward P. LeProhon, *Voluntary Abortion, or, Fashionable Prostitution, with Some Remarks upon the Operation of Craniotomy* (Portland: B. Thurston & CO., 1867), pp. 4-5.

[19] Ibid., p. 12.

[20] Ibid., p. 3.

[21] Ibid., p. 9.

[22] Ibid., p. 13.

[23] Ibid.

[24] Ibid., p. 12.

[25] "The Social Crime as Affecting Our Native Population." *Medical Record* 2 (March 15, 1867): 37-38, 37.

[26] Ibid.

[27] Nathan Allen, "Vital Statistics of Massachusetts," *New York Observer* (October 4, 1866): 1, 1.

[28] Ibid.

[29] "The Decay of New England," *BMSJ* 75 (November 1, 1866): 287-91, 287.

[30] "The Social Crime as Affecting Our Native Population," p. 38.

Chapter 13

[1] "Criminal Abortion," *Northwestern Christian Advocate* 15 (March 13, 1867): 82-83.

[2] "Who Hath Believed our Report?," *Northwestern Christian Advocate* 15 (March 27, 1867): 100.

[3] "Criminal Abortion," *Northwestern Christian Advocate*, p 82.

[4] Ibid.

[5] Ibid.

[6] Ibid.

[7] Ibid.

[8] Ibid.

[9] Ibid.

[10] Ibid., p. 83.

[11] Ibid.

[12] "Who Hath Believed our Report?," p. 100.

[13] "We have received a copy…," *BMSJ* 76 (March 21, 1867): 145-46, 145-46.

[14] "We are glad to notice …," *Medical Record* 2 (April 15, 1867): 87.

[15] "Criminal Abortion and the Public Press," *Buffalo Medical and Surgical Journal* 6 (April 1867): 358-62.

[16] Ibid., p. 358n.

[17] John Todd, *Serpents in the Dove's Nest* (Boston: Lee and Shepard, 1867), p. 5.

[18] "Editorial Notes," *JGSB* 2 (March 1870): 188.

[19] HRS, "On Self Abuse in Women: Its Causation and Rational Treatment," p. 455.

[20] Minutes, 1866 Annual Meeting, *TAMA* 17 (1866): 41.

[21] "Vermont Medical Society—Semi-Annual Session," *BMSJ* 76 (July 11, 1867): 478-80, 479.

[22] Lucius Castle Butler, "The Decadence of the American Race, as Exhibited in the Registration Reports of Massachusetts and Vermont: Causes and Remedy," *BMSJ* 77 (September 5, 1867): 89-99.

[23] Ibid., pp. 89-92.

[24] Ibid., pp. 94-95.

[25] Ibid., pp. 96-97.

[26] Ibid., pp. 97-98.

[27] Ibid., p. 98.

[28] Ibid., p. 99, The "he or she is a criminal …" came originally from HRS's quotation of the letter from the Catholic Bishop of Boston in his May 1859, "Its Victims." Rev. John Todd reproduced it in his *Serpents in the Dove's Nest* and added the italics.

[29] "A Move in the Right Direction," *Medical Record* 2 (October 15, 1867): 384.

Chapter 14

[1] HRS, *Is It I? A Book for Every Man*.

[2] HRS to Thomas Addis Emmet, June 3, 1867, *Is It I? A Book for Every Man*, p. iv.

[3] "Publishers' Note," *Is It I? A Book for Every Man*, pp. vii-xix. Reprinted in *A Proper Bostonian on Sex and Birth Control* (New York: Arno Press, 1974). Also see Dyer, *Champion*, pp. 236-239.

[4] HRS, *Is It I? A Book for Every Man*, p. 8.

[5] Ibid., pp. 9-10.

[6] Ibid., p. 57.

[7] Ibid., pp. 89-90.

[8] Ibid., p. 92

[9] Ibid., p. 93.

[10] Ibid., pp. 95-96.

[11] Ibid., p. 96. Gray's comments from the asylum report were given in "Abortion and Insanity," *Medical Record* 2 (July 15, 1867): 240.

[12] Ibid., p. 111.

[13] Ibid., pp. 115-16.

[14] Ibid., p. 117

[15] Ibid., p. 125.

[16] Ibid., p. 147.

[17] Fordyce Barker, "Remarks Made Before the Medical Society of the County of New

York, Feb. 3, 1868," *Medical Record* 3 (May 15, 1868): 151-54, 151-52.

[18] "Medical Society of the County of New York," *Medical Record* 3 (May 15, 1868): 164-65, 164-65.

[19] M.M. Eaton, "Four and a-Half Inches of Whalebone in the Uterus.—Abortion.—Narrow Escape from Death," *Chicago Medical Examiner* 9 (April 1868): 218-19.

[20] Ibid., p. 219.

[21] Montrose Anderson Pallen, "Foeticide, or Criminal Abortion," *Medical Archives* 3 n.s. (April 1869): 193-206.

[22] "Pallen, Montrose Anderson," In Howard A. Kelly and Walter L. Burrage, *Dictionary of American Medical Biography* (New York: Appleton, 1928), pp. 931-32.

[23] Pallen, "Foeticide, or Criminal Abortion," p. 194.

[24] Ibid., p. 196.

[25] Ibid., p. 204.

[26] Ibid., pp. 198-99.

[27] Ibid., p. 206.

[28] "Procured Abortions, and Criminal Advertisements," *MSR* 18 (June 13, 1868): 517-18.

[29] Wm. C. Todd, "Criminal Abortion," *MSR* 18 (June 6, 1868): 501-2.

[30] "Abortions—Actions of the Essex (N.J.) District Medical Society," *MSR* 18 (January 18, 1868): 62.

[31] "Abortion," *MSR* 18 (April 11, 1868): 332.

[32] "Punishment of Abortionists," *MSR* 18 (April 18, 1868): 350-51, 351.

[33] "Criminal Abortion," *MSR* 19 (August 15, 1868): 133-34.

[34] Nathan Allen, "Changes in Population," *Harper's New Monthly Magazine* 38 (February 1869): 386-92, 390.

[35] Elijah Franklin Howe, *Ante-Natal Infanticide* (Terre Haute: Allen & Andrews, 1869); Reprinted in *Abortion in Nineteenth Century America* (North Stratford, N.H.: Ayer, 1974).

Chapter 15

[1] HRS and Franklin Fiske Heard, *Criminal Abortion: Its Nature, Its Evidence, and Its Law* (Boston: Little, Brown, and Co., 1868). Mohr (*AIA*, p. 159) claimed that Storer attended law school "in part at least to prepare himself for the collaboration [with Heard] on *Criminal Abortion.*" Storer attended law school four years earlier in 1864 to prepare himself for teaching medical jurisprudence (See Dyer, *Champion*, p. 175).

[2] Ibid., p. vi.

[3] Ibid., p. 2n. Italics added to both sentences.

[4] Ibid., p. 3n.

[5] Ibid., p. 60n.

[6] Ibid., pp. 42-47.

[7] Ibid., pp. 56-57, 56n.

[8] Ibid., p. 74n.

[9] Ibid., p. 3n.

[10] Ibid., p. 147n.

[11] See Dyer, Champion, pp. 268-69; 275; 279-81.

[12] Although Storer was actively involved with antiabortion efforts until his serious illness early in 1872, Mohr indicated (*AIA*, p. 159): "By the end of the 1860s Storer's health began to fail badly and in 1872 he finally left the country for sunnier climates abroad." Mohr also claimed that this removed Storer "from medical politics in the United States."

Storer returned in 1877 and was active in national, Boston, and Newport medical politics, even hosting the AMA annual meeting in his home city of Newport in 1889.

[13] GSB. Proceedings, meeting of April 6, 1869, *JGSB* 1 (October 1869): 195-208, 203.

[14] GSB. Proceedings, meeting of April 20, 1869, *JGSB* 1 (October 1869): 210-23, 221.

[15] Mohr, *AIA*, p. 216.

[16] Ibid., p. 217.

[17] "Editorial Notes," *JGSB* 1 (September 1869): 180-92, 184-85. Stress added.

[18] "Editorial Notes," *JGSB* 1 (September 1869): 189-90.

[19] "Editorial Notes," *JGSB* 2 (January 1870): 51-64, 63-64.

[20] GSB. Proceedings, meeting of June 21, 1870, *JGSB* 3 (December 1870): 357-73, 369.

[21] Ibid.

[22] Ibid., p. 373. At the August 2, 1870 meeting of the Society, Horatio reported that the Governor promised cooperation in preventing abortionists from going free.

[23] "Editorial Notes," *JGSB* 3 (August 1870): 106-19, 119.

[24] Massachusetts Medical Society. Minutes, meeting of Councillors, October 5, 1870, Countway Library.

[25] "Editorial Notes," *JGSB* 3 (October 1870): 253-72, 269-70.

Chapter 16

[1] A. Cleveland Coxe, *Moral Reforms Suggested in a Pastoral Letter with Remarks on Practical Religion*, (Philadelphia: J.B. Lippincott, 1869), p. 10.

[2] Ibid., p. 30.

[3] Ibid., pp. 39-41.

[4] "The Crime of Abortion," *MSR* 20 (May 29, 1869): 415.

[5] *Pastoral Letter of the Most Rev. Archbishop ... May 1869* (Baltimore: John Murphy & Co., 1869), p. 24.

[6] Ibid., p. 11.

[7] Bishop Rene H. Gracida, "A Pastoral Letter on Abortion and Excommunication," (Corpus Christi, Texas: Diocesan Press, September 8, 1990).

[8] Orson Squire Fowler, *Creative and Sexual Science: Or, Manhood, Womanhood, and Their Mutual Interrelations; ... Etc., As Taught By Phrenology and Physiology* (Cincinnati: Cincinnati Publishing, Co., 1870), p. 871.

[9] Archbishop Martin J. Spalding to Bishop James Gibbons, March 4, 1869, Archives of the Archdiocese of Baltimore (71-U-1).

[10] Personal correspondence with Fr. Paul K. Thomas, Archivist, Archdiocese of Baltimore, November 14, 2001.

[11] Personal correspondence with Professor Thomas W. Spalding, author of *Martin John Spalding: American Churchman*.

[12] "Extravagance and Excesses of the Times," *Catholic Mirror* (February 20, 1869): 4.

[13] According to Thomas W. Spalding: "Spalding was in the habit of calling the Roman authorities' attention to just about everything of importance he wrote." (Personal communication, November 5, 2001.) Archbishop Spalding would visit the Vatican to attend the Ecumenical Council, but face-to-face discussion with the Pope was not a factor in the October Papal Bull, since Spalding arrived in late November 1869.

[14] Hugh Lenox Hodge, *Fœticide, Or Criminal Abortion: A Lecture Introductory To The Course On Obstetrics And Diseases Of Women And Children, University Of Pennsylvania, Session 1839-40* (Philadelphia: Lindsay and Blakiston, 1869). Reprinted in *Abortion in Nineteenth Century America* (North Stratford, N.H.: Ayer, 1974).

[15] Ibid., p. 6.

[16] Ibid., p. 4.

[17] Ibid., pp. 9-10.

[18] Ibid., pp. 38-39.

[19] Ibid., p. 43.

[20] "Conviction and Suicide of an Abortionist," *MSR* 21 (July 24, 1869): 87.

[21] "Abortionists," *Canada Lancet* 21 (March 1889): 217-18, 218.

[22] Andrew Nebinger, *Criminal Abortion; Its Extent and Prevention* (Philadelphia: Collins, Printer, 1870). Reprinted in *Abortion in Nineteenth Century America* (North Stratford, N.H.: Ayer, 1974).

[23] Ibid., p. 29.

[24] Ibid., pp. 27-28.

Chapter 17

[1] John Cowan, *The Science of a New Life* (New York: J.S. Olgivie, 1918).

[2] Ibid., p. 275.

[3] Henry Clarke Wright, *The Unwelcome Child, or, the Crime of an Undesigned and Undesired Maternity* (Boston: B. Marsh, 1858).

[4] Cowan, *Science of a New Life*, 276-77.

[5] Ibid., p. 278

[6] Ibid., p. 280.

[7] Ibid.

[8] Ibid., pp. 300-1.

[9] Ibid., p. 301.

[10] Ibid.

[11] Ibid., pp. 301-2.

[12] Ibid., p. 304.

[13] Augustus Kinsley Gardner, *Conjugal Sins Against the Laws of Life and Health and Their Effects upon the Father, Mother and Child* (New York: J.S. Redfield, 1870). Reprinted (New York: Arno Press, 1974).

[14] Ibid., pp. 111-12.

[15] Ibid., pp. 130-32.

[16] Fowler, *Creative and Sexual Science*, p. 868.

[17] Ibid.

[18] Ibid., p. 870.

[19] Ibid.

[20] Ibid., pp. 869-70.

[21] Ibid., pp. 870-71.

[22] Ibid., p. 871.

[23] Ibid.

[24] George Henry Napheys, *The Physical Life of Woman: Advice to the Maiden, Wife and Mother* (Philadelphia: David McKay, 1890).

[25] Ibid., pp. xxiv-xxv.

[26] Ibid., pp. 138-39.

[27] Ibid., p. xxvi.

[28] Ibid., pp. 137-38.

[29] Nicholas Francis Cooke *Satan in Society: By a Physician* (Cincinnati: C.F. Vent, 1876). Reprinted (New York: Arno Press, 1974), p. 24.

[30] Ibid., p. 118.

[31] Ibid., p. 119.

[32] Ibid., pp. 122-23.

[33] Ibid., pp. 125-26.

[34] Ibid., pp. 130-31.

[35] Franklin Wayne Intrikin, *Woman's Monitor* (Cincinnati: C.F. Vent, 1871).

[36] Ibid., p. 380.

Chapter 18

[1] Obed Chester Turner, "Criminal Abortion," *BMSJ* 5 n.s. (April 21, 1870): 299-301.

[2] "Obituary: Dr. O.C. Turner," *BMSJ* 107 (November 9, 1882): 456.

[3] Turner, "Criminal Abortion," p. 299.

[4] Ibid.

[5] Ibid., pp. 299-300. The Editors' footnote read: "*We are astounded that any regular practitioner should have dared to make such a confession! We say, show him up, and let him be expelled from the Massachusetts Medical Society."

[6] Ibid., p. 300.

[7] Ibid.

[8] "Obituary: Dr. O.C. Turner," p. 456.

[9] Addison Niles, "Criminal Abortion," *Transactions of the Illinois State Medical Society* (Chicago: 1871), pp. 96-101, 96. Described as a leading physician of Quincy in his wife's obituary: *Quincy Daily Whig* (April 26, 1902).

[10] Ibid., pp. 100-1.

[11] Minutes, 1870 Annual Meeting, *TAMA* 21 (1870): 1-67, 35. Information on Dominick O'Donnell came from Joseph Ryan's dissertation, *Wresting with the Angel:* ...(See Bibliography).

[12] Minutes, 1870 Annual Meeting, p. 35.

[13] Nathan Allen, "On the Physiological Laws of Human Increase," *TAMA* 21 (1870), 383-407, 387.

[14] Dominick A. O'Donnell and Washington Atlee, "Report on Criminal Abortion," *TAMA* 22 (1871): 239-58. Mohr (*AIA*, p. 159) claimed that the 1871 report reflected the AMA's concern that "its recommendations had not been enacted in every state," and thus it "renewed its campaign to win tougher anti-abortion statutes in another major report on the subject in 1871. However, no such concern was expressed in the 1871 report or in the 1870 resolutions that led to it and only a single sentence in the long 1871 report mentioned the need for "more rigorous laws." What is more, there were no calls for legislation in the six Resolutions appended to the Report.

[15] See Dyer, *Champion*, pp. 374-76.

[16] Ibid., pp. 323-25.

[17] O'Donnell and Atlee, "Report on Criminal Abortion," p. 244.

[18] Ibid., p. 251.

[19] Ibid., p. 241.

[20] Ibid., pp. 248-49.

[21] Ibid., pp. 257-58.

[22] Ibid., p. 258.

[23] "Killing no Murder," *MSR* 25 (August 1871): 195-96.

[24] Ibid., p. 195.

[25] Ibid., p. 196.

Chapter 19

[1] "The Reputable Doctors' Opinion of Lookup Evans," *New York Times* (hereafter *NYT*) (May 23, 1871), p.2. "Concerning the Crime of Abortion," *Medical Record* 6 (June 15, 1871): 181-83, 181.

[2] "Trial of Dr. Wolff," *NYT* (Jan 26, 1871), p. 3.

[3] "Close of the Trial of Dr. Wolff," *NYT* (Jan 27, 1871), p. 3.

[4] "Lookup Evans Again," *NYT* (May 13, 1871), p. 2.

[5] "Lookup Evans Convicted and Sentenced," *NYT* (May 19, 1871), p. 6.

[6] Mohr, *AIA*, pp. 178-80.

[7] Described in articles in the *NYT* (August 27, August 29-September 3, 1871).

[8] "Law for the Abortionists," *NYT* (September 7, 1871).

[9] "Prevention of Abortion," *Medical Record* 6 (September 15, 1871): 325-26, 325.

[10] Ibid., p. 326.

[11] GSB. Proceedings, meeting of September 26, 1871, *JGSB* 6 (January 1872): 2-8, 5-6.

[12] "New York Academy of Medicine," *BMSJ* 8 (November 16, 1871): 326-327, 327.

[13] Marvin N. Olasky, *The Press and Abortion, 1838-1988* (Hillsdale, N.J.: Lawrence Erlbaum, 1988), pp. 30-31.

[14] "The Alleged Prevalence of Criminal Abortion," *MSR* 25 (September 30, 1871): 306-7, 306.

[15] Ibid., p. 307.

[16] Thomas Davison Crothers, "Report of a Criminal Abortion with Death," *MSR* 25 (October 14, 1871): 331-33.

[17] Ibid., p. 333.

[18] "The Abortion Business," *MSR* 25 (October 14, 1871): 348-49, 348-49.

[19] "Editorial Notes," *JGSB* 5 (October 1871): 251-56.

[20] Ibid., p. 256.

[21] East River Medical Association, *Report of Special Committee on Criminal Abortions* (New York: S.W. Green, 1871).

[22] Ibid., p. 3.

[23] Ibid.

[24] Ibid., pp. 3-4. Stress added.

[25] Ibid., p. 4.

[26] Ibid., pp. 5-6.

[27] Mohr, *AIA*, p. 160.

[28] Ibid.

[29] Ibid., pp. 240-43.

[30] Ibid., p. 238.

[31] Ely Van de Warker, *The Detection of Criminal Abortion and a Study of Foeticidal Drugs* (Boston: James Campbell, 1872), p. iv.

[32] GSB. Proceedings, meeting of February 6, 1872, *JGSB* 7 (August 1872): 97-113, 103.

[33] GSB. Proceedings, meeting of February 20, 1872, *JGSB* 7 (September 1872): 161-76, 163.

[34] Ibid., p. 164.

[35] Ibid., pp. 174-75.

[36] "The Medico-Legal Society," *Medical Record* 6 (February 1, 1872): 543-44, 543.

[37] Ibid.

[38] Mohr, *AIA*, pp. 218-219.

[39] Cyril J. Means, "The Law of New York Concerning Abortion and the Status of the Foetus, 1664-1968: A Case of Cessation of Constitutionality," *New York Law Forum* 14

(Fall, 1968): 411-515, 478.

[40.]"Editorial Notes," *JGSB* 6 (May 1872): 393-400, 394.

[41] Dyer, *Champion*, pp. 394-408.

Chapter 20

[1] J.C. Stone, "Report on the Subject of Criminal Abortion," *Transactions of the Iowa State Medical Society* (Davenport: Griggs, Watson & Day, 1871), pp. 26-34, 29.

[2] Ibid., pp. 30-31.

[3] Ibid., pp. 33-34.

[4] P.S. Haskell, "Criminal Abortion," *Transactions of the Maine Medical Association, 1871-1873* 4 (Portland: 1873), pp. 465-73.

[5] Ibid., p. 466.

[6] Ibid., p. 467.

[7] Ibid., p. 468.

[8] James S. Whitmire, "Criminal Abortion," *Chicago Medical Journal* 31 (July 1874): 385-393.

[9] Ibid., pp. 386-87.

[10] Ibid., p. 389.

[11] Ibid., p. 390.

[12] Ibid., p. 393

[13] "'Abortion Not a Crime,'" *Chicago Medical Journal* 31 (September 1874): 569-71, 569.

[14] Ibid., p. 571.

[15] John W. Trader, "Criminal Abortion," *Saint Louis Medical and Surgical Journal* 11 n.s. (November 1874): 575-590.

[16] Ibid., pp. 575-76.

[17] Ibid., p. 583.

[18] Ibid., p. 587.

[19] Alfred A. Andrews, "On Abortion," *Canada Lancet* 7 (June 1, 1875): 289-91.

[20] Ibid., p. 289.

[21] Ibid., pp. 289-90.

[22] Ibid.

[23] Ibid.

[24] Homer O. Hitchcock, "Report on Criminal Abortion," *Fourth Annual Report of the Secretary of the State Board of Health of the State of Michigan* (Lansing: W.S. George & Co., 1876), pp. 54-62.

[25] Ibid., pp. 59-61.

[26] Edward Cox, "Criminal Abortion," *Transactions of the Michigan State Medical Society* (Lansing: W. S. George & Co., 1877), pp. 369-82, 369-71.

[27] Ibid., p. 371.

[28] Ibid., p. 372.

[29] The *Transactions of the Michigan State Medical Society* that included this paper apparently had a large distribution. At least 22 libraries currently have these 1877 *Transactions* in their collections, whereas only 8 report the *Transactions* for earlier years.

[30] Ibid., p. 373.

[31] Ibid., p. 374.

[32] Ibid., p. 375.

[33] Ibid., p. 376.

[34] Ibid.

[35] Ibid., p. 377.

[36] Ibid., pp. 377-78.

[37] Ibid., p. 379.

[38] Ibid.

[39] Ibid., pp. 379-80.

[40] Ibid., p. 380.

[41] Ibid.

[42] Ibid., pp. 380-81.

[43] Ibid., p. 382.

[44] John Harvey Kellogg, *Plain Facts for Old and Young* (Burlington: I.F. Segner, 1889), pp. 516-17.

[45] Ibid., pp. 518-20.

[46] Ibid., p. 515.

[47] John Harvey Kellogg, *The Home Hand-Book of Domestic Hygiene and Rational Medicine* (Battle Creek: Modern Medicine, 1903), p. 357.

[48] See Browder, *The Wickedest Woman in New York: Madame Restell, The Abortionist*, pp. 158-83.

[49] Nicholas Francis Cooke, *Licensed Foeticide* (Detroit: American Observer, *1879*). The date was not given on the publication but Cooke indicated he was speaking exactly 25 years after obtaining his M.D. He obtained it in 1854.

[50] Ibid., pp. 13-14.

[51] Edwin Moses Hale, *An Open Letter to the Medical Profession; Being a History and Defense of Dr. Hale's Pamphlet, Entitled, "On the Homoeopathic Treatment of Abortion ..."* (Chicago: J. Millikan, 1877) This included "an exposure of the animus of the attacks upon its author by Dr. G.D. Beebe and others."

[52] Cooke, *Licensed Foeticide*, p. 15.

[53] Edward Hazen Parker, "The Relation of the Medical and Legal Professions to Criminal Abortion," *TAMA* 31 (1880): 465-471.

[54] Ibid., pp. 465-67.

[55] Ibid., pp. 469-70.

[56] Ibid., p. 470.

[57] Ibid., p. 471.

[58] "Minutes of the Section on State Medicine," *TAMA* 31 (1880): 411-12.

[59] "Proceedings of the Suffolk District Medical Society," *BMSJ* 104 (April 14, 1881): 347-52, 349.

[60] "A Conviction for Criminal Abortion," *BMSJ* 106 (January 5, 1882): 18-19.

[61] Ibid., p. 19.

[62] Ibid.

[63] Edward Cox, Homer O. Hitchcock, and Simeon S. French, "Report of the Special Committee on Criminal Abortion," *Report of the State Board of Health, Michigan 1881* (Lansing: W.S. George, 1882), pp. 164-68.

[64] Ibid., pp. 165-66.

[65] Ibid., p. 166.

[66] Ibid., p. 167.

[67] Ibid.

[68] Ibid.

[69] Ibid., pp. 167-168.

[70] Jno. S. Pearson, "Criminal Abortion," *Saint Louis Medical and Surgical Journal* 42 (March 1882): 237-39, 237.

[71] Ibid., p. 238.

[72] Ibid., p. 239.

[73] J. Miller, "Criminal Abortion," *Kansas City Medical Record* 1 (January 1884): 295-98, 295.

[74] Ibid.

[75] Ibid., p. 296.

[76] Ibid., p. 297.

[77] Ibid.

[78] Ishbel Ross, *The Life Story of the First Woman Doctor* (New York: Harper and Brothers, 1949), p. 88.

[79] Ibid., p. 206.

[80] Mohr, *AIA*, p. 73.

[81] Caroline Dall, "Diary when in Rhode Island," unspecified date between 16 May and 14 June 1870, Caroline Wells Healey Dall papers 1811-1917 (Box 22, Folder 4). MHS

[82] Several sources indicate that this came from *The Revolution* 4 (December 2, 1869): 346.

[83] Alice B. Stockham, *Tokology: A Book for Every Woman* (Chicago: Sanitary Publishing Co., 1885).

[84] Ibid., pp. 227-29.

[85] Ibid., p. 232.

Chapter 21

[1] James E. Kelly, "The Ethics of Abortion, As a Method of Treatment in Legitimate Practice," *JAMA* 7 (November 6, 1886): 505-509.

[2] James E. Kelly, "Causality in Disease, Applied to the Phenomenon of Vomiting in Pregnancy," *BMSJ* 114 (April 15, 1886): 337-41, 337.

[3] Kelly, The Ethics of Abortion, p. 505.

[4] Ibid., p. 506.

[5] Ibid., p. 507.

[6] Ibid., pp. 507-8.

[7] Ibid., p. 509.

[8] GSB. Transactions, Meeting of September 9, 1886, *JAMA* 7 (November 6, 1886): 529

[9] Kelly, The Ethics of Abortion, p. 509.

[10] "Criminal Abortions," *JAMA* 8 (March 12, 1887): 298.

[11] Ibid.

[12] James W. Hoyte to HRS, March 20, 1857, Countway Scrapbook of letters on abortion.

[13] John Bryan Ward Nowlin, "Criminal Abortion," *Southern Practitioner* 9 (May 1887): 177-82.

[14] Ibid., pp. 178-179.

[15] Ibid., p. 180.

[16] Ibid., p. 181.

[17] Ibid., p. 182.

[18] Isaac N. Quimby "Introduction to Medical Jurisprudence," *JAMA* 9 (August 6, 1887): 162-67.

[19] Ibid., p. 164.

[20] "Minutes 39th Annual Meeting," *JAMA* 10 (June 2, 1888): 690-700, 699.

[21] Ibid., p. 700.

[22] A.K. Steele, "The Medico-Legal Aspect of Criminal Abortion," *JAMA* 9 (December 10, 1887): 762-64.

[23] Ibid., p. 763.

[24] "A Promised Investigation," *Chicago Times* (December 17, 1888): p. 5, col. 2.

[25] Steele, "The Medico-Legal Aspect of Criminal Abortion," p. 763.

[26] Ibid., p. 764.

[27] Ibid.

[28] Ibid.

[29] Henry Clay Ghent, "Criminal Abortion, or Foeticide," *Transactions of the Texas State Medical Association* (1888): 119-46.

[30] Ibid., p. 120.

[31] Ibid., p. 128. Stress added.

[32] Ibid., pp. 141-42.

[33] Ibid., pp. 144-45.

Chapter 22

[1] Henry C. Markham, "Foeticide and Its Prevention," *JAMA* 11 (December 8, 1888): 805-6.

[2] Ibid., p. 805.

[3] Ibid., pp. 805-6.

[4] Ibid., p. 806

[5] Ibid.

[6] Ibid.

[7] Ibid.

[8] "Seeking the Remedy," *Chicago Times* (January 1, 1889): p. 1, col. 3.

[9] "N.C.M," (Should have been H.C.M.), *Chicago Times* (December 22, 1889): p. 5; "Seeking the Remedy," *Chicago Times* (January 7, 1889): p. 2, col. 7.

[10] "Infanticide," *Chicago Times* (December 20, 1888): p. 5, col. 5.

[11] "The Medical Society Acts," *Chicago Times* (December 19, 1888): p. 4, col. 2.

[12] "The Doctors Will Investigate," *Chicago Times* (December 18, 1888): p. 2, col. 3.

[13] John Floyd Banton, *Revolution in the Practice of Medicine* (Chicago: Review, Printing and Pub. Co., 1885).

[14] "Infanticide," *Chicago Times* (December 16, 1888): p. 1, col. 1.

[15] Ibid.

[16] "Infanticide" *Chicago Times* (December 17, 1888): p. 1, col. 1.

[17] Ibid.

[18] "Infanticide" *Chicago Times* (December 18, 1888): p. 1, col. 1.

[19] "Infanticide," *Chicago Times* (December 19, 1888): p. 1, col. 3.

[20] "Infanticide," *Chicago Times* (December 21, 1888): p. 1, col. 1; (December 23, 1888): p. 1, col. 1.

[21] "Infanticide," *Chicago Times* (December 19, 1888): p. 1, col. 2.

[22] "Infanticide," *Chicago Times: Supplement* (December 23, 1888): p. 3, col. 4.

[23] "The Remedy," *Chicago Times* (December 28, 1888): p. 1, col. 1.

[24] "Dr J. H. Etheridge Wouldn't Do It Himself, but Recommended Another," *Chicago Times* (December 16, 1888): p. 1, col. 4.

[25] "Dr. Etheridge's Plan," *Chicago Times* (December 18, 1888): p. 2, col. 3.

[26] "Infanticide," *Chicago Times* (December 16, 1888): p. 1, col. 3.

[27] "Thurston is Expelled," *Chicago Times* (January 8, 1889): p. 1, col. 4.

[28] Ibid.

[29] Hobart tribute mentioned December 20, 1888: p. 1, col.3; Tributes to Belfield, Guinne, and Gilman mentioned on December 22, 1888: p. 1, col. 2; p. 5, col. 1; p. 5, col. 4, respectively.

[30] "Infanticide," *Chicago Times* (December 16, 1888): p. 1, col. 4.

[31] Ibid.

[32] "Infanticide," *Chicago Times* (December 19, 1888): p. 7, col. 3; (December 21, 1888): p. 3, col. 6.

[33] "The Remedy," *Chicago Times* (December 29, 1888): p. 1, col. 3.

[34] "Infanticide," *Chicago Times: Supplement* (December 23, 1888): p. 3, col. 5.

[35] "Closer Preaching Needed," *Chicago Times* (December 25, 1888): p. 4, col. 1.

[36] "The Remedy," *Chicago Times* (December 27, 1888): p. 1, col. 2.

[37] "Infanticide," *Chicago Times: Supplement* (December 23, 1888): p. 3, col. 5.

[38] "Infanticide," *Chicago Times* (December 22, 1888): p. 5, col. 2.

[39] "Seeking the Remedy," *Chicago Times* (January 2. 1889): p. 5, col. 2.

[40] "Talk about the 'Times,'" (December 21, 1888): p. 4, col. 6.; "Talk about the 'Times'" (Editorial pages), for December 23-24, 1888 and December 26, 1888.

[41] "Professional Abortionists," *Journal of the American Medical Association* 11 (December 29, 1888): 912-13, 912.

[42] T. Gaillard Thomas, *Abortion and Its Treatment, From the Stand-Point of Practical Experience* (New York: Appleton and Company, 1892).

[43] Ibid., p. 102.

[44] Ibid., pp. 104-12.

[45] Denslow Lewis, "Criminal Abortion and the Traumatisms Incident to Its Performance," *Chicago Clinical Review* 5 (October 1895): 9-25, 9.

[46] Ibid., pp. 10-11.

[47] Ibid., p. 11.

[48] Ibid., pp. 11-12.

[49] Ibid., p. 12.

[50] "Abortionists," *Canada Lancet* 21 (March 1889): 217-18.

[51] Ibid., p. 217.

[52] Ibid., pp. 217-218.

[53] Ibid., p. 218.

Chapter 23

[1] Anonymous, "Abortion," *Medico-Legal Journal* 7 (September1889): 170-87.

[2] Ibid., p. 176.

[3] Ibid., p. 177.

[4] Ibid., p. 181.

[5] Ibid., pp. 182-83.

[6] Ibid., pp. 183-84.

[7] Ibid., pp. 184-85.

[8] Ibid., pp. 185-86.

[9] Ibid., p. 187.

[10] Junius C. Hoag, *Medico-Legal Journal* 8 (March 1890): 116-26, 118.

[11] Ibid., p. 118.

[12] Ibid., p. 121.

[13] Ibid., p. 122.

[14] Ibid., p. 123.

[15] Ibid., p. 124.

[16] Ibid., p. 125.

[17] Ibid., pp. 125-26.

[18] Charles H. Harris, "Special Operation of Abortion," *New York Journal of Gynaecology and Obstetrics* 1 (September 1892): 842-45.

[19] James Coffee Harris, *The Personal and Family History of Charles Hook and Margaret Monk Harris* (Georgia: J.C. Harris, 1911).

[20] Seale Harris, "The Abortionist," *Journal of the Medical Association of the State of*

Alabama 4 (December 1934): 222-24.

[21] Harris, "Special Operation of Abortion," p. 842.

[22] Ibid.,

[23] Ibid., p. 843.

[24] Ibid., pp. 843-45.

[25] Ibid., p. 845.

[26] Mary Amanda Dixon Jones, "Criminal Abortion, Its Evils and Its Sad Consequences," *Medical Record* 46 (July 7, 1894): 9-16,

[27] Ibid., p. 9.

[28] Ibid., p. 10.

[29] Ibid., pp. 10-11.

[30] Ibid., p. 12.

[31] Ibid., p. 15.

[32] Ibid., pp. 15-16.

[33] Ibid., p. 16.

[34] Regina Morantz-Sanchez, *Conduct Unbecoming a Woman* (New York: Oxford, 1999), pp. 179-180.

[35] Francis W. Higgins, "Abortion and Manslaughter," *Gaillard's Medical Journal* 56 (March 1893): 217-223, 218.

[36] Ibid., p. 221.

[37] Ibid.

[38] Ibid., p. 222.

[39] J. Milton Duff, "Chairman's Address," *JAMA* 21 (August 26, 1893): 290-93, 291.

[40] Newspaper clipping, Francis W. Higgins file, Cortland County New York Historical Society.

Chapter 24

[1] William Henry Parish, "Criminal Abortion," *MSR* 68 (April 29, 1893): 644-49, 645.

[2] Ibid.

[3] Ibid.

[4] Mohr, *AIA*, pp. 240-241.

[5] Parish, "Criminal Abortion," p. 648.

[6] Ibid.

[7] "Abortion Socially, Medically and Medico-Legally Considered," *BMSJ* 134 (June 4, 1896): 566-67, 566.

[8] Ibid.

[9] Ibid., p. 567.

[10] Ibid., pp. 567-68.

[11] Ibid.

[12] Ibid.

[13] Mohr, *AIA*, pp. 241-242.

[14] Lewis, "Criminal Abortion and the Traumatisms Incident to Its Performance," p. 9. Stress added.

[15] Joseph Taber Johnson, "Abortion and Its Effects," *American Journal of Obstetrics and Diseases of Women and Children* 33 (January, 1896): 86-97

[16] Ibid., pp. 90-91.

[17] Ibid., p. 93.

[18] Ibid., p. 92.

[19] Ibid., p. 96.

[20] James Foster Scott, "Criminal Abortion," *American Journal of Obstetrics and Diseases of Women and Children* 33 (January, 1896), 72-86, 72. Stress added.

[21] Mohr, *AIA*, p. 240. Stress added to show that Scott was not saying most members of the profession were claiming times were "not so impure."

[22] Scott, "Criminal Abortion," p. 73.

[23] Ibid.

[24] Ibid., pp. 79-80.

[25] Ibid., p. 82.

[26] James Foster Scott, *The Sexual Instinct: Its Use and Dangers as Affecting Heredity and Morals: Essentials to the Welfare of the Individual and the Future of the Race* (Chicago: Login Brothers, 1930), p. 230.

[27] Ibid., pp. 260-61.

[28] Ibid., p. 272.

[29] Ibid., p. 294.

[30] Ibid., pp. 296-98.

[31] Ibid., p. 298.

[32] Ibid., pp. 303-304.

[33] Joseph Waggoner, M.D. "Criminal Abortion and Its Relation to the Medical Profession," *Cleveland Medical Gazette* 11 (February 1896): 268-272.

[34] Ibid., p. 269.

[35] Ibid., p. 270.

[36] William McCollom, "Criminal Abortion," *JAMA* 26 (February 8, 1896): 257-59, 257. The near identical claim by Vermont's William McCollom in 1865, suggests that the Vermont physician had moved to Brooklyn.

[37] Ibid.

[38] Ibid.

[39] Ibid., p. 258.

[40] Ibid., pp. 258-59.

[41] H.B. Smith, "Criminal Abortion," *Transactions of the Indiana State Medical Society* (1898): 235-239, 235-236.

[42] Ibid., p. 236.

[43] Ibid., pp. 236-37.

[44] George A. Phillips, "Criminal Abortion: Its Frequency, Prognosis and Treatment" *Transactions of the Maine Medical Association for 1895-1897* 12 (1897): 302-309.

[45] Ibid., pp. 302-4.

[46] Ibid., p. 306.

[47] Ibid., p. 307.

[48] Ibid., p. 308.

[49] Ibid., pp. 308-9.

[50] Ibid., p. 309.

[51] Ibid.

[52] "Criminal Abortion," *BMSJ* 125 (October 22, 1896): 417.

[53] HRS, "Criminal Abortion: Its Prevalence, Its Prevention, and Its Relation to the Medical Examiner Based on the 'Summary of the Vital Statistics of the New England States for the Year 1892' By the Six Secretaries of the New England State Boards of Health," Microfiche #AN 0320 in the Adelaide Nutting Historical Nursing Microfilm Collection which is a microfiche of an offprint of the article in *Atlantic Medical Weekly* (Providence, R.I.) 8, (October 2, 1897): 209-218. pp. 1-2 of the offprint.

[54] Ibid., pp. 6-7.

[55] Ibid., p. 10. The passage about the Nashville American Medical Association meeting

where Horatio was selected to lead the Committee on Criminal Abortion, apparently led James Mohr to incorrectly report that Horatio was in attendance at that meeting. Mohr wrote (*AIA*, p. 155): "at the AMA meeting in 1857, when Storer called for action, ..."

[56] Ibid., pp. 12-13.

[57] Ibid., p. 14.

[58] Ibid., p. 25n.

[59] Ibid., pp. 25-26.

[60] Ibid., p. 33.

[61] Ibid., pp. 33-34.

[62] Newport Medical Society to "medical societies and otherwise," August 21, 1897, part of accession number Acc. 2001-063, Boston Medical Library in the Francis A. Countway Library of Medicine. Reproduced in Dyer, *Champion*, p. 467.

[63] Dyer, *Champion*, pp. 467, 589. The advertising flyer included "Medical Press Notices" for Horatio's 1897 pamphlet, quoting praising passages from the *Texas Medical News*, "*Medical Council, Philadelphia*," *JAMA*, and *New England Medical Gazette*.

Chapter 25

[1] WorldCat indicated that the key words *medical* and *journal* produced twice as many serials for the decade 1900-1909 as for any previous decade. As with the last four or five decades of the nineteenth century, only a fraction of the physician papers opposing criminal abortion are discussed in this book.

[2] Mrs. John Van Vorst and Marie van Vorst, *The Woman Who Toils* (New York: Doubleday, Page & Co., 1903), p. 2.

[3] Denslow Lewis, "Facts Regarding Criminal Abortion," *JAMA* 35 (October 13, 1900): 943-47, 943-44.

[4] Ibid., p. 944.

[5] Ibid.

[6] Ibid., pp. 944-45.

[7] Ibid., p. 947.

[8] Minnie C.T. Love, "Criminal Abortion," *Colorado Medicine* 1 (December 1903): 55-60.

[9] Ibid., p. 55.

[10] Ibid., p. 58.

[11] Ibid.

[12] Ibid.

[13] Ibid.

[14] Ibid., p. 57.

[15] Ibid., p. 59.

[16] Ibid., p. 60.

[17] Ibid.

[18] Thomas W. Barlow, "Medicolegal Aspects of Criminal Abortion," *Medical News* 84 (May 21, 1904): 1007-8. Also published in *JAMA* 42 (May 21, 1904): 1375-76.

[19] Ibid., p. 1007.

[20] Ibid., pp. 1007-8.

[21] Ibid.

[22] Ibid., p. 1008.

[23] Ibid.

[24] Ibid.

[25] Louis G. LeBeuf, "The Attitude of the Medical Profession Towards Race Suicide and

Criminal Abortion," *New Orleans Medical and Surgical Journal* 57 (July 1904): 3-18, 3-4.
[26] Ibid., p. 7.
[27] Ibid., p. 9.
[28] "The Writhing of a Scotched Snake," *American Medicine* 8 (November 19, 1904): 867-68.
[29] Theodore Roosevelt, *An Autobiography* (New York: Macmillan, 1913), p. 305.

Chapter 26

[1] Charles Sumner Bacon, "The Duty of the Medical Profession in Relation to Criminal Abortion," *Illinois Medical Journal* 7 (June 1905): 18-24, 18.
[2] Ibid., p. 19.
[3] Ibid., p. 21.
[4] Ibid., pp. 21-22.
[5] Peter J. O'Callaghan, "The Moral and Religious Objections to Inducing Abortion," *Illinois Medical Journal* 7 (June 1905): 24-26, 25.
[6] Charles B. Reed, "Therapeutic and Criminal Abortion," *Illinois Medical Journal* 7 (June 1905): 26-29, 26.
[7] Ibid.
[8] Ibid., pp. 27-28.
[9] Ibid., p. 29.
[10] Rudolph Wieser Holmes, "Criminal Abortion; A Brief Consideration of Its Relation to Newspaper Advertising. A Report of a Medico-Legal Case," *Illinois Medical Journal* 7 (June 1905): 29-34, 29-30.
[11] Ibid., p. 30.
[12] Ibid.
[13] Ibid., pp. 31-32.
[14] Ibid., pp. 35-36.
[15] J.M. Sheean, "The Common and Statute Law of Illinois," *Illinois Medical Journal* 7 (June 1905): 37-39, 39.
[16] Harold M. Moyer, "The Privileged Communication …," *Illinois Medical Journal* 7 (June 1905): 39-40, 40.
[17] "Symposium Discussion," *Illinois Medical Journal* 7 (June 1905): 40-45, 40-41.
[18] Ibid., p. 43.
[19] Ibid., p. 45.
[20] Ibid., p. 44.
[21] Inez C. Philbrick, "Social Causes of Criminal Abortion." *Western Medical Review* (hereafter *WMR*) 10 (1905): 102-10. Also published in *Medical Record* 66 (September 24, 1905): 489-92.
[22] Ibid., p. 102.
[23] Ibid., pp. 105-6.
[24] Ibid., pp. 109-10.
[25] A. B. Somers, "Measures for prevention of criminal abortion" *WMR* 10 (1905): 110-13, 110.
[26] Ibid., p. 113.
[27] Ibid., p. 111.
[28] Ibid., pp. 112-13.
[29] W.O. Henry, "The Pathology and Treatment of Criminal Abortion," *WMR* 10 (1905): 86-93.
[30] William A. De Bord, The Nebraska Law," *WMR* 10 (1905): 93-97.

[31] W. B. Ely, "The Ethics of Criminal Abortion," *WMR* 10 (1905): 97-102.

[32] Ibid., p. 102.

[33] Henry Schwarz, "Diseases of the Kidneys as Indications for the Interruption of Pregnancy," *Interstate Medical Journal* 13 (November 1906): 863-65.

[34] Ibid.

[35] Louis M. Warfield, "Tuberculosis as an Indication for the Interruption of Pregnancy," *Interstate Medical Journal* 13 (November 1906): 866-69, 868.

[36] Ibid., pp. 868-69.

[37] W.H. Vogt, "The Indications for the Interruption of Pregnancy in Reference to Heart Disease," *Interstate Medical Journal* 13 (November 1906): 869-74.

[38] Bernard W. Moore, "Hyperemesis as an Indication for the Interruption of Pregnancy," *Interstate Medical Journal* 13 (November 1906): 874-78, 876.

[39] Frederick Joseph Taussig, "The Ethics and Laws Regarding the Interruption of Pregnancy," *Interstate Medical Journal* 13 (November 1906): 878-79.

[40] Ibid., p. 878.

[41] Ibid., p. 879.

[42] Ibid.

[43] Alexander Russell Simpson, "Criminal Abortion," *The Scottish Medical and Surgical Journal* 17 (December 1905): 481-96.

[44] Alexander Russell Simpson, "Criminal Abortion from the Ethical Point of View," *Clinical Review (Chicago)* 23 (1904-5): 333-50.

[45] Ibid., p. 333.

[46] Ibid., pp. 333-34.

[47] Ibid., pp. 334-35.

[48] Ibid., pp. 335-37.

[49] Ibid., pp. 341-42.

[50] Ibid., pp. 342-43.

[51] Ibid., pp. 343-44.

[52] Ibid., p. 347.

[53] Ibid., p. 346.

[54] Ibid., pp. 347-48.

[55] Ibid., p. 348.

[56] Ibid., p. 349.

[57] HRS, "Reminiscences of J. Y. Simpson," *Edinburgh Medical Journal* 7 (July 1911): 12-17. Much of the letter is included in Dyer, *Champion*, pp. 70-73.

Chapter 27

[1] J.M. Doleris, "Statistics Concerning Abortion," *Annals of Gynecology and Pediatry* 18 (August 1905): 401-417.

[2] "The Prevalence of Abortion," *Annals of Gynecology and Pediatry* 18 (August 1905): 422-25, 422.

[3] Ibid., p. 424.

[4] Ibid.

[5] Ibid., p. 425.

[6] William P. Pool, "Some Indications for Inducing Abortion and Premature Labor," *Brooklyn Medical Journal* 17 (August 1903): 365-68.

[7] Ibid., p. 365.

[8] Ibid.

[9] Frank A. Higgins, "The Propriety, Indications and Methods for the Termination of Preg-

nancy," *JAMA* 43 (November 19, 1904): 1531-35.

[10] Ibid., p. 1531.

[11] Ibid., p. 1532.

[12] Ibid., p. 1534.

[13] Ibid.

[14] Henry W. Cattell, "The Propriety, Indications and Methods for the Termination of Pregnancy," *JAMA* 43 (December 31, 1904): 2044-45, 2044-45.

[15] Ibid., p. 2045.

[16] Frank A. Higgins, "The Propriety, Indications and Methods for the Termination of Pregnancy," *JAMA* 44 (January 7, 1905): 48-49.

[17] Henry W. Cattell, et al., "Criminal Abortionists in Philadelphia," *The Pennsylvania Medical Journal* 8 (September 1905), 786-87.

[18] Henry W. Cattell, "Some Medico-Legal Aspects of Abortion," *Bulletin of the American Academy of Medicine* 8 (October 1907): 334-52.

[19] Ibid., p. 336.

[20] Ibid., The paper referred to was John M. Grant, "Criminal Abortion," *Interstate Medical Journal* 13 (June 1906): 513-18.

[21] Ibid., p. 337.

[22] Ibid.

[23] Ibid., p. 341.

[24] Ibid., p. 347.

[25] Ibid., p. 352.

[26] Francis A. Harris and William F. Whitney, "Criminal Abortion, Perforation of the Uterus with Passage of the Fetus into the Abdominal Cavity, and Prolapse of the Intestine. Death. Dismemberment," *BMSJ* 155 (December 20, 1906): 739-741.

[27] William H. Sanders, "The Physiologic and Legal Status of the Fetus in Utero," *JAMA* 46 (February 24, 1906): 551-53. Sanders read the identical paper before the Medical Association of the State of Alabama six years later and the paper was published in *Pediatrics* in September 1911.

[28] Ibid., p. 551.

[29] Ibid., pp. 551-52.

[30] Ibid., p. 552.

[31] Ibid.

[32] Thomas G. Atkinson, "Sociological Status of the Fetus in Utero," *Medical Standard* 29 (April 1906): 182-86.

[33] Ibid., p. 182.

[34] Ibid.

[35] Sanders, "The Physiologic and Legal Status of the Fetus in Utero," p. 551.

[36] Atkinson, "Sociological Status of the Fetus in Utero," p. 183.

[37] Ibid.

[38] Ibid., p. 184.

[39] Ibid.

[40] Ibid.

[41] Ibid.

[42] Ibid., p. 185.

[43] Ibid.

[44] Ibid., p. 186.

[45] Thomas G. Atkinson, "Is a Fetus a Person?," *Medical Standard* 33 (December 1910): 445.

[46] Charles Sumner Bacon, "The Legal Responsibility of the Physician for the Unborn

Child," *JAMA* 46 (June 30, 1906): 1981-84.
[47] Ibid., p. 1983.
[48] Ibid., p. 1984.

Chapter 28

[1] Albert VanderVeer, "Spontaneous and Criminal Abortion from a Medico-Legal Point of View," *American Journal of Surgery* 20 (July 1906): 201-4, 201-3.
[2] Ibid., p. 204.
[3] Ibid.
[4] R.H. McDonnell, "What Shall the Medical Profession Do To Prevent Abortions?," *Journal of the Kansas Medical Society* 6 (July 1, 1906): 278-82.
[5] Ibid., pp. 278-79.
[6] Ibid., p. 281.
[7] Ibid.
[8] "AMONG OURSELVES WE FREELY DISCUSS IT," *Journal of the Michigan State Medical Association* 5 (April 1906): 221-22.
[9] Ibid., p. 221.
[10] Ibid.
[11] Ibid., p. 222.
[12] Henry Orlando Marcy, "Education as a Factor in the Prevention of Criminal Abortion and Illegitimacy," *JAMA* 47 (December 8, 1906): 1889-90, 1890.
[13] Ibid.
[14] Ibid.
[15] H.A. Pattison, "Abortion," *Illinois Medical Journal* 11 (June 1907): 652-58.
[16] Ibid., p. 655.
[17] Ibid.
[18] Ibid.
[19] J.H. Lyons, "The Moral Qualifications of the Physician," *Northwest Medicine* 5 (October 1907): 289-96, 290.
[20] Ibid., p. 291.
[21] Ibid.
[22] Ibid., pp. 294-95.
[23] Ibid., pp. 295-96.
[24] Ibid., p. 296.
[25] C.N. Suttner, "A Plea for the Protection of the Unborn," *Northwest Medicine* 5 (October 1907): 305-10, 305.
[26] Ibid., p. 306.
[27] Ibid., pp. 306-7.
[28] Wilhelm Becker, "The Medical, Ethical and Forensic Aspects of Fatal Criminal Abortion," *Wisconsin Medical Journal* 7 (April 1909): 619-35.
[29] Ibid., p. 620.
[30] Ibid., p. 619.
[31] Ibid.
[32] Ibid., pp. 624-25.
[33] Ibid., pp. 625-26.
[34] Ibid., p. 626.
[35] Ibid.
[36] Ibid., pp. 627-28.
[37] Ibid., p. 629.

[38] Ibid., p. 635.
[39] Walter B. Dorsett, "Criminal Abortion in Its Broadest Sense," *JAMA* 51 (September 19, 1908): 957-61.
[40] Ibid., p. 957.
[41] Ibid.
[42] Ibid., p. 958.
[43] Ibid.
[44] Ibid.
[45] Ibid., pp. 958-59.
[46] "Resolutions on Abortion," *JAMA* 50 (June 13, 1908): 2008.
[47] Ibid.
[48] "Supplementary Report from the Reference Committee on Hygiene and Public Health," *JAMA* 50 (June 13, 1908): 2011.
[49] E.F. Fish, "Criminal Abortion," *Milwaukee Medical Journal* 17 (April 1909): 106-9.
[50] Ibid., pp. 107-8.
[51] "Resolutions on Criminal Abortion," *Journal of the Medical Society of New Jersey* 6 (June 1909): 38.
[52] A.B. Davenport, "Criminal Abortion," *Lancet-Clinic* 102 (September 25, 1909): 331-36.
[53] Ibid., p. 331.
[54] Ibid., p. 332.
[55] Ibid.
[56] Ibid.
[57] Ibid., p. 333.
[58] Ibid.
[59] Ibid.
[60] Ibid.
[61] Ibid.
[62] Ibid., pp. 333-34.
[63] Ibid., p. 335.
[64] "Does It Pay? No!," *Canada Lancet* 42 (May 1909): 648-49.
[65] Ibid., p. 649.
[66] John Hunter, M.B., "Medicine Versus a Criminal Act," *Canadian Journal of Medicine and Surgery* 27 (February 1910): 77-81.
[67] Ibid., p. 79.
[68] Ibid., p. 80.
[69] Ibid., p. 81.
[70] Ibid.
[71] Frederick Joseph Taussig, *The Prevention and Treatment of Abortion* (St. Louis: C. V. Mosby, 1910).
[72] Ibid., pp. 78-79.
[73] Ibid., p. 79.
[74] Ibid., pp. 79-80.
[75] Ibid., p. 81.
[76] Ibid., p. 163.
[77] Ibid., p. 165.
[78] Ibid.
[79] Frederick Joseph Taussig, "The Control of Criminal Abortion as Influenced by the Present War," *Interstate Medical Journal* 23 (1916): 772-78. Frederick Joseph Taussig, "Abortion in Relation to Fetal and Maternal Welfare," *American Journal of Obstetrics*

and Gynecology 22 (1931): 868-77.

[80] Frederick Joseph Taussig, *Abortion—Spontaneous and Induced: Medical and Social Aspects* (St. Louis: C. V. Mosby, 1936), p. 401.

[81] National Committee on Maternal Health, Inc., *The Abortion Problem* (Baltimore: Williams & Wilkins Co., 1944), p. 46.

Afterword

[1] Seale Harris, "The Abortionist," *Journal of the Medical Association of the State of Alabama* 4 (December 1934): 222-24.

[2] Samuel A. Cosgrove and Patricia A. Carter, "A Consideration of Therapeutic Abortion," *American Journal of Obstetrics and Gynecology* 48 (September 1944): 299-309. Samuel A. Cosgrove, "Therapeutic Abortion," *Journal of the Michigan State Medical Society* 55 (September 1955): 795-98.

INDEX

rates for different cities and states, 137

real and apparent objections to discussion of, 58

reason for decrease of rate of population increase, 56

regular physicians and, 70

regular physicians implicated in, 115, 144

state laws against, 2, 61, 72, 123, 223

Criminal Abortion: Its Nature, Its Evidence, and Its Law, 140, 151, 209, 216, 248

Crothers, Thomas Davison, 176

Cushing, Ernest Watson
"great crop of abortionists in Boston and in all our cities", 234
factor in criminal abortion was a "strike of the womb", 267
women stopped seeking abortions after quickening, 234
wondered why Charles Harris had not been expelled from his medical society, 234

Dall, Caroline, 112, 131, 200
letter praising *Why Not?*, 112

Dana, Israel Thorndike
"Report of Committee on the Production of Abortion", 109
abortion "prevails chiefly amongst married and otherwise respectable women", 110
need to correct moral sense of community, 243
physician can do "nothing but pity", 110
physician who practices abortion does the most harm, 110

Davenport, A.B.
criminal abortion "the most cowardly and debasing of murders", 290
decried the giving of placebos to women requesting abortion, 289
described multiple instances where women were persuaded to have their babies, 291
knew woman who had ten criminal abortions in five years, 288
praised the Catholic clergy, saw Protestant clergy silence as cowardice, 289
regular physicians "most active of all in committing the crime", 289

Davis, Nathan Smith, 123, 162, 208, 212, 213

"there is no reason why Dr. Hale should not be convicted", 215
abortionists "unfit for citizenship", 220
disagrees with Brainard about danger of abortion, 47

Davison, John L., 176, 221, 222
physician who refused to provide the abortion charged with it., 222
physicians should report requests for abortion to authorities, 222

Divorce, 124, 134

Dix, John H., 87

Dixon Jones, Mary Amanda, 202, 234, 235, 244, 268
"Criminal Abortion, Its Evils and Its Sad Consequences", 228
"physician stands as a preserver of life", 231
"What if the mother of Washington, of Shakespeare, of Lincoln, or of Milton had so acted?", 229
abortion has destroyed "uncounted number of children", 228
abortionist's "work the blackness of darkness, by whomsoever performed?", 229
convinced at least 12 of 21 abortion requestors to bear their children, 229
showed fallacy of Charles Harris' views, 230

Doctress Emma Burleigh, 176

Doering, Edmund J., 214
strong supporter and possible instigator of *Times* expose, 214

Dorsett, Walter B.
called for AMA Committee on Abortion to improve abortion laws, 286
clergymen unwilling to shock congregations by mentioning abortion, 285
described the "fashionable or fad doctor" and his work, 285

Draft abortion statute, 35, 37, 73

Duff, J. Milton, 232
physician abortionists should be "stamped as villains", 232

Duty of the "clerical, legal, and medical" professions, 135

Duty of the profession, 24, 28, 31, 33, 46, 51, 57, 59, 65, 73, 77, 106, 116, 127, 135, 152, 159, 166, 170, 188, 210, 232,